CONTENTS

The Work of Hospitals

GLOBAL MEDICINE IN LOCAL CULTURES

EDITED BY WILLIAM C. OLSEN
AND CAROLYN SARGENT

RUTGERS UNIVERSITY PRESS
New Brunswick, Camden, and Newark, New Jersey, and London

LIBRARY OF CONGRESS CATALOGING-IN-PUBLICATION DATA

Names: Olsen, William C., editor. | Sargent, Carolyn F., 1947- editor.
Title: The work of hospitals: global medicine in local cultures / edited by
   William C. Olsen and Carolyn Sargent.
Description: New Brunswick: Rutgers University Press, [2022] |
   Includes bibliographical references and index.
Identifiers: LCCN 2021015670 | ISBN 9781978823037 (paperback; alk. paper) |
   ISBN 9781978823044 (hardcover; alk. paper) | ISBN 9781978823051 (epub) |
   ISBN 9781978823068 (mobi) | ISBN 9781978823075 (pdf)
Subjects: MESH: Hospitals | Global Health | Anthropology, Medical
Classification: LCC RA963 | NLM WX 100 | DDC 362.11—dc23
LC record available at https://lccn.loc.gov/2021015670

A British Cataloging-in-Publication record for this book is available
from the British Library.

References to internet websites (URLs) were accurate at the time of writing. Neither the author nor Rutgers University Press is responsible for URLs that may have expired or changed since the manuscript was prepared.

⊖ The paper used in this publication meets the requirements of the American National Standard for Information Sciences—Permanence of Paper for Printed Library Materials, ANSI Z39.48-1992.

www.rutgersuniversitypress.org

Manufactured in the United States of America

The Work of Hospitals

The Work of Hospitals

Introduction

William C. Olsen and Carolyn Sargent

The hospital will save you if you suffer . . .
—*Patient in rural West Africa, 1989*

ANTHROPOLOGISTS HAVE CONTRIBUTED to the vast scholarly literature on global health, demonstrating that globalization includes the dissemination of health care institutions, medications, medical procedures, biotechnologies, and concepts of caretaking. The hospital is perhaps the core component in the world of biomedicine, now accessible to some extent to most rural and urban populations. *Hospital*, like *clinic* or *health care center*, is a term that is widely used and has entered common parlance. Yet anthropological analysis suggests the complexity of the hospital as institution.

By exploring hospitals as both domains of science and manifestations of sociality, this collection expands the existing literature on hospital ethnography. In this volume, we build on groundbreaking work by such scholars as Finkler (2001); Finkler and Van der Geest (2004); Kaufman (2005); Long, Hunter, and Van der Geest (2008); Wendland (2010); Livingston (2012); and Street (2014). We supplement their efforts to demonstrate how particular hospitals are linked to local histories of healing and health care institutions. In addition, we show how hospitals play a significant role in the social production of health and disease, and how power relations at the community and state levels, and with global stakeholders are reflected in hospital functioning or dysfunction.

We define the hospital as a place or space of medical practice, a site of social relations and production of moral order, an institution shaped by a broader modernity project. The hospital mission, at its most abstract, is uniform: to cure the sick, to enhance well-being, to provide preventive health care, to attend to suffering, to stave off death (Sobo 2011). But as ethnographic research on hospitals has shown, this idealistic vision may be far from the reality of hospitals in everyday life. Hospitals are shaped by historical trajectories, political dynamics, and economic trends. Hospitals are sources of hope, but they also generate unanticipated negativity, uncertainty, and despair.

Chapters in this book take into account the rapid pace of globalization, transnational migration, and perturbations in the global economy, together with numerous sites of social unrest and violence, which have consequences for implementing the theoretical mission of "The Hospital," especially in resource-poor settings. Accordingly, scholars have argued that hospitals will be limited in achieving idealized goals "so long as they function as institutions only for curative care, detached from the larger social, economic, cultural, and political context of the people's lives which largely determines their health" (Bajpai 2014, 1).

Similarly, WHO (the World Health Organization), in a statement on the capacity of hospitals to fulfill patient needs, notes that hospitals as local institutions are shaped by macro structures and forces external to the health sector, such as privatization, national policies and politics, and decentralization (https://www.who.int/health-topics/hospitals#tab=tab_2). Moreover, hospitals and health care are postcolonial projects linked to neoliberal policies of development (Pfeiffer and Chapman 2010; Pfeiffer and Nichter 2008). As numerous scholars observe (Pfeiffer 2003; Pfeiffer and Chapman 2010; Foley 2008; Biehl 2016; Mishtal 2010), in the context of neoliberalism, many low-resource countries have experienced increasing privatization, dependency on nongovernmental organizations (NGOs), dysfunction of public sector institutions such as hospitals, and growing withdrawal of funding for nonprofit organizations that have compensated for the decline in hospital capacity building. Chapters in this book provide examples of the need to restore or introduce person-centered functionality. We ask what policies, national or global, are adapted and implemented in particular hospital settings, and which remain beyond reach?

Hospital research presents familiar topics: biomedicine, disease, technologies, medical space, the sick patient, the concerned family, and the care providers. Looking closer, each area leads to wider conversations on the body in political economic context. Biomedicine builds its premise upon the diseased body. In this process, the body also becomes an apparatus of state power. Chapters in this volume extend support of fundamental premises laid out by Foucault (1994), whose argument was that the clinic is a device for state supervision and regulation. In addition to substantiating this contention, our authors illustrate how measures for health care are deeply affected by economic flows and deliberative politics. In hospitals, health, wealth, and the state are inseparable. Foucault's well-known concept of *biopower* asserts that the state uses medical data on persons to oversee and regulate bodies and lives, routinized within contemporary capitalism.

As the state historically asserted its domain over medical practice, it also assumed the right to transform human lives. The hospital became a pivotal place for health transformation and maintenance. As John M. Janzen (chapter 5, this volume) observes, the shaping of health care with its particularities and variations—hospitals, clinics, pharmacies, and research—is nowhere more pronounced than in Africa. Private sector investment and the proliferation of NGOs, while state structures deteriorate due to limited national backing, has left health systems, particularly hospitals, in disrepair in Africa and globally. In many circumstances, it is patients and their communities who bear the largest burden of this uneven distribution of institutional biomedicine. Joao Biehl (2005), for example, provides a disturbing example of health inequality in which hospitals in Brazil serve as dumping grounds for the impoverished who are sick and without family support, thus some hospitals become "zones of social abandonment."

A common theme in hospital ethnography questions how hospitals can function while they lack the medications, equipment and technologies, and sufficient personnel normally assumed to be available and necessary. This collection of ethnographies demonstrates how hospital administrators, clinicians, and other staff work to confront innumerable risks, including civil unrest, widespread poverty, endemic and epidemic disease, and supply chain instability (Wendland 2010, 135). Livingston (2012) and Wendland (2010) both eloquently refer to improvisation as a key strategy for managing the hospital as clinical and social institution in low-resource environments. In spite of the assumption that hospitals are intrinsically "biomedical" (Clark et al. 2010, 396), our authors provide compelling ethnographic evidence that for patients and staff in hospitals worldwide, illness represents a complex set of social, political, and economic issues, in which social facts may be as pertinent as clinical diagnosis and treatment.

Moving beyond the construct of the hospital as place (but see Gilmour 2006; Whittaker and Chee 2015), we consider populations engaged in the work of hospital therapeutic practice as social formations and communities. Patients, family members, doctors, pharmacists, nurses, laboratory technicians, psychologists, and social workers, to name a few, all constitute the social milieu in which multiple stakeholders interact with one another, within the broader contexts of community and state. As institution, the hospital is a "liminal space," where "questions about ultimate concern and encompassing meaning present themselves with more urgency than in the routine of everyday life" (Long, Hunter, and Van der Geest 2008). Hospital practices and procedures become meaningful within national and local health care modalities, and within forms of behavior and modes of thought, which provide context to actions regarding health and treatment of the body. Nevertheless, at the same time, hospitals, as sites of biomedical practice, are at least partially shaped by science. At the core, the hospital is the "the site of the construction and treatment of the medicalized body" (B. Good 1994, 85).

Hospital ethnography foregrounds familiar themes of medical anthropology. One premise is that concepts of the body are not universal. For example,

African concepts of diseases of god versus diseases of man (J. M. Janzen 1978) illustrate where applications of science and those of local cultures may diverge. Wider powers of divinity may be invoked at important moments of clinical endeavors, such as where practitioners in Ecuadoran in vitro clinics understand how reality integrates Catholic cosmology, medical instruments, professional skills, prayer, and human anatomy to treat infertility and promote conception in resource-poor communities (Roberts 2012). This same duality is found in fistula hospital surgery theaters in Ethiopia, where patients perceive doctors' skills to be the result of formal education but also of divine powers; doctors became instruments of God's will (Hannig 2017; and chapter 2, this volume). Chapters in Part I show how hospital biomedicine resolves enigmas raised by science and through medical technologies. Yet, these treatments often combine with alternative modes of therapy—those rarely seen or legitimized within medical schools—as individuals and communities also engage in local medical options that recognize alternative configurations of the body and thereby imply that other modes of healing are at least as valuable in treating illness symptoms. Chapters by Hannig and by Olsen, for example, show how biomedical procedures in hospitals are recognized and sought after for the power and capacity for bringing about a cure for fistula disorders and for epilepsy, respectively. Yet, mystical powers found in orthodox religion (Hannig, Ethiopia) and in the healing of charismatic Christian pastors and divination (Olsen, Asante) are also commonly accepted and widely legitimized. Part I also shows how hospital procedures give context to the place of ethnic identity within a larger cosmopolitan population (see Mattingly [chapter 3], Los Angeles) and also how state maneuvers impact upon the hospital patient (Hoke and Leatherman [chapter 1] in the Andes and Janzen [chapter 5] on the Democratic Republic of Congo [DRC] and Uganda). Chapters complement a well-known premise of medical anthropology: that the meanings of sickness affirm associations between the sick person and the wider community. They also show how hospital procedures are commonly articulated through local cultures and practices.

Hospitals everywhere have deep impacts on healing constructs, perceptions of the body, reliance on medical technologies, and use of pharmaceuticals. Hospital staff are arbiters of how the body works, of a life in pain, and how bodily malfunctions are diagnosed and addressed. The chapters in this book raise provocative questions regarding the global variability of practices labeled biomedical. Comparing hospital procedures and conceptualizations of the body, its functions and malfunctions in diverse settings, gives an even closer look at variations in clinical practice in hospital contexts. Hospital personnel take as their responsibility the diseased body, the trauma victim, or the dysfunctional mind. Yet worldwide, class, ethnicity, and knowledge of the body as understood by patients, kin, and clinicians are not only dissimilar but also may be at odds. This means patients participate in care that comes from providers who are strangers to them, both as people but perhaps even as adherents to fundamentally different ontological systems. These differences generate diverse understandings and tensions regarding how to define the patient's disorder and how to treat it.

The language of biomedicine and the use of diverse primary spoken languages can also be barriers to communication necessary for patient–provider interactions and, ultimately, to the patient's search for healing, as examples from our chapters indicate. Olsen observed such constraints among staff at Mampong Government Hospital in central Ghana, which consist of clinicians including six medical doctors (MDs). Two Ghanaian doctors are English and Twi-speakers, while three or four Cuban doctors have very little English and no Twi. The Cuban physicians communicate with nurses and patients often via sketches or by pointing to a body part and making sounds of discomfort in limited Spanish or English. Hospital patients may be local Twi-speakers; but they may also have no Twi and are Mamprusi, or Wala, or Fulani, or from other northern areas. In such cases, patient, nurse, and doctor may speak no common language. One Cuban doctor explained, "We get to be pretty good at guessing what the problem is." Other chapters (e.g., chapter 10, by Carolyn Sargent) show serious misunderstandings that arise when immigrant patients and oncologists try to exchange perspectives on complex aspects of diagnosis and treatment, in the absence of interpreters.

Analyzing symptoms and deciphering diseases are, at least in theory, central components of hospital procedure. Yet in some hospital settings, the lack of diagnostic precision and subsequent ambiguity may muddle results of biomedical therapy while also providing space for other forms of social and clinical improvisation. In an idealized representation of the hospital, clinicians (doctors, nurses, lab techs, aides) perform routine and specialist labor and they seek to maintain patient protocol. They render diagnoses or participate in the act of sustaining the façade that diagnosis is possible, listen to and communicate with patients regarding their disorders, examine the body, prescribe drugs, and invoke a plan of wellness for patients and their families. Medical encounters involve diagnoses of a person's general health, compromised by bacteria, genetics, viruses, or trauma, among other possible causes. There may also be counseling about past and future modes of care, family and personal lifestyles, and performance as a community member and as kin. Such exchanges may involve highly technical information and suggestions for medical regimens or, in other settings, they may include supposition and best guesses gleaned from the senses and interactions in the absence of medications, diagnostic equipment, and medical certainty. This information becomes specialized as it passes through doctors and nurses, often representatives of authority, prestige, and power but whose authority is incomplete and contested in many settings. Ultimately, global ethnography demonstrates a vast gulf between the idealized mission of the hospital and the implementation of this mission in everyday practice.

Part II indicates how hospitals are commissioned with medical supervision of patients. However, realities of care do not always accommodate such a biomedical charge. State health mandates in many parts of the world guarantee free or low-cost health coverage. Yet, patients in many global hospital locations encounter practices that fall short of wider national expectations. Underfunding in places such as Mexico, Guatemala, and Peru require concerted efforts by patients and their families to provide food and supplies. Labor and routines of hospital staff are also impacted by institutional hierarchies and by fiscal limitations of the state. Rural African hospitals are often examples of the gap found between promised health care and care actually provided. This difference can be critical at times of both serious and also routine care, as is noted for Tanzania by Strong (chapter 8) and the DRC by Janzen (chapter 5).

Depending on the extent of state authority, infrastructure, resources, and adherence to national regulations, hospitals may experience a serious deficit of qualified personnel (e.g., Strong [chapter 8] and Varley [chapter 13], in this book), which is often experienced most intensely by the patient but also produces stress and tensions among clinicians and staff. We pursue the important issue of how varieties of medical practice, knowledge of the body, access to resources, and the pursuit of treating pathologies and malfunction differ according to community, national, and global contexts from which we draw case studies. Since physicians and patients may understand symptoms differently, we also show how manifestations of medical pluralism arise within a contested platform of scientific orthodoxy and regional medical practices.

Smith-Oka and Hurd (chapter 9) and Chary and Rohloff (chapter 7) describe the economically challenging circumstances presented to hospital patients where resources are scarce. Using *Hospital Salud* (public) and *Hospital Piedad* (private) in Puebla, Mexico, Smith-Oka and Hurd demonstrate how hospital spaces shape human identities by reflecting the economic hierarchies of the wider society. All patients in their study viewed the economy and government resistance to investing in the health sector as significant barriers to enhanced quality of care in Mexico. Lack of funding is a direct result of the relatively low priority given to medicine and hospitals compared to other social concerns and government responsibilities. As one patient observed, "there are hospitals but they don't have physicians nor supplies." With a low doctor/patient ratio, patients often experience insufficient attention from clinical personnel; with inadequate supplies, procedures are often delayed or impossible to carry out.

Accordingly, the realities of hospital functioning often contrast with national and global health care policies and objectives. Hospitals thus become "contested space" between policy and practice. For example, in chapter 7 Chary and Rohloff describe limits on use of medication, devices, and procedures in the *Instituto de Cancerologia* (INCAN) in Guatemala City. A waitlist for radiation therapy may exceed 1,000 patients—resulting in delays lasting for months. Patients often expect to purchase their own supplies from private pharmacies, due to the financial deficits plaguing public institutions. The inability of many patients or family members to obtain these materials diminishes the quality of care and may even result in otherwise unnecessary deaths.

Hoke, Stumo, and Leatherman, in chapter 1, address hospital space and the growing impact of economic inequality on the goal of providing wide access to health care in Peru. Public health programs in Peru since 2000 served to reduce maternal deaths and levels of infant mortality. Yet, funding for aid programs is distributed unevenly because of racial profiling and favoring of urban centers. Distribution biases and forces of neoliberalism have resulted in ineffective programing in impoverished areas of the country. Consequently, hospital assistance for women is inadequate, inefficient, and often suspect, sometimes nonexistent. Women's narratives tell the tale of discrimination, neglect, and state marginalization of indigenous peoples' medical needs.

Part III addresses the social and cultural conditions of patients in hospitals. Chapters address modes of social differentiation as found within health and clinical settings. Modes of social differences include ethnicity, gender, class, and race. Chapters in this part illustrate how hospital conditions reflect those in society at large. However, the added realities of medical care may provide an even sharper focus on each of these forms of social inequality.

Marginalization of ethnic minorities is also problematic in hospitals across Europe. Georges (chapter 12, in this book), for example, observes that widespread beliefs among Greeks emphasize short labor is necessary for the safety of the baby. As a result, most obstetric care in Greece is located in hospitals and the country's high number of obstetricians are largely engaged in performing planned cesarean sections in private hospitals. For recent immigrants, Roma women, or other economically disadvantaged groups without a cultural predilection for surgical birth, midwife-supervised public hospital births have become common. Clinicians contend that immigrants differ from Greek women in their needs during childbirth and are less likely to require cesarean births. At the same time, midwifery is sustained by opportunities to engage in independent practice, without supervision by an obstetrician, in public hospital settings.

Janzen's chapter illustrates the impact of state public health programs on therapeutic efficacy in two central African rural hospitals in Uganda and the DRC, and the consequences for hospitals when the state collapses. Hospitals in Kinshasa, and elsewhere, functioned at only minimal levels, despite the financial input of local and international NGOs. Yet circumstances of despair in hospitals of the DRC contrast with those found in northern Uganda, despite a history of civil war and deprivation in both states. St. Mary's Lacor Hospital in Uganda illustrates how the state's rapid development and distribution of vaccines for Ebola and active cooperation with NGOs and drug companies resolved emergencies during the outbreak and helped to contain a larger epidemic. These cases identify ways in which the role of the state is clearly implicated in hospital outcomes.

Mattingly's chapter (chapter 13) explores a cosmopolitan hospital ethnographically situated in the heart of Los Angeles. It draws upon a fifteen-year study of African American families caring for children with significant illnesses and disabilities and the clinicians who serve them. Conceptually, the chapter considers the urban hospital as a cultural borderland, a space of perilous travel for those who must visit it. Encounters between health professionals and staff and patients are very often sites of cultural and racial Othering. If hospitals are cultural borderlands, if they are spaces of Othering, if they demand (at least of patients who travel there) the cosmopolitan capacity to communicate in foreign tongues, including the idioms of biomedicine, it is obvious that clinical encounters can readily produce (and reproduce) mistrust. In this chapter Mattingly asks: how, concretely, is mistrust produced in this border place? But, perhaps more interesting, how is it challenged? That is, how do actors attempt to create bonds of social connection in the face of this resilient mistrust, to counter its production and create a space of mutuality? How do they attempt to create communities of care that span clinic and home worlds in the face of enormous class and race divides? Can a theoretical framing of border zones and an ethnographic insistence on looking at processes at a micro level have something to contribute here? The primary ethnographic material that addresses these questions is focused on a single encounter between a mother whose daughter has been diagnosed with brain cancer, and the oncologist who treats her.

The ambiguities of health care shape patient trajectories in the District Headquarter Hospital in Gilgit Town, northern Pakistan. Varley (chapter 13) generates the notion of "night side medicine" to describe alarming moments of clinical neglect, misuse of medications, and routinized mistreatment—all to the detriment of patient care. Structural violence leads to understaffed hospitals and inadequately supervised or performed clinical procedures. Maternity patients suffer from iatrogenic complications, including acquired diseases and infections, childbirth injuries, and all too frequently, death. Varley confronts the crisis of maternity care in the Gilgit Town regional hospital by addressing the combined perils of structural inequalities and clinical irregularities. The intentionality of such irregularities poses particular challenges for intervention. In a reflexive assessment of ethnographic responsibility, she questions the potential for anthropologists to engage in team research that would enhance the likelihood of productive advocacy for improved patient care.

As our chapters illustrate, the goals of caregiving may be at odds with state and local economic constraints and the tensions associated with hospital budgetary management. Containing costs contrasts with the "moral, emotional, religious, and aesthetic expressions of patients and caregivers" (Kleinman 2012, 2550). In reality, hospital expenditures may well prohibit patients and their families from receiving care, and constrain caregivers' interventions, regardless of potential harm to the patient.

Hospitals may be regarded as icons of clinical practice where staff routines are regulated by professional, social, and legal codes of conduct. In the United States, the discourse of public relations depicts hospitals as living entities functioning in a realm of knowledge, skill, and competency and set apart from quotidian values and concerns of the world around them. For example, on its website, the American Hospital Association speaks of how "hospitals know" and how "hospitals understand," and even that "hospitals are determined" to engage in the communities around them. Hospitals historically became caregiving institutions as they also delineated the "natural history of particular syndromes in life and death" (Rosenberg 1987, 150). But what caregiving means in the everyday life of hospital staff varies considerably in diverse global settings.

Here, we frame caregiving as theory by invoking the model of intersubjectivity outlined by Michael D. Jackson. Jackson asserts that analyzing the intersubjective relations of persons (Jackson 1998, 35) best enables our understanding of sociality and living in the world. Intersubjective hospital encounters are dependent on the manifestations of care as practice in any particular time and place; care "implies a negotiation about how different goods might coexist in a given, specific, local practice" (Mol, Moser, and Pols 2010, 13). As patients seek better care and better health, and health care providers work to accomplish these mutual goals, care is constantly in flux, the object of "tinkering" in a quest to deliver wellness (Mol, Moser, and Pols 2010).

Anthropology of hospitals shows us a logic of care as manifest in a "collective moral imagination" (Livingston 2012). In Botswana, for example, empathy and procedure are "predicated on a kind of inter-subjectivity that is often effaced by or pushed to the background of biomedical ideas and practice," but which are rediscovered in the common Setswana term for therapeutics (Livingston 2012, 111). This concept assumes a social foundation of the human body, which acknowledges thoughts, feelings, and actions and how these impact another person. As one medical doctor in Malawi's Queen Elizabeth Hospital confessed, "working in the hospital for me is not just working with sick people as a healer, to heal them. But many times it's as if I'm participating in their suffering" (Wendland 2010, 190). In this case, medical doctors become like traditional healers in that they endure the suffering of patients and thus "materialize the patient's interiority in and on their own bodies" (Livingston 2012). Medical staff acknowledge pain and discomfort. They then transform the suffering by adjusting their own "bodily consciousness." Hospital ethnography takes us into the clinical world where biomedical constructs of normal and sick become contextualized within an apparatus of societal responses to disease. Hospitals provide technical and often emotional care: bathing, feeding, providing medication, consoling, drug regimens, and minimizing pain. Caregiving can be a defining moral experience, a "practice of empathic imagination, responsibility, witnessing, and solidarity with those in great need" (Kleinman 2009, 293). But although caregiving ought to protect those who are vulnerable and in distress, through intent—as when nurses seek to sanction noncompliant patients—or structural impossibility, this form of caregiving is not always realized in settings across the globe (Hull 2017; Strong 2020; Varley, this book).

Caretaking is a changing variable, which challenges limits of local medical staff to respond to patient needs, in the absence of necessary resources. A recent study of Fann psychiatric hospital in Dakar, Senegal, shows the presence of caregiving family members as a vital asset in patient recovery due to a lack of staff (Kilroy-Marac 2019, 87). This full-time service was mandated but not compensated. In Africa and elsewhere, family caregiving may result from the low numbers of doctors and staff. Patient care demands in Kenyatta National Hospital's cancer ward in Nairobi "challenged the ward doctor and nurses many times" due to understaffing; and this was the result of the "low status of the cancer ward" (Mulemi 2010, 56).

In contrast, Nichter, Sopoh, and Johnson (chapter 6) illustrate that increased funding together with patient-centered programming may produce positive consequences in diverse ways. Nichter and colleagues address innovations in caring for patients with Buruli ulcer (BU) in Benin. Increased government funding for treatment and public education forums on BU avoidance through sanitation procedures were critical to the initiative, which calls for restructuring of staff–patient relations to increase patient satisfaction, staff efficiency, and administrative policies. Another benefit of the project was improvement of patient and caretaker participation in improving hygiene and sanitation within the center. Patients and families became more aware of causes of BU and treatment rationales. The authors identify the role of social scientists in transforming the hospital into a community, in which patient narratives improved interactions with staff and led to enhanced patient satisfaction with ulcer treatment. The study concludes that rural African hospitals are more likely to be transformed into efficient therapeutic communities as staff and administrators engage in problem-solving regarding patient suffering, and when social awareness of diseases includes recognition of patient illness experiences.

Anita Hannig's chapter also discloses the impact of caregiving and active doctor–patient relations in the Bahir Dar Fistula Center in Addis Ababa. In the center, science and religion comingle as active forms of caregiving and treatment for fistula patients. Readings of sacred texts and prayer are fundamental steps preceding surgery. In this setting, medical knowledge is itself a manifestation of God's knowledge; doctors' knowledge and skills are blessed by God. As such, doctors and patients believed physicians had "special powers" in their ability to care for and cure patients. Patients thereby submit to hospital procedures and doctor prognoses much like a parishioner may submit to the directives of a priest. Patients recognize an undeniable connection between divine will and therapeutic success.

Unfortunately, social, political, and economic constraints often limit the extent to which individual providers and their institutions can achieve the ideals of technical–affective caring. This reality is evident in the chapters by Strong, by Sobo, and by Olsen. Adrienne Strong writes of nursing and modes of health care in Mawingu Regional Referral Hospital in Rukwa, Tanzania, as these have changed after the end of the Nyerere presidency in the mid-1980s. Broader national economic shifts and health sector restructuring have led to declining public confidence in the nursing profession. Older nurses argued that a lack of intrinsic vocational calling to nursing leads to poorly motivated, disengaged nurses who often did not fulfill either technical or emotional caring ideals. Combined with increasing patient loads and persistent supply shortages, younger nurses retreated from the emotionally and physically dirty world of nursing care and into the escapism of social media and cell phones.

In high-tech, well-resourced hospitals in the United States, patients and caregivers may still confront challenges in treatment decision-making. In the Children's Hospital in San Diego, California (CHSD), E. J. Sobo describes how parents deal with uncertainties they experience during the provision of care for their children. Drawing on three studies—one focusing on children with cancer, the second on anesthesia risk, and the third on choosing experimental modes of medical care such as cannabis—Sobo shows that parents maintain confidence in the hospital as ultimate authority, even in the presence of errors or medication failure. Parents who chose to administer cannabis to their children when other medications had not been successful nonetheless conceptualized their efforts as contributing to the hospital's efforts to provide best practices. Even parental acts of refusal (considered noncompliance by clinicians) were intended to help biomedicine live up to its culturally constructed promise to make their children better. Sobo's research demonstrates that hospital medicine everywhere—even in the Global North—is subject to experimentation by nonspecialists in the interest of patients and their families.

Similar to Sobo's work, practices in African hospitals sometimes fall into the hands of nonspecialists. Olsen reviews modes of care for patients with epilepsy in Mampong Government Hospital (MGH), in central Ghana. As in much of Africa, the cause of onset of epilepsy is often associated with supernatural modes of attack, including witchcraft. Public health literature claims that because of beliefs in spirits patients avoid the hospital. Reality of witchcraft-induced illness is affirmed. Even so, public health presumptions are misplaced since most patients do seek care in hospitals for epilepsy symptoms

despite public scrutiny over stigma. Moreover, for the Asante, stigma is a prohibitive marker in social situations such as marriage and choice of marital
partner. Three psych-ward nurses at MGH demonstrated considerable levels
of listening and attentive nurturing for their patients while also encouraging
the use of pharmaceuticals.

In chapter 10, Carolyn Sargent describes barriers for treatment of West
African immigrant women for breast cancer in two Paris public hospitals situated in the northern region of Seine St. Denis. These hospitals target populations, including patients from Senegal, Mali, Mauritania, Guinee and Cote
d'Ivoire. For many patients, cancer is a disease that cannot be cured. Such
interventions as chemotherapy and radiation therapy are often unfamiliar to
patients and their families. Patients also experience challenges to accessing
care because of economic precarity, immigration status, and civil rights.
Patients often become disengaged from hospital procedures given language
barriers and dissonance in ethical constructs concerning illness and death,
which affect adherence to treatment. Nonetheless, despite demanding working conditions, physicians continue to demonstrate commitment to the
women who consult with them and, indeed, to learn from them regarding
concepts of appropriate interventions, caretaking, and ethics in their societies
of origin.

Chapters in this volume document the global variation in hospital missions,
structures, and clinical practice. In the context of neoliberalism and global
austerity measures, health care services confront numerous challenges in
attempting to meet the needs of local populations. Our overview of hospitals
in diverse settings foregrounds the tensions between the public and private
sectors, as resource-poor states are constrained in supporting hospitals, lacking budgetary means to do so. NGOs may attempt to substitute for dysfunctional public institutions, but in the long run this serves to produce even
greater lack of capacity in the public sector. Ethnographic research presented
in this book shows the improvisation and commitment clinicians demonstrate
while working without adequate materials, personnel, and financial means.

Medical anthropology has shown how health and illness are realities best
described, and more fully understood, within historic and cultural frames.
As our chapters substantiate, the human body, with its manifestations of
irregularities and wellness, is subject to alternative modes of interpretation,
intervention, and management at the levels of the individual, family, and
community. This volume pursues a sharper focus to these dynamics by providing original research on clinical practice and caretaking within hospital
settings in locations on five continents. The collection illustrates how hospital
interventions for cancers, reproductive health, infectious diseases, chronic illness, and myriad other conditions become part of routines that occur within
specific social, economic, and political infrastructures—the product of the

global proliferation of biomedicine. Hospitals, as core institutions within bio-medicine, take on diverse forms and meanings in specific local settings. The imagined and idealized hospital, as we show, may diverge considerably from the reality of the hospital in action, in everyday life.

This volume asserts four foundational premises for continued research in medical anthropology. First, hospitals are themselves institutions of power. Hospitals are usually regulated by the state, at least in some manner. Proce-dures, instruments, and medicines are regulated by normative professional bodies, which limit and expand medical applications according to what is considered medically viable in a particular context. Second, related to this point is the mandate of authority given to and practiced within hospitals. In the abstract, biomedicine positions doctors and other medical staff as final arbiters on medical matters, but the work of this volume serves to probe the boundaries of their authority, as patients and practitioners themselves recog-nize the limits of biomedicine in particular settings. Third, for nearly two centuries, hospitals have provided caretaking in order to improve health, facilitate wellness, and give transition to dying. Hospital staff are expected through personal and professional norms and ethics to exhibit care of clients' body and mind; yet staffing limitations or indifference alter that ideal. Fourth, hospital procedures and personnel are not disconnected from wider forms of social differentiation, including factors such as age, class, gender, and ethnic-ity. In fact, hospitals are often sites at which broader social inequities are made visible through differential access to treatments and resources or differing lev-els of affective care demonstrated by hospital staff members.

Hospital ethnography's specific focus on health institutions contributes insight into social dynamics, as well as state and global processes. It is in this capacity that the chapters in this volume contribute to conversations ranging well beyond medical anthropology. The ethnography we present here includes attention to power relations within the state, which impact medical outcomes, and how the ebb and flow of global economies influences institutional capac-ity to deliver medical care. Working specifically within hospitals also reveals new forms of understanding about the partial power of institutions and bureaucracy. Confrontations between patient need and the harsh limitations or absence of supplies, instruments, and other resources requisite to complete their hospital therapy reveal improvisation and instability in the institutional setting. Likewise, confrontations and frictions between health care workers and their patients, or among health care personnel, open a window onto how actors reinvent norms and create new spaces for personal and professional needs, as well as access to power, meaning, and caring.

PART ONE

 *Global Medicines in
Local Cultures*

CHAPTER 1

Global Health Goals and Local
Constraints in a Rural Peruvian Clinic

Morgan K. Hoke, Samya R. Stumo,
and Thomas L. Leatherman

IN ITS EFFORTS to meet the United Nations Millennium Development Goals (MGDs) of reducing maternal and under-five child mortalities, Peru developed initiatives intended to make health care more accessible for poor mothers and infants, to increase the number of births attended by trained health care professionals, and to close the gap between rich and poor in terms of basic health indicators. Two key initiatives included a national insurance program, *Seguro Integral de Salud* (SIS), for the poor and a conditional cash transfer social assistance program aimed at poverty alleviation (*JUNTOS*). Both of these efforts locate significant power and responsibility within regional and local clinics, which are part of a largely decentralized health care system. Rural clinics serve as the access point of care for SIS beneficiaries and sites for the monitoring and surveillance of women and children beneficiaries of *JUNTOS*. As seen in the work of Smith-Oka (2009, and this volume) and others (e.g., Guerra-Reyes 2016; Jacay 2012), the way such programs operate under the control of medical establishments can have "unintended" consequences, particularly in terms of the quality of care for women. Despite best intentions and improved outcomes in health indicators (see below), observations in clinics and reports from patients suggest much of the care they receive is callous, disrespectful, and even contrary to promoting better health. The clinic is thus an ideal site for ethnographic examinations of the cultures of care that emerge from the implementation of national and regional health policies and programs.

Our objective in this chapter is to convey results of ethnographic work on the provision of care in a rural clinic in the southern highlands of Peru. This rural clinic is in many ways a distinct site from those other hospital-based ethnographies in this volume. However, we believe that the power of hospitals to reflect the core values and beliefs of a given culture, as argued by van der Geest and Finkler (2004), is still very much present and arguably even more so in the context of rural health clinics, making their examination relevant for this volume. We draw on surveys, clinic observations, and interviews with both providers and health care recipients to examine a culture of care within a decentralized and neoliberal national health care system. We argue that the dual effects of decentralization and neoliberalization—specifically the linkage between decentralization, metrics of care, "flexible" labor, and funding of clinics and personnel—create the context for disjunctures between health policy in the abstract, local practices of implementation, and consequent effects on the quality of care for local populations.

BACKGROUND

In 2016, an article in *Lancet Global Health* highlighted Peru's success in addressing millennial development goals of lowering infant and neonatal mortality and reducing maternal mortality and childhood stunting (Huicho et al. 2016). Between 2000 and 2013, Peru boasted a 4.2 percent per year reduction in maternal mortality and a 6.2 percent per year reduction in infant mortality. Maternal deaths were halved between 2000 and 2015 (from 140 to 68 per 100,000 live births), and infant mortality rates were reduced from 33 to 17 per 1,000 births during the same period. Stunting, which had remained relatively stagnant in Peru (30–40%) between 1992 and 2007, declined precipitously to 17.5 percent by 2013 (Huicho et al. 2016). These strides are even more impressive when we consider that in the year 2000, the health system, the economy, and the most vulnerable populations were recovering from a protracted twenty-year civil war and severe cutbacks in health services due to structural adjustment policies enacted during the presidency of Alberto Fujimori. These public health accomplishments are understood by politicians and health officials alike to be the result of new policies and programs targeting the poor, specifically the SIS insurance program, intended to provide basic health care to vulnerable segments of the population, and *JUNTOS*, a conditional cash transfer (CCT) program targeting families living in poverty. In addition, a series of policy directives promoting "intercultural" birthing practices were passed to provide more culturally appropriate maternal health care and to increase use of health care services and the number of births attended by a skilled birth attendant, especially among rural indigenous women. The structure and implementation of these programs is key to our argument about disjunctures between policy and practice, and the juxtaposition of positive health outcomes and poor quality of care.

EXPANSION OF PUBLIC HEALTH CARE

In the decades preceding our research, the Peruvian health system had suffered greatly due to a protracted civil war (1980–2000) and draconian structural adjustment policies of President Fujimori ("Fujishock") implemented in the early 1990s. During this period, social spending was dramatically cut and many social services including health care were restructured under market principles and increasingly privatized. By 2000 and the collapse of the Fujimori presidency, health indicators placed Peru among the poorest performing of Latin American countries, and as one of the least funded as a percentage of gross domestic product (GDP; Physicians for Human Rights [PHR] 2007).

A significant restructuring of the health care system began in the early 2000s with a major decentralization of the public health system (Supreme Decree 052-2005-PC 2005) and, eventually, the creation of SIS. Under this model of decentralization, all health care outside of Lima was directed by regional health authorities (DIRESAs). In essence, the Ministry of Health (MINSA, or *Minsterio de Salud*) set policies while budgeting and implementation are devolved to the DIRESAs, which also set local performance measures (basis for quotas) required to meet policy goals. These regional centers supervise a number of *Redes de Servicios Salud* (health care networks) that administer local *Microredes de Salud*, which in turn oversee a number of local *postas* (small, rural health posts). The *microredes* have at least one clinic that provides primary care, referring more complicated cases requiring greater specialization and technical care to a regional hospital located at the center of the *Redes de Salud*. Our ethnography focuses on the Microred de Nuñoa in the southern highlands.

Along with a decentralized system of care, the ministry enacted a deeper "flexibilization" of the labor force as part of the neoliberalization of the public health care system. Within the public sector's health workforce two contrasting labor regimes dominate: There are permanent employees (*nombrados*) with job security and benefits (e.g., paid holidays, retirement benefits, and social security covering health care) and temporary employees (*contratados*) on short-term contracts of usually one year but as short as three months, and without benefits and job security (their position can be withdrawn at any time by the employer). Many rural health centers are staffed by contracted physicians on a temporary placement through SERUM (*Servicio Rural y Urbano Marginal en Salud*), the Rural and Marginalized Urban Health Service. This service is one of the strategies used by MINSA to increase primary care coverage in rural and marginal urban areas, and a requirement for those health professionals who would like to work in the public sector. A recent report by World Bank (Carpio and Bench 2015) noted that over 30 percent of the health workforce was employed on temporary contracts, which were highly unstable and varied widely in wages and benefits. Nationally, 11 percent of physicians were serving through SERUM, with levels up to 25 percent in more rural departments (Carpio and Bench 2015).

Evaluation and funding of centers and staff by DIRESAs under the increasingly neoliberal health system hinges on their ability to meet various performance measures (*metas* or quotas) (PHR 2007). Hence, the centers and the health care workforce, especially the large number of contracted laborers, work under the pressure of meeting these performance goals to maintain employment and funding for the center. Despite growth in the numbers of hospitals, health centers, and posts over the past decades, the public health care system remains underfunded. According to a 2013 World Bank report, only 5 percent of the GDP is spent on health and of that only 54 percent on the public system (Francke 2013). Thus, centers and staff are asked to meet productivity measures in a climate of inadequate funding and significant job precarity.

JUNTOS—Conditional Cash Transfer Program

In the early 2000s, several social assistance programs were initiated, including nutritional supplementation programs (*Qali Warma*, *Vaso de Leche*), support for senior citizens (*Pensión 65*), and a conditional cash transfer program (*JUNTOS*), designed to address extreme poverty and help ameliorate effects of a twenty-year civil war that hit rural indigenous groups the hardest. *JUNTOS* ("together") began in 2005 and provides a bimonthly stipend of 200 soles (about US$60) to impoverished households with children under nineteen years of age. Mothers (or other guardians) must meet the conditions of school attendance for their children, complete vaccinations and regular health checks for children, and for women to attend pre- and postnatal care checks. Eligibility can be suspended for six months for failure to comply with any of these requirements, or permanently for repeated failures. The clinic that oversees many of the eligibility requirements has power over household participation in *JUNTOS*. It has been widely reported that clinic staff regularly use their power to determine eligibility in *JUNTOS* as a means to control rural women, thus ensuring their compliance with a variety of productivity goals used to evaluate staff and clinic performance.

"Intercultural" Reproductive Care

Peru has adopted several policies and decrees stating that women have a right to adequate care, births, privacy, respect, dignity, and freedom from coercion. Adopting broad international recommendations, it has also advanced policies of promoting "intercultural" birth and reproductive care (Camacho, Castro, and Kaufman 2006; Guerra-Reyes 2016) intended to support customary, culturally appropriate, and baby- and mother-friendly birth practices of indigenous groups in health care institutions. Many centers have constructed *Casas Maternales* ("mothers' houses") designed to facilitate birth in clinics where women can come with their family and live for days or weeks before birth. It is suggested that centers add birthing poles or ropes to facilitate vertical birth, create birthing rooms that are warm, allow family to be present at births, and keep vulnerable areas of mothers covered to prevent exposure to cold and other environmental elements during and after birth—the latter being consistent with local health beliefs. Like other aspects of the decentralization of MINSA policies, the implementation of these practices has been highly uneven. For example, Guerra-Reyes (2016) notes how in a clinic designated as a model for intercultural birth (e.g., including birthing poles and a *Casas Maternales*), that buy-in and compliance on the part of clinic staff was lacking, indicating the continuing hegemony of the biomedical birthing model.

SIS, JUNTOS, Intercultural Care, and Clinic Use

The degree to which expansion of SIS, *JUNTOS,* and "intercultural" reproductive care are singularly or collectively responsible for changing indicators of clinic use and maternal and infant mortality is unclear. However, a consensus among some is that these programs have led to reductions in infant and maternal mortality (Huicho et al. 2016), in part due to enhanced use of medical facilities for birth. In 2000, 24 percent of births in rural areas and 58 percent in urban zones took place in medical facilities (Franke 2013). However, by 2012 over 58 percent of rural and 85 percent of urban births occurred in medical facilities, an increase of 34 percent and 27 percent, respectively (Huicho et al. 2016). What remains less clear is whether these shifts have come at a cost to patient-focused care. The case studies we present in this chapter suggest that the decentralized nature of the health care system and the drive to achieve quotas transforms rural indigenous women from recipients of enhanced care into the objects of surveillance, control, and even coercion to achieve local and regional performance goals and national and international development goals.

Ethnography in the Clinic: Nuñoa Region and Health System

Located in a rural district in the south-central highlands of Puno, Nuñoa remains relatively poor and isolated, with over 80 percent of the population living below the poverty line and 50 percent living in extreme poverty (INEI 2015). Infant mortality in the Department of Puno, in which Nuñoa is situated, decreased significantly (about 30%), from around 71 to 50 infant deaths per 1,000 live births between 1995 and 2015. Yet, the 2015 levels of infant mortality of 50 per 1,000 remained almost twice that of the country overall (27 per 1,000) and were the third worse among departments nationally (National Institutes of Statistics and Computing 2021).

A well-developed social hierarchy characterizes the region, including a small, relatively wealthy elite class of large landowners, a large lower class made up of farmers and pastoralists who speak Quechua as their first language, and a small but growing middle class made up of Spanish-speaking professionals. Indigenous residents have long suffered the exploitation of their land and labor along with racial and class-based discrimination that often surfaces within the health system.

The Nuñoa *Centro de Salud* (CS) was opened in 1960 as a "sanitary outpost" (Calderón Sanchez 2012), and the original health center—a small, dark, cold, and altogether uninviting place—was built in 1970 (Morse and Stoner 1986). A new health center was built in 2009, with rooms designated for X-rays, dentistry, and even minor operations with hopes to expand equipment, staff, and level of authorized care. Yet, the funding to equip these rooms never materialized and much of the new center remains unused (Stumo 2015). The *Centro Salud* (CS) in Nuñoa is staffed by three physicians. It is the central hub of the *Microred* of the District of Nuñoa and oversees six satellite health posts, typically staffed by a nurse or an auxiliary health worker (the largest is staffed by a physician, a nurse, and a health worker). The *Microred* of Nuñoa reports to the *Red de Servios de Salud* of Melgar, with a central hospital in the province capital of Ayaviri located an hour away by car. The CS refers cases requiring specialized care such as obstetric complications or other emergencies to a hospital in Ayaviri. The CS staff conduct mobile visits to rural communities, often setting up in a nearby health post or school to provide care to local populations, including checkups for *JUNTOS* participants. The physicians and staff echoed the charges mentioned earlier by Francke (2013), that health centers and staff are asked to meet the health needs of the local population, and the productivity measures established by regional DIRESAs, in a climate of inadequate funding and significant job precarity.

The quality of care provided in Nuñoa is highly variable due to the impermanence of clinic staff and irregular hours of attendance. The clinic is staffed by one to three physicians, providing rural service as part of their post-medical school obligation (SERUM). Most physicians do not speak Quechua, do not like the highlands, and are dissatisfied with their posting in what they consider a cold, desolate, and culturally foreign locale. Doctors are generally repositioned within one to two years of arriving, leading to high overall turnover. In addition, the physicians at the center double as clinic administrators managing resources, paperwork, and the constant battles with regional oversight and expectations. A few nurses and obstetric nurses are *nombrados* though the majority are *contratados* on temporary appointments.

The clinic primarily serves the poor, rural, and indigenous population through the SIS program. Others visit private physicians, the hospital in Ayaviri, or frequently travel to the larger cities of Arequipa and Cuzco. The majority of visits involve child monitoring as mandated by the JUNTOS program. Hours of attendance are often unclear, and it is common to see a line of patients waiting at the gate to see whether they will receive attention that day. On days when care is provided, women may wait all day, including periods when a physician might disappear for several hours and without any clear indication if and when they might return.

The case studies presented below are derived from interviews with women attending the Nuñoa clinic (*Centro de Salud*) and with health care staff (doctors, nurses, technicians), as well as from observations in the primary clinic in Nuñoa and in satellite clinics and/or health promotion activities of teams visiting rural communities in the district. We also interviewed administrators of the JUNTOS program and parents and schoolteachers involved in the *Qali Warma* (school lunch) programs. Interviews took place in individuals' homes, in markets, and in clinic settings. The case studies were collected in the summer of 2014, though many insights into clinic and health worker attitudes and practices were gleaned from years of earlier research beginning in the 1980s, and especially in the summer of 2013 when one of us (MKH) accompanied health workers to a series of rural clinics and health promotion visits across the district. The interviews with clinic staff dealt with the organization, structure, and operation of the health care system in Nuñoa, the system of *nombrado* versus *contratato* positions, funding, and attitudes toward the rural communities they serve. Interviews with women focused on different aspects of their birth experience, available health care and health resources, and other interactions with the clinic and clinic staff. Interviews were conducted in semi-structured and open-ended/unstructured formats.

EXPERIENCE OF REPRODUCTIVE CARE IN NUÑOA

We present three different case studies of reproductive care taking place in and around the local health center in Nuñoa, Peru. These vignettes demonstrate how national policies and programs, enacted at the local level within a decentralized neoliberal health system, can produce conflicting outcomes and experiences of care.

Nelida's Story: Flexible Rigidity in Decentralized Health Care

Nelida sighed while holding her six-month-old son, Leoncio. We were resting after having hauled dozens of buckets of water from a dug well in the ground to water her cows while Leoncio had slept on a blanket nearby. Between buckets, Vicky and I had been asking her about why she insisted upon carting her young son Leoncio over an hour and a half to the provincial capital of Ayaviri for his checkups rather than to the health post located just a short walk away in the community center. "They suspended me from JUNTOS there," she replied. She glanced to her son, adjusting the hand-knit cap he was wearing. "And it wasn't even my fault," she exclaimed. She then explained how Leoncio had been born prematurely at the larger hospital in Ayaviri. The doctor who delivered Leoncio gave her explicit instructions that he should not follow the normal vaccination schedule and that he should receive just one or two vaccinations at a time rather than the normal four or five that are administered around the age of two months.

When Leoncio's two-month appointment rolled around, Nelida, who had since returned home from the hospital, took him to her local health post. The doctor normally on duty at the post was on holiday and the nurse was the only staff member performing the monthly *JUNTOS* checkups during which children's growth is closely monitored and routine vaccinations are administered (both required conditions). When Nelida refused the vaccinations as instructed by the doctor from the regional hospital, the nurse became frustrated, accusing her of lying to avoid the vaccinations. The nurse insisted that Leoncio receive the vaccinations according to the normal schedule despite his small size due to prematurity. Nelida, continued to plead her case but had no records to show from the regional doctor to prove that she was only trying to follow his instructions. Despite the growing anger of the nurse, Nelida remained firm in her refusal of the vaccinations, having been warned of the potential harm to her son. Finally, Nelida decided to leave, taking Leoncio with her after having only received two vaccinations. The following month, when Nelida went into town to retrieve her *JUNTOS* transfer, she found herself on the list of suspensions for noncompliance and was forced to return home empty-handed. After that, she began seeking Leoncio's care in Ayaviri, but she did not seek reinstatement in *JUNTOS*.

One of the key ways that health center staff meet their quotas is through the regular provision of services in the course of their administration of "controls" or required monthly checkups for the *JUNTOS* program. The formal conditions for participation in *JUNTOS* include attendance at prenatal and postnatal health checks, registration of infants in the national identification system, as well as immunization, health and nutrition controls, and regular school attendance for children. All conditions but school attendance are evaluated by clinic staff, giving them great power when it comes to informing program participants of the conditions and determining their compliance. Compliance with program requirements is generally assessed on just a couple of days a month when the "control" appointments are scheduled. This limited availability is due in part to the infrequency of mobile clinic visits, when additional staff from the health center come to the satellite health posts to provide vaccinations and additional personnel to complete the "controls." There is very little flexibility in scheduling, so women must make the trip to the health post on the scheduled day in order to maintain their *JUNTOS* eligibility.

One of the supposed benefits of the decentralization of health care administration is that when decisions are made locally by those most knowledgeable of local contexts, care can be tailored to the population. In theory, this should allow for the customization of care in a way that is beneficial to the patients. Unfortunately, as we see in the case of Nelida, the intended effect of decentralization is turned on its head. The meeting of quotas within the neo-liberal accounting of care provisioning provides perverse incentives for the health workforce to demand compliance of their patients. While the decen-tralized nature of this system allows for flexibility on the side of health center staff, it does not allow for flexibility on the patient/client side. For Nelida, a problem emerged due to a lack of communication between the regional hospi-tal, the CS, and the small health post where she received her controls. There was no communication between the branches of care provision that would protect the nurse from not making her quota or Nelida and her son from a burdensome vaccination schedule. Thus, rather than work with Nelida to find another time to complete the vaccinations, as a decentralized system should theoretically allow, the nurse simply suspended her from the program.

This restricted flexibility is also due in part to the limited number of days that the nurse actually offers care at the rural health post. Care is not available on a daily basis. Rather, there are only a certain number of days a month when health post staff are actually present and provisioning care. While regu-lar hours are posted at the front of the health post, they are rarely maintained. The staff of many of the rural clinics rely on word of mouth and radio announcements to let people know when they are available at the health post. Most of the care provided is offered on just a few days a month corresponding with either the prenatal and monthly child checkups required by *JUNTOS* or on days where additional activities are scheduled, such as a visit from the nutritionist or a team of doctors and nurses from the main health center. As such, for the nurse, creating an alternate vaccination schedule for Nelida and Leoncio represented a significant obstacle that she was unable to overcome.

Claudia's Story: Coercion and the Casa Maternal

Claudia, a pregnant mother of four, had birthed all of her children at home comfortably and without complications. This was before the *Centro de Salud* had begun to enforce institutional births, requiring mothers to give birth in the CS. Often this meant women had to spend extended stays in the *Casa Maternal*, a small outbuilding on the CS's property, which contained a few rooms with single beds, a central area with a small table and stove, and a dilapidated bathroom, while they waited to give birth. Claudia had not wanted to bring her four other children into town to stay in the *Casa Maternal* as it would disrupt their schooling. Further, she would need her husband to come with them to help her cook for herself and the children and manage their care and this was impossible as someone needed to remain with their animals in the countryside. Thus, she remained at home in the later stages of her pregnancy. When she went into labor suddenly one cold June night, she worried about the newly initiated rules mandating that women give birth in the clinic. She and her family were in their small cabaña in the rural commu-nity where they lived. She sent her husband to find the technician in charge of the small health post in the community center. After seeing that the local post was dark and empty, he continued on his motorbike to the main health center in Nuñoa, about thirty minutes away. After pounding on the gate with no response, he returned home.

He arrived at the house and was greeted by the cries of his new son. In his absence, Claudia had given birth alone and with no complications. The following day they informed the CS of the birth to try to register the child and explained that they had attempted to find someone who could bring her to the Centro by ambulance but nobody was around. The next day three staff members arrived at Claudia's rural home and began chastising her for not trying harder to get to the clinic and for not presenting herself earlier for internment in the *Casa Maternal*. They demanded to see her placenta to prove that she had successfully expelled it and forced her to accept two injections that were "to stop bleeding." Several days later they returned with a police officer and demanded that the couple pay the S/.700 fine[1] for failing to give birth at the CS. Initially protesting, the couples' story of their attempts to seek help at both the health post and the CS fell on deaf ears. Claudia and her husband gave up trying to convince the health center staff and just sat still, stared straight ahead, and refused to respond to further demands that the fine be paid. Eventually the staff became weary of trying to elicit a response from the stoic couple. When the police officer told the CS staff there was nothing he could do to enforce the fine, the group finally left the couple alone.

Claudia's story and the pressure to pay a fine for failing to give birth in the clinic demonstrate the extreme end of the "creative" and arguably coercive ad hoc measures put in place by staff in Nuñoa to achieve their goals. When questioned about the inception of the fine, the clinic staff reported it was a decision made at the district level "for their own good." They argued that the fine "incentivized" women to give birth in the clinic where biomedical intervention would be possible in the case of complications. As an added bonus, the funds obtained from the fines could be used for health center expenses that could not be covered with their limited allocation from the regional health ministry. Additionally, by increasing the proportion of women giving birth in the clinic, the CS staff are more likely to meet the quotas of in-clinic births. While the presence of the police officer at the home when the CS staff sought to retrieve the fine lent gravity to the threat, his inability to enforce the policy ultimately points to the tenuous legality of such "creative" informal conditions. To our knowledge, the fine is not a policy that is widely practiced in the region or the Peruvian health care system at large and its legality is highly suspect.

While the fine represents one extreme, there are significantly more subtle and regular ad hoc conditions that are illustrative of the underlying culture of care and the sentiments that surround social aid programs like *JUNTOS*. We have observed health center staff setting conditions ranging from attending activities and classes, to providing food to health center staff, to the production of artisanal crafts. A technician in charge of one of the rural health posts boasted about how he regularly requires the mothers in *JUNTOS* to bring in weavings or other handcrafts or to work on one while they wait so that "they know they have to do some work" to receive their benefits. The operating assumption is that because these women have incomes low enough to qualify to receive *JUNTOS*, they do not work. This type of thinking erases the countless hours of domestic work, child care, and at times back-breaking agricultural labor that women in Nuñoa undertake on a daily basis.[2]

The mandate that Claudia present herself at the *Casa Maternal* prior to giving birth represents another sort of ad hoc condition, something that is not legally required but which CS staff can use to leverage patients into care. As previously noted, to support the effort to reduce maternal and neonatal mortality through increasing births attended by a trained medical professional, *Casas Maternales* or mothers' houses were set up in association with rural health centers like that in Nuñoa. Like the health center, the *Casa Maternal* is minimally equipped. The rooms where women sleep offer a simple wooden bed and a barren mattress pad, with the more well-furnished rooms boasting an additional chair or a table. A gas stove for cooking is provided in the common area shared between the three or four rooms, but it is often unaccompanied by gas. In a separate but nearby building, a *fogon* (or traditional wood stove) is available for cooking, but it is necessary for women and their families to supply their own fuel. Women are not provided any additional care or services while they stay at the *Casa Maternal* and are responsible for supplying their own bedding, food, and fuel, and for performing the cooking and cleaning. Thus, women must often bring another family member with them in order to assist them while they wait to give birth in the *Casa Maternal*.

For many women, residence in the *Casa Maternal* is an impossibility. As in the case of Claudia, she and her husband could not manage care for herself, their children, and their animals if they were separated with her having to remain in the *Casa Maternal*. For many rural women, internment in the *Casa Maternal* is incompatible with the realities of daily life. This is especially true among the most marginalized segments of Peruvian society, families with little income and poor social networks who are less able to buffer against the loss of labor that may come with hospitalization or internment. Indeed, such losses resulting from pregnancy and birth, like illnesses, may represent spaces of vulnerability (Leatherman 2005), wherein families experiencing them find themselves at greater risk for experiencing poverty and/or diminishing socioeconomic status.

Marleny's Story: Delivering Babies without Delivering Care

Marleny returned to her natal home of Nuñoa to be with her mother and sister for the birth of her second child. Though she and her husband live in

Cusco, just over five hours away, she felt the support of her mother and sister would be necessary in managing her young son, then four years old, and the birth. Marleny's mother had extensive knowledge of ethnomedicinal practices and provided her with the culturally specific prenatal care, including herbal baths and *sobadas*, or massages, necessary for an uncomplicated birth. While she would have liked to deliver at home with her mother and sister, on the morning when Marleny's contractions began, she and her family gathered their things and headed to the health center. Upon arriving, Marleny's mother and sister furnished the bed in the birthing room with sheets and blankets. They brought new blankets and clothes for the baby as well as towels and a sheepskin to catch and clean the afterbirth.

According to her mother's knowledge of labor, Marleny should have been permitted to walk around and to drink hot chocolate, which is thought to strengthen the mother and move the labor along. Instead, the health center staff insisted that she remain lying on her back in bed without anything more than water. The labor progressed slowly throughout the morning. Nurses would periodically check on Marleny in the brightly lit but frigid windowless delivery room in the back of the CS. Her mother and sister gently pressed coca leaves to her forehead and soothed her through the contractions. The labor was progressing normally, and it looked like her dilation would be complete at any moment. Nevertheless, when it came to the end of regular clinic hours at 2:30, the majority of the staff left for lunch. Before leaving, the on-duty obstetrician, a middle-aged man who held one of two coveted *nombrado* obstetric positions, briefly examined Marleny and promptly left, calling over his shoulder as he walked out the door that he thought it would be a few hours more. A single nurse technician was left on duty to attend to Marleny.

When it became apparent that the birth was imminent, the remaining nurse repeatedly called the obstetrician to return for the birth. While she was calling, Marleny and her mother looked around the room for the birthing pole that should have been installed to allow women to give birth standing or kneeling, as was common practice prior to the medicalization of birth in Nuñoa, but it was nowhere to be seen. Despite having significantly less experience than Marleny's mother who had successfully delivered countless babies, including four of her own, the nurse insisted that Marleny lie on her back and begin pushing. When the baby emerged, it was Marleny's sister and mother who caught the baby and tended to him. After the labor was complete, the nurse insisted that Marleny remain on the bed, uncovered below the waist, until the obstetrician or doctor returned to inspect her for complete expulsion of the placenta. She lay there, uncovered in the cold, cavernous room for over an hour before the general physician on call arrived to evaluate the situation and cut the baby's umbilical cord. The on-call obstetrician did not return until the following day.

In many ways, Marleny's birthing story is not unique. Women who give birth in the CS rarely consider it to be a pleasant experience. Many Quechua women in Nuñoa experience gruff treatment and disregard for their beliefs and practices when it comes to birthing. The Nuñoa health center contains a large sign stating that they respect traditional birthing practices and depicting an indigenous woman laboring in several positions, including kneeling and using a birthing pole. Indeed, the installation of birthing poles was recommended alongside the establishment of *Casas Maternales* to facilitate institutional birthing among rural, indigenous populations throughout Peru (MINSA 2005; Guerra-Reyes 2016). Despite the national-level recommendations and the promotional material stating support for traditional birthing practices, Marleny faced significant pressure to give birth according to biomedical norms rather than her own, laboring in bed on her back instead of standing or kneeling.

Beyond the practices associated with birth itself, there are also specific cultural guidelines about how pregnant women should be cared for before and after birth that conflict with health center practices (Camacho et al. 2006; Guerra-Reyes 2016; MINSA 2005). For example, women should be kept away from very bright lights and should remain warm and covered at all times. When Marleny was left exposed on the bed for over an hour, at 4,012 meters above sea level in the altiplano, she was left in an extremely vulnerable position, literally and figuratively. Exposure of orifices, especially during birth, invites illness from and risk for several culturally bound syndromes such as "*sobreparto*" (Larme 1998; Larme and Leatherman 2003). Cold and malevolent winds can enter the body and leave a woman weak, preventing her from recovering normally after the birth and potentially causing her recurring health problems for the rest of her life (Larme 1998; Larme and Leatherman 2003). By dismissing or ignoring the culturally salient beliefs of their patients around birth, health center staff deliver babies without delivering care.

Marleny's case is somewhat exceptional in that most births are attended by an obstetrician, a nurse, and a technician, usually with a doctor available in case of emergencies. It is not rare for the CS staff to take meals together, leaving a single technician on watch. However, by most accounts, staff are generally attentive to calls to return to the center and do so promptly. Marleny's story highlights a source of significant problems with the current structure of health care provision: the nature of employment for health center staff. In her case, the obstetrician's "named" position allowed him to be derelict in his duties with few if any consequences. Indeed, the "untouchable" nature of named positions simultaneously represents a goal and source of annoyance for all contracted workers. They regularly complain about the lazy nature of their *nombrado* colleagues who show up late, ignore their paperwork, and seem to be absent or call in sick. Thus, Marleny's case demonstrates the issues with both labor regimes present in health care service in Peru: quotas set for clinics and contracted staff leads them to enforce requirements of clinic-based births, and the more permanent or tenured positions allow CS staff to provide poor-quality care because there are few incentives for doing so.

DISCUSSION

Our findings echo those of other scholars working in clinical settings in Peru and other places in Latin America (Smith-Oka 2009; Guerra-Reyes 2016; PHR 2007; Samuel 2015). Most of these studies document the presence of discriminatory practices, acts of overt racism, and negative attitudes of health care providers toward their clients, which often result in poor quality of care. Though we also observed these kinds of issues, they are not the primary focus of this chapter. As Andersen (2004) noted of differential treatment of villages in Ghanaian hospitals, the blaming of staff attitudes are incomplete and insufficient explanations. There are resource stresses, poor working conditions, and service in foreign and unwelcome locales; it is important to remember that physicians and staff are themselves under surveillance. Thus, we also seek to analyze structural conditions that shape the practice of care in the context of the "friction" between global and national-level policies intended to reduce maternal and neonatal mortality and the local realities of the rural clinic.

Our discussion focuses on three points. First, there is a culture of care shaped by larger cultural and social dynamics where racial, class, and gender biases are rather transparent and inform treatment regimens and rationalities. Second, care is provided within the structures of a neoliberal health system that imposes mandates on a contingent workforce that are not easily met but are crucial for jobs and funding. Finally, these structures coupled with the power to determine eligibility for social assistance programs creates the conditions for badgering and even coercive practices on the part of health staff to force compliance from mothers in meeting clinic goals.

In the introduction to a 2004 collection on Hospital Ethnography in *Social Science and Medicine*, van der Geest and Finkler argue that "biomedicine and the hospital as its foremost institution is a domain where the core values and beliefs of a culture come into view. Hospitals both reflect and reinforce dominant social and cultural processes of their societies." Drawing on our observations, hospitals (or in this case health centers) do indeed reflect dominant core cultural values and beliefs. Hence, when the locus of power of care is centered in a culture and social system that discriminates against poor, and indigenous members in particular, it is not surprising to see emergent issues of care. A phrase uttered more than once from health care staff was that demands for compliance were "for their own good" (Stumo 2015), harkening to common paternalistic attitudes embedded in class and racial ideologies, that view indigenous groups (or any poor and less educated) as incapable of "rational" decisions about their fertility and health (Ewig 2010; PHR 2007). Ewig (2010) takes it a step further by noting that the public health system in Peru from its earliest inception has not been so concerned with providing care as monitoring and regulating women's bodies and their fertility. In this sense she states that a "woman's experience in a health center with disparaging *mestizo* doctor reflects a longer policy history in which the state has never viewed poor indigenous patients as rights-bearing citizens deserving of health services" (Ewig 2010, 7).

A key concern frequently reported by the staff in Nuñoa was the increasing number of *metas* or productivity goals issued by the DIRESAs that filter down to the *Redes* and *Micro-Redes* to implement. Indeed, a 2007 study by Physicians for Human Rights in Peru noted how

> Peru's health sector is highly autocratic and vertical. . . . This autocracy is reproduced within the Regional Directorates of Health (DIRESAs) as well. Health professionals who work in establishments have little control as to how funds are to be spent or what policies their establishments follow. . . . For example, the MINSA still imposes quotas autocratically for institutional births and prenatal visits on front-line health workers in the name of promoting "productivity." In addition to the women in the population who bear the consequences of the perverse incentives created by such policies, it is the health professionals who are on short-term contracts without benefits who suffer most from such quotas. (PHR 2007, 10)

While health care workers are under surveillance of the DIRESAs, they in turn have been given the power of surveillance and control over rural indigenous women through the structure of *JUNTOS*. The ability to issue birth certificates, determine eligibility of participation in this "conditional cash transfer program" and then suspend mothers from the *JUNTOS* rolls, creates opportunity and incentive to pressure mothers into meeting whatever conditions will best help them meet quotas. The decentralization of care—with attention to numbers but no oversight of how they are reached—means that the "conditions" for conditional cash transfer can be well outside the original intent of national policy.

As we have seen in all three case studies, the two forms of labor, either extremely contingent or virtually life-appointed, can both lead to the provision of poor-quality care, particularly when combined with the neoliberal model of accountability. For contingent workers, they are judged solely by the numbers and thus feel the need to adhere strictly to certain guidelines that help them meet their metrics. As we saw in the case of Nelida, the precarious position of the contracted technician led her to be inflexible about the immunization schedule to ensure that she was following the guidelines by which she would be evaluated. In contrast, the named obstetrician in Marleny's story demonstrated significant disregard for his patient when he left Marleny during her labor and failed to return for the birth, knowing he would face little consequence for doing so. While his actions were not directly influenced by a need to achieve a given set of goals, had quality of care been a consideration it is likely that this kind of behavior would not be tolerated, even from other permanently contracted health care providers. Overall, the reliance on limited metrics that center on coverage and quantity of care rather than quality of care poses a significant problem for the Peruvian health care system, but when combined with a system reliant on highly contingent labor or tenured labor, it produces a situation that is highly exploitative of its workforce and exposes its patients to poor care. Our ethnographic work in Nuñoa demonstrates the unintended but significant costs borne by those seeking care from and working within the national health care system—costs brought about by structures of employment in the national health care system and the value placed on quantity rather than quality of care.

Not only does the current provision of care in Nuñoa rely on a tradeoff between quantity and quality, but it also suffers from the regular use of coercive practices. Many of these practices emerge as a product of the decentralized nature of the health care system fueling the use of ad hoc measures to achieve local, regional, national, and even international health goals. The 700 *sol* fine represents a significant financial burden and serves as a strong deterrent for home births. In some cases, fines achieve the intended outcome of compliance with health center demands, and sometimes fines are used to cover unmet clinic expenses. Yet, it represents a coercive and ethically questionable practice that targets the most disempowered and marginalized families with limited resources and social capital to avoid or contest the practice. While Claudia and her husband were unintimidated by the health center staff and the police officer, countless families ultimately do acquiesce to the demand that they pay the fee for failing to give birth in the CS, even when they made a good faith effort to do so but were unable to locate CS staff. Claudia's case illustrates one of the more moderate examples of the creative requirements imposed by health center staff to exert pressure on their patients to adhere to their instructions. In the course of our ethnographic work, a number of women indicated that they had been bullied into using injectable birth control after a pregnancy when they were told by health center staff that it was one of the requirements for remaining eligible for *JUNTOS*.

The efforts and success in decreasing poverty, improving child nutrition, and lowering infant and maternal mortality rates in Peru are to be applauded. Expanded health coverage with a target of universal care, poverty alleviation programs, and the promotion of intercultural birth practices are evidence of a national commitment to improved health outcomes for the Peruvian population. Yet, as we have illustrated through our analyses, policies and programs conceived on a global and national stage can look very different at rural sites of implementation. The structural realities of a neoliberal and decentralized health care system transform the clinic into a mechanism of state surveillance and control used to manage indigenous patients, long seen by policymakers and clinic workers as an unruly population in need of control. These structural realities merge with longstanding social hierarchies, and discriminatory and paternalistic attitudes toward indigenous patients, to create a culture of care that, despite improving indicators, is detrimental to the health of the residents in Nuñoa.

Notes

1. Approximately US$230 at the time that the incident occurred.
2. The rhetoric of welfare queens has taken on new life in the context of this conditional cash transfer program and is deployed regularly by health center staff and townspeople who are not beneficiaries of the program.

CHAPTER 2

Science and Sanctity

BIOMEDICINE AND CHRISTIANITY AT
AN ETHIOPIAN HOSPITAL

Anita Hannig

IN THEORY AS much as in practice, science and religion have
frequently been conceptualized as opposite epistemic systems or mutually
exclusive ways of understanding the world. The other day, I saw a greeting
card in a store in Portland, Oregon, that read: "Dear Religion, pictures or it
didn't happen. Love, Science." In hospital settings, the apparent dichotomy
between science and sanctity can feel even more pronounced. In the United
States, for instance, many Catholic hospitals decline to participate in interventions that violate their religious convictions, such as abortions or medically assisted deaths (which are legal in Oregon). In these situations, it is
tempting to pit the concept of progressive, value-free scientific objectivity—
the idea that science reflects an empirical, universal reality—against the idea
of conservative religious subjectivism.

Critical observers have long challenged and complicated this model,
through theory and ethnography, and shown that medicine and religion are
fields whose boundaries are often less discrete and rigid than commonly
assumed (Comaroff and Comaroff 1997; Cooper 2006; Donham 1999; Klassen 2011). They have demonstrated, for example, that biomedical healing
often requires the same kind of faith in its efficacy that is demanded of religious adherents, and that biomedical authority can be just as dogmatic as the
teachings of some religious traditions. In his classic work *Magic, Science, and
Religion and the Scope of Rationality* (1990, 10), Tambiah explains how science
became a belief system in its own right:

> A commitment to the notion of nature as the ground of causality, of
> nature as a uniform domain subject to regular laws, can function as a
> belief system without its guaranteeing a verified "objective truth" as
> modern science may define it. In other words, the appeal to "nature" or

"science" can serve as a legitimation of a belief and action system like any other ideological and normative system.

And yet, anthropologists have also found that there is a lot at stake ideologically (and otherwise) at upholding the apparent distinction between science and religion, and at rendering religion as falsifiable and unempirical, as based in "belief" rather than "knowledge" (Good 1994; see also V. Adams 2001; Pigg 1996).

When religion constitutes an integral part of the world of hospital medicine—when the holy and the clinical wrestle daily for the attention of patients, families, and doctors—we are faced with fascinating conundrums. In the context of rapidly advancing biomedical innovation, such as in vitro fertilization, organ transplants, or end-of-life technology, this duality can lead to competing agendas and frictions, based on diverging ideas of suffering, personhood, and the value of life. Despite the potential for antagonism in these situations, technological interventions rarely work in direct opposition to religious orthodoxy and, more often than not, eventually become folded into its very fabric (Hamdy 2012; Inhorn 2006; Kahn 2000; Lock 2002; Roberts 2012; Scheper-Hughes and Ferreira 2007).

In other words, the intersections between medicine and religion in clinical spaces cannot escape our notice and deserve critical analysis. What do the overlaps between these ostensibly disparate epistemic systems reveal about contemporary hospital work? How do actors in these spaces envision the work of healing in ways that are much more complementary than they are opposed? And why does it matter to arrive at a more nuanced understanding of these processes?

In the Ethiopian hospital where I conducted the majority of fourteen months of ethnographic research, religion and hospital medicine did not occupy separate domains. They constantly permeated each other to the point of becoming indistinguishable. Biomedicine came to be seen as a profoundly religious endeavor, and religion inflected surgical treatment each step of the way. Neither patients nor surgeons saw biomedicine as an isolated realm that could escape divine influence. In Amharic, the primary language spoken by patients and doctors at this hospital, the verb "to heal" (*adane*) means both "to cure" and "to save." Similarly, the term for medicine (*medhanit*) and for Savior (*medhané*) derive from the same root, suggesting that healing has long been understood in both a medical and a religious register, and that physical and spiritual healing go hand in hand. In a world where patients shuttled back and forth between churches and clinics to find healing, biomedicine and religion were tightly interwoven.

Female patients who came to this hospital, the Bahir Dar Fistula Center in northwestern Ethiopia, had all incurred obstetric fistula, a maternal childbirth

injury that leads to chronic incontinence. Obstetric fistula results from prolonged, obstructed labor that is unrelieved by an emergency medical intervention, such as a cesarean section. The protracted pressure of the stuck fetus against
the mother's pelvic tissues produces a hole in her bladder and sometimes her
rectum wall, rendering her incontinent of urine or feces, and sometimes both.
The baby almost never survives the multiday ordeal of labor. Whereas obstetric
fistula is extremely rare in resource-rich countries, where access to emergency
obstetrics is taken for granted, it affects an estimated one million women in the
Global South, most of whom live in sub-Saharan Africa. At specialized fistula
hospitals all across Ethiopia, women can access free surgeries to attempt to
repair these injuries and regain their continence.

I carried out the majority of my research at the regional fistula repair center
in Bahir Dar, the capital of the northwest Amhara region. There, I inserted
myself into the daily routines of the ward and, with the help of local research
assistants, interviewed individual patients in private, groups of patients, teachers,
and medical personnel. In the mornings, I usually attended patient education
classes, where they learned about hygiene, the alphabet, mother–child health,
nutrition, and Jesus. I shadowed practitioners during ward rounds and operations, observed patient discharge procedures, and socialized with staff over lunch
and outside of work. On weekends and during religious holidays, I joined staff at
Ethiopian Orthodox Church services at various neighborhood churches. When
possible, I also accompanied the health officer on rural outreach visits. By and
large, however, I focused my studies on the personal histories, bodily practices,
and quotidian clinical lives of patients and staff inside this medical institution.

The center was run by a faith-based international nongovernmental
organization (NGO), Hamlin Fistula International. Nearly all patients there
identified as Orthodox Christians, except a small number of Muslims. By
contrast, the expatriate management staff who ran the main fistula hospital in
Addis Ababa (Ethiopia's capital) and some of the satellite centers (like the one
where I worked) were almost exclusively Protestant. Conflicts between these
religious forms and efforts to convert Orthodox patients to a more "enlight-
ened" form of Christianity abounded, but they are not the focus of this chapter. What I am interested to show here is that, for both patients and expatriate
doctors, the project of surgery—which Rachel Prentice (2013, 6) has called
"biomedicine's most distinctive and technologically intensive means of treating bodies"—took on markedly religious qualities.

In this chapter, I shine a light on the perspectives of two distinct populations at this Ethiopian hospital—expatriate surgeons and local fistula
patients—to elucidate the profound entanglements of medicine and religion
in this clinical space. One of my goals is to show that the work of healing is
often as much a medical project as it is a religious one. Once we begin to see
medicine and religion as not invariably opposed and irreconcilable, we may
gain a much better sense of how they work together.

Surgery and Salvation

From the beginning of fistula repair in Ethiopia in the 1960s, surgery was seen as an act of salvation that would reverse the social death sentence to which fistula sufferers had allegedly been condemned, on account of their incessant leaking (cf. Hannig 2017). Their Protestant faith gave expatriate surgeons an ideological foundation for the enterprise of surgery, which they saw as a kind of biblical rebirth rich with redemptive potential.

Reginald and Catherine Hamlin, the hospital's cofounders, were born in New Zealand and Australia, respectively. As obstetrician-gynecologists, they spent the majority of their early professional lives working in maternity wards in Australia, London, and Hong Kong. Both devout Anglicans, they came to Ethiopia in 1959 in response to an invitation by Haile Selassie, advertised in the *Lancet*, to found a midwifery school at the Princess Tsehai Memorial Hospital in Addis Ababa. The emperor's call for foreign professionals was part of his plan to boost Ethiopia's medical and educational facilities in the wake of the country's postwar reconstruction period. Even though the midwifery project ultimately failed to get off the ground, during the course of their work in obstetrics and gynecology the Hamlins encountered their first fistula patients, whom they soon started treating. Years later, in 1975, the Hamlins opened a specialized hospital in Addis Ababa that would cater solely to their needs.

The Hamlins—and many of the expatriate staff they would hire later—thought about their mission in Ethiopia in terms of a divine calling: their religious faith anchored their day-to-day clinical work and provided a moral compass that would guide them through an array of professional and personal challenges over the years. Catherine and Reginald both came from families of missionaries who had proselytized around the world; Catherine's grandfather had been a major financial backer of the Sudan Interior Mission (Hamlin 2001, 11–16). In her first memoir, Catherine explains that it was God who first brought her and her husband to Ethiopia:

> I am sometimes asked how I have come to spend the greater part of my life in Ethiopia. The answer is simple. I believe that Reg and I were guided here by God. It is not inconceivable that the call was uttered long ago, before either of us were born. There is a verse in the Psalms which says, "For you have heard my vows, O God; you have given me the heritage of those who fear your name." (Hamlin 2001, 11)

In his fundraising pleas for fistula surgery, Reginald routinely referred to women with fistula as "fistula pilgrims." As part of his donor correspondence, he would often enclose a black-and-white photograph of two fistula patients, who had each traveled three hundred miles to reach the hospital, along with a picture of one of them who left the hospital three weeks later, "going home in joy, cured, to life anew." In using the term "pilgrims," Reginald made a direct comparison between the healing quests of fistula patients and religiously inspired travels to places of worship, thus rendering patients' voyages in search of healing as experiences of a religious kind. In an early letter dated June 12, 1964, Reginald presented surgery as the ultimate release from a life of despair. "We have now cured over 330 women suffering from the most miserable birth injuries, and if you in Birmingham could only see the joy radiating the face of just one of them, as she goes home cured and a normal woman once more, you would have your reward." It is hard to overlook the central motif of biblical rebirth that grounds rhetoric about fistula repair—that is, the idea that fistula surgery returns women to a life worth living. Take, for instance, this passage from Catherine Hamlin's biography: "Before [surgery] she [the patient] had been downcast and miserable; now she was reborn as a beautiful, smiling woman" (2001, 86).

Worse off than the oldest archetype of human suffering (the "leper"), women who sustained fistula in "the rugged, remote, and roadless mountainous provinces of Ethiopia," the Hamlins suggested, were the social pariahs of the modern age. Surgery promised to be much more than a technocratic solution to a physical ailment: it entailed the wholesale transformation of a woman into a social entity once more. This transformation was reinforced symbolically by outfitting her with a new dress on her release from the hospital, a practice that has continued to this day.

In a 1977 letter to his friend Chassar, medical professor at the Nuffield Department of Obstetrics and Gynecology in Oxford, Reginald thanked him for his support in helping to "create this surgical and humanitarian haven for very brave, charming, gravely-injured, young Ethiopian women," who arrived at the hospital "in shame and wretchedness, but go home restored to life anew." In a 1976 postscript to a newspaper article the Hamlins used for fundraising purposes, Reginald noted along similar lines, "Our free Addis Ababa Fistula Hospital, 40 beds, was opened on May 24th 1975. Since then it has been *making ten new lives each week* for women reduced to wretchedness and poverty by childbirth injuries of the vagina and bladder. Every benefactor who sees their joy and their gratitude as they go home cured, once again citizens of the world, is profoundly moved" (emphasis mine).

The transformative aspect of fistula surgery—its ability to "make new lives"—stood in a symbiotic relationship to a foundational narrative of social pariahdom: surgery would lift women with fistula out of situations of misery and isolation and reinstate them as human beings. The symbolic and material efficacy of fistula surgery, it seemed, had no limits.

The religious commitment that drove the Hamlins to do God's work in Ethiopia was the same conviction that buoyed them during times of adversity. In one of his early letters to the Queen's National Birthday Trust (a charitable organization based in London), Reginald wrote that he often pondered the biblical verse Mark 14:31, which he had affixed on the wall above his desk.

The verse reads: "But Peter kept saying emphatically, 'Even if I have to die with you, I'll never deny you!' And all the others kept saying the same thing." Like Peter, who vowed to never betray Jesus, Reginald had made a solemn promise to treat any fistula patient who arrived at the hospital for treatment, even if he had to pay for the surgery out of pocket. Both his letters and Catherine's own writings contain this motif of self-sacrifice. "With the fistula pilgrims he found the great cause he had been seeking," she recalls in her memoir (Hamlin 2001, 89). "He was drawn to them because he loved them. We found that looking after them was never a hardship and never once did we feel we wanted to do something else. We both knew that this was work that God wanted us to do and we were thankful that we so enjoyed doing it."

Similar to liberal Protestants in North America who, according to Klassen (2011, 7), approached healing "not solely as a form of bodily repair or cure, but as an expansive concept and practice," the Hamlins used fistula patients' hospital stays to furnish them with spiritual training. Since the hospital's inception, patients who awaited or convalesced from surgery have been invited to attend literacy and Bible study classes. Even during times when the Hamlins had to be careful about disclosing that aspect of their work, such as under the Socialist Derg regime (1974–1991) when both local and expatriate Protestants across the country faced religious persecution, missionary friends helped them to continue their Bible study classes. "[The classes] included some literacy as well," Catherine writes about Bible classes during the Derg era (Hamlin 2001, 174), "so we could truthfully say we were fulfilling the government's education policy if any questions were asked." Before the Derg formally banned the importation of Bibles to Ethiopia, the Hamlins distributed Protestant Bibles in vernacular languages to patients who were being released from the hospital by secretively placing them "in their small bundles of clothing when they left to go home" (Hamlin 2001, 174).

It would be a mistake, however, to think of the literacy classes solely as a smokescreen for Bible study. Literacy has always been a vital aspect of Protestant Christianity's orientation toward biblical exegesis. It was through the act of making Scripture accessible to the laity that the monopoly of biblical knowledge could be wrested away from trained clergy (Donham 1999; Cooper 2006). The cultivation of patients' reading abilities at the hospital was thus, in large part, designed to give them access to biblical texts. At the Bahir Dar Fistula Center, the handful of women who arrived with prior reading knowledge were all given a copy of the New Testament while their peers studied the alphabet.

Until today, Catherine thinks the hospital owes much of its success to God's favor. "We must say that we're a Christian organisation here, John," she tells her biographer John Little (2010, 117). "That's why we've prospered. God has been behind the work. He's the one that's been sustaining all these trusts and so on. We must keep Him at the head of our work and must remain nominally Christian, at any rate. That's really important in our charter—that we're trying to show our Lord's compassion for these people."

Several scholars have commented on the special affinity between Protestant Christianity and notions of healing. As Klassen (2011) observes, "Many Christian traditions of interpretation have portrayed Christianity as a religion with healing at its core" (14). In some Protestant circles, healing even came to be seen "as the birthright of Christianity," at the heart of which stood Jesus Christ as healer par excellence (15). "The naturalizing power of both religion and biomedicine," Klassen points out (65), "has been constituted in intimate combination." When Protestants found employment as doctors, they would frequently merge physical and spiritual healing. For example, among colonial missionaries in South Africa, "the provision of medical care was clearly consistent . . . with a rhetoric of salvation" (Comaroff and Comaroff 1997, 340). As pious Anglicans, the Hamlins saw their medical work with fistula patients in Ethiopia first and foremost as God's work.

Protestantism permeated many aspects of daily clinical life at the main fistula hospital in Addis Ababa. Staff would attend daily prayers and Bible readings at the start of each day at the chapel (Béte Misgana—House of Praise) on the hospital grounds. Reading and prayer gatherings occurred simultaneously at various times during the day around the hospital—in the main ward, kitchen, and laundry facilities. Each fistula surgery was also preceded by a short prayer. At this hospital, nearly all the national staff in executive positions were Protestants, many of whom took an active role in conducting the morning prayer sessions. The expatriate management staff who had been hired to run the fistula hospital in Addis Ababa, the midwifery college, and some of the satellite centers were almost exclusively Protestant as well. Before he came to Ethiopia, the CEO at the time of my research had worked as a missionary for the Church Mission Society in Egypt for ten years. Among the expatriates who ran the Addis Ababa hospital, only the medical director, Dr. Jamison, was a non-Christian, much to the chagrin of the hospital's board of trustees.

At the Bahir Dar Fistula Center, the presence of Protestant Christianity was much more subdued and harder to spot: it centered primarily on the figure of Dr. Radford, the Australian chief surgeon and director of the center. Dr. Radford was an Anglican like the Hamlins, and since his childhood he had wanted to become a missionary doctor. Before arriving in Ethiopia, he had served at various missionary hospitals across Africa. His wife, also from Australia, had grown up in Tanzania where her parents were posted as missionaries. The Radfords understood their work in Ethiopia as a divine obligation. They would go wherever God needed them to carry out His good works, Dr. Radford's wife told me, and where He needed them the most was Africa. Bahir Dar's small Protestant community, which included a sizable proportion of foreigners, became their new spiritual home. On Sundays, the Radfords would sometimes hold church services in their own living room.

Dr. Radford ran communal morning prayers on the ward at the beginning of each week day. Doctors, nurses, and nurse aides would drop whatever they were doing and gather at the nurses' station when the doctor's booming voice echoed through the ward before morning rounds ("*Nu!*"—"Come!"). They would face the Orthodox cross at the far end of the ward and listen silently to Dr. Radford recital of a passage from the New Testament. Solomon, the health officer, or Dr. Mesfin, the other Ethiopian surgeon, subsequently read the Amharic translation of the verses Dr. Radford had selected. After the Bible reading, Dr. Radford would pronounce a public prayer, which was then followed by the staff's private prayers, uttered under their breaths while they crossed themselves three times (to represent the Orthodox Trinity of Father, Son, and Holy Spirit). The director wrapped each prayer session up with a loud "Amen."

A closer look at the style and content of Dr. Radford's morning prayers conveys how he viewed his role as a surgeon. "Father, we give thanks for this morning's reading, Father, and for this reminder that we should be living as children of the Lord," he would usually begin. He then thanked God for furnishing him with the grace and skills to perform his work and pledged that he would continue to serve God in his capacity as a doctor. Next, he listed the difficult surgical cases that lay ahead of him and his team that day. "Father, we ask for Your assistance as we operate today," he announced one Monday, "especially on the first lady we have operated on so many times. May You be able to grant her some sort of improvement this morning." The doctor's prayers would then conclude with a variant of the phrase, "We ask for all these things in Your holy, most precious name. Amen."

In his prayers, Dr. Radford's positioned himself as God's humble son and servant who was enabled by God's grace to carry out his work. An effective surgery owed its success as much to the doctor's surgical skill and medical training as to the personal favors God had granted him; in fact, these things were inseparable in the doctor's mind. Similar to the North American Protestants that Klassen (2011) writes about in her work, who "insisted that the science behind biomedicine was itself a gift of divine wisdom" (xi), Dr. Radford in large part credited God for his surgical skills. As a medical student in Australia he had learned a saying that still stuck with him: "God heals and doctors get paid for it." That was why the doctor would frequently single out especially challenging surgical cases and ask for their improvement. Because, at the end of the day, what happened in the operating theater was an upshot of God's will.

One Wednesday morning in February 2010, Dr. Radford brought up the cases of two patients whose healing trajectories gave him reason to worry:

Father, thank You for the graces You have given to us. . . . We ask for the lady there from Oromo. She is breaking now and [we pray] that she won't be discouraged, and that we will be able to help her in the future and provide her with some sort of cure. And the little girl, may she continue to get better and be discharged and improve and get some sort of good result from the operation. Father we thank You for all the patients that are arriving now and [pray] that we can send them home again. We give thanks for all these things in Your holy, most precious name. Amen.

In underscoring difficult surgical cases during his prayers, the surgeon sought to enlist God's assistance not just during surgery but throughout patients' period of convalescence. If the stitches held, the doctor wouldn't alone take credit for that; at the same time, the surgeon wasn't alone responsible if a surgery failed.

At the fistula hospital, Protestantism functioned as a primary motivational and ideological force that allowed surgeons like the Hamlins and Dr. Radford to carry out their everyday clinical work—their faith filled them with a deep sense of calling and purpose. From the start, God was seen to stand behind the work of the hospital, overseeing every suture.

OF DOCTORS AND PRIESTS

Like surgeons, Orthodox Christian patients experienced and gave order to their hospital stay through religious registers of various kinds. Many patients saw access to hospital doctors' knowledge as restricted not just because it rested on a complicated body of scientific facts, but because they understood that God had explicitly authorized such knowledge. And because most lay-people had limited access to this type of specialized knowledge, patients tended to be rather deferential in their interactions with senior medical staff, especially doctors. They hardly ever asked them any questions and would often exaggerate their reverence by trying to prostrate themselves in front of them. Incidentally, the hierarchies of expertise patients found at the hospital were similar to the gradated hierarchies of knowledge and access they were accustomed to from church (on which more below).

Some might argue that this submission to figures of authority is not that surprising in a society that scholars have generally characterized as hierarchical (Levine 1965; Hoben 1970; Messay 1999; Malara and Boylston 2016). But there is more to the story. Patients' deference vis-à-vis doctors also had to do with their concrete sense that hospital doctors were sanctioned by divine power very specifically—that they sat just a few tiers below God. Across the area of my research, biomedical doctors' divine legitimacy was a popular cultural truism. "Doctors are beneath God and they can cure you," an instructor at the fistula center would routinely tell patients. "Their knowledge comes from God. That is why it is better to be assisted by doctors."

Unlike other types of healers, the instructor suggested, hospital doctors were directly authorized by God to administer their medicine. They therefore didn't present a challenge to divine power but glorified it. Similar to some of the more devout Orthodox Christian patients, who considered *bahilawí med-hanít* (traditional medicine) an anathema to the Orthodox Church, the instructor forbade patients from frequenting any nonbiomedical practitioners. Educators went to great lengths to convince patients to steer clear of the services of rival forms of medical authority and assured them that the hospital was the only place that could offer a cure. "Even if you don't understand [hospital medicine]," one instructor pleaded with them, "you have to go to a doctor."

Instructors liked pointing out that patients had physical, tangible proof of the efficacy of hospital doctors as many of them had been cured at their hands. "You have seen the treatment at this hospital," they would urge, "so we are not expecting you to go back to traditional healers." And yet, the rivalry between traditional medicine and biomedicine wasn't solved by such simple appeals to logic. Instructors didn't elevate hospital medicine on the basis of its "superior" science alone. Hospital doctors had an additional advantage: they had God on their side. What separated biomedical knowledge from other types of knowledge was that God had blessed it. In an effort to highlight the scientific efficacy of surgical treatment for fistula, instructors moved away from scientific discourse and brought in an authority of a different order—the divine.

In general, specialized knowledge in Ethiopian medicinal systems is distributed unevenly. Whereas patients may know some things about a certain illness and its recommended course of treatment, they usually expect experts to understand the deeper layers of meaning behind their symptoms. Because of this epistemological discrepancy, patients usually surrender to technical forms of authoritative knowledge (though they may remain distrustful of such knowledge or of the curer's intention). The power of expert knowledge, as Malara (2011) argues, stems from the fact that the person on which power is meant to work has no access themselves to the genesis of such power. Because hospital medicine has the ability to handle aspects of human physicality that go beyond those of other medical experts, people often regard it as especially powerful. At the fistula center, many of the patients I talked to spoke about their impression that biomedical doctors possessed a remarkable amount of power. And they viewed this power as an indication of God's favor. For Ethiopian Orthodox Christians, Messay (1999, 185) writes, power is "the most visible manifestation of the will of God, its favored language. Accordingly, those who have power in this world appear as those to whom God lends power."

Patients and nurse aides at the Bahir Dar Fistula Center frequently insisted that hospital doctors had "special powers." Liyu, a woman in her late twenties, was at the fistula center for a second operation when I met her. She suffered from a congenital abnormality of the urethra that had caused her to become incontinent. She told me that doctors derived their powers directly from God. Since her early childhood, Liyu had been leaking urine, but her parents delayed bringing her in for treatment because they were afraid that they wouldn't be able to afford the cost. Liyu was dismayed about her parents' initial reticence to find a solution for her incontinence. "Why wouldn't they sell one cow for me?" she asked me. Eventually, Liyu found out about the fistula center through a radio spot, heard that the treatment was free, and managed to locate a ride there through a local NGO. Though her first surgery slightly reduced the severity of her leakage, as soon as she drank more water she couldn't control her urine. Yet her parents were delighted about the changes. "I don't blame you for hating me," her mother said to her. "We almost killed you. The doctors are your family now." When we spoke, Liyu had just undergone her second operation; she was still unsure about whether it had worked. Nonetheless, her faith in the abilities of hospital doctors was unshaken. "I believe that God gives doctors power and teaches them everything they know," she said, "so they can cure us."

On one of my visits to a patient's home on Lake Tana, an animated discussion ensued among her and her neighbors about the efficacy of hospital doctors. Yashume, a seventy-year-old woman with fistula, had just returned to her village to recover from her second operation. The surgery had lessened the volume and regularity of her incontinence, to the point where she would only leak in her sleep and when she stood up abruptly after sitting for a long time. In the course of this conversation, while everyone was sitting in Yashume's house drinking coffee, one woman declared: "Doctors are special, they see *everything*. You have to tell them your secrets, even those secrets you wouldn't tell your husband; otherwise you might not be cured." Everyone nodded in agreement. Her remark and its favorable reception suggest that she and her neighbors perceived biomedical doctors as omniscient figures who knew about and had access to the most private crevices of a person's body. Doctors saw things others couldn't see; you told and showed them things you would never dream of sharing with anybody else.

For example, even though Amhara women felt extremely modest about disrobing fully in front of anyone other than their close kin, they had to acquiesce to presenting their bodies to doctors at the hospital. Abenet, a middle-aged patient from East Gojjam, was among those who approached the issue pragmatically. "I am here to be cured," she told me. "I don't have a choice, I let them see me. This is a hospital and not my house." Unlike her house, where she would never display her naked body to strangers (especially not if they were male), the hospital was a space that necessitated a suspension of ordinary conventions of undress. Other women articulated a tension between a cultural system that values privacy and concealment (Hannig 2013) and the open exposition of their bodies as objects legible to biomedicine. And yet, to put an end to their leaking and achieve bodily closure, women had to agree to having a very intimate part of their body unveiled.

Patients' intuition around not keeping anything from their doctors exposes a striking parallel between disclosing your bodily secrets to a medical expert and confessing your sins to a priest. If you wanted a shot at being healed, it was best to not keep anything from either one of them. To appreciate the full meaning of this comparison, it deserves mentioning that Orthodox Christians in Ethiopia experience the sacred through a variety of mediators—most prominently, priests, Mary, and the saints—and graded layers of access. As Tom Boylston (2012, 107) has pointed out, Ethiopian Orthodox Christianity is built on a "division of religious labor and the labor of knowledge." Commanding and interpreting biblical doctrine are seen as the exclusive province of the ordained clergy, who spend much of their teen and adult lives being trained in religious texts, whose mastery becomes the sole source of their income. An Ethiopian Orthodox religious disposition thus doesn't depend on a layperson's familiarity with Scripture. Rather, Orthodox Christians "regard the priesthood as a repository of knowledge and arbiter on the reasoning behind questions of religious practice" (Boylston 2012, 126). Trained clergy act as critical intermediaries between lay believers and the divine, a relationship that extends even beyond a believer's lifetime. After someone dies, relatives pay money to a priest so that he may facilitate the deceased person's soul's entry into heaven through his prayers and hold a set number of mourning feasts on behalf of the deceased. That is why laypeople typically defer to priests in most religious matters. Boylston notes that it is precisely "the limited access to holy and occult texts and to esoteric knowledge" that "makes them powerful" (2012, 151).

Patients' submission to doctors as repositories of the art of biomedicine was analogous to their reliance on priests as principal vessels of divine knowledge. Like priests, hospital doctors had access to knowledge that was seen as restricted. And, similar to priests, biomedical doctors were privileged tools in the hands of God who mediated many aspects of human physicality, if not spirituality. For both hospital doctors and priests, a professional hierarchy guaranteed that only those who had been appropriately trained could advance to a special status replete with special privileges (see also Foucault 1994).

The idea of sacrifice in disrobing in front of a doctor also surfaced elsewhere, in a similar act of surrender. I once asked Yashume if she had been afraid of her first surgery. "No," she told me. "I *gave* my body to this surgery to be cured." For her, surrendering her body to surgery was akin to consigning herself to a higher power. In other words, there was something virtuous about submitting her body to the doctor, who had the power of reversing its lack of containment. As Yashume saw it, to give her body over to the doctor was to surrender to God. In this respect, it is noteworthy that the only time patients were permitted to fast at the fistula center was the day preceding their surgery (to prevent solid waste from interfering with the operation). Given the significance of fasting to an Ethiopian Orthodox disposition (Hannig

2014), this detail may well have added to patients' impression of surgery as a project of spiritual import.

At the same time, patients' asymmetric understanding of the doctor–patient relationship didn't necessarily mean that they trusted the powers of hospital doctors unconditionally nor that they believed in the efficacy of hospital medicine in the abstract. Fistula patients knew of too many people who had died at the hands of doctors, who were rumored to have an unnervingly low threshold when it came to slicing into bodies. Nor was hospital medicine considered to be suitable for all manner of afflictions. For those who had succumbed to illness in the wake of being attacked by *buda* (the evil eye), a clinical injection would almost certainly result in death. Moreover, some patients blamed incompetent clinicians for their fistulas in the first place. According to estimates by the Addis Ababa Fistula Hospital, at least 11 percent of all fistulas in Ethiopia are caused by doctor malpractice, mainly by attempted cesarean sections that puncture the laboring woman's bladder. In our interviews, these patients were indignant in telling me that, "A doctor killed my bladder." Abbaynish, a nurse aide at the fistula center who had herself incurred fistula during labor, put it this way: "People say it is safe to give birth in a hospital or a clinic, but women are even getting fistula in these places now. These women, they went to hospitals and clinics to give birth, but after their delivery they got fistula, too."

Sometimes, fistula patients' medical treatment interfered directly with their religious values, especially when it came to fasting. For Ethiopian Orthodox Christians, fasting involves a prohibition against consuming any meat, dairy, and tobacco products. In addition, a proper fast means refraining from eating and drinking altogether until about noon or 3 P.M. on weekdays and 9 A.M. on weekends (the time when church services end). The liturgical year consists of about 250 fasting days, of which the laity is expected to observe approximately 180. The remaining days are obligatory only for members of the clergy. Women suffering from fistula drew significant spiritual strength from fasting during periods of ill health; those were precisely the times when they felt they were most in need of God's good will. Submitting themselves to an exacting routine of fasting was a personally controllable expression of their devotion to God. But once women arrived at the fistula center, they were asked to suspend their fasting schedules.

From the hospital's standpoint, the consumption of fluids and food was critical in preparation for and during recovery from surgery. Conversely, rather than impeding their healing process, women told me that fasting would actually accelerate their journey to health; it was through fasting that they could please and obey God. Nearly all of them talked about their urgent desire, once they returned home, to compensate for the fasting days they had lost at the hospital. But since most fistula patients had, by the time they arrived at the hospital, come to think of surgical treatment as an appropriate solution for their leaking, they were usually prepared to compromise on some of their values. By pausing their fasting and agreeing to disrobe in front of doctors, they submitted themselves to the exigencies of hospital treatment, extending to doctors a similar degree of deference as they showed to priests.

Patients saw a clear relationship between divine will and therapeutic success. Kidist, for example, a woman of eighteen from the North Gondar zone, had undergone two unsuccessful surgeries for her fistula and was left sorely disappointed. Despite her obvious frustration, she didn't fault the doctor who had performed the surgery. After all, it wasn't just up to him to bring about her cure. "I believe doctors have the power to heal us," she said to me, her voice firm. "They won't say, 'We should hurt this one or kill this one.' But if God doesn't help them, things will turn out poorly. We came here believing in doctors more than we believe in our parents." Echoing both Dr. Radford's conception of his medical agency and popular ideas about doctors' intimate relationship with the divine, Kidist knew that the success of her operation depended in large part on God's willingness to assist the doctor. If no such help was forthcoming, the most skilled and dedicated surgeon might have nothing to show for their efforts. Patients like Kidist folded the event of surgery into their existing concerns with a properly pious disposition. In doing so, they came to interpret the act of surgery as a religious experience that channeled God's will through the operating doctor.

Conclusion

This chapter taps into a growing concern in medical anthropology to produce accounts of illness that take the hospital as the primary site of ethnographic inquiry. Despite temporal and spatial markers that define the hospital as a liminal space, what goes on inside the hospital constantly gestures to the world outside of it. In this way, the hospital becomes a place that always and already points beyond itself. Recent ethnographies have directed our attention to the permeable, porous nature of hospitals, which—rather than constituting a world apart—are firmly embedded in their surroundings (Anderson 2009; Livingston 2012; Street 2014). In Papua New Guinea, Alice Street (2014, 22) takes the public hospital as a "crucial site of production for the everyday state, a place where people engage with, imagine, and contest forms of state power."

An anthropology of hospitals can attune us to concerns, dynamics, and motivations that exceed a narrow clinical context and allow us a glimpse into the world that lies beyond. This world never entirely stays outside hospital walls or operating theaters—it continually converges onto clinical space. In the case at hand, this world is one where medicine and religion are always and already intertwined instead of being at odds with one another. In the set of Ethiopian hospitals that I studied, religious convictions and practices infused the work of healing through and through. Even the most technocratic aspect of biomedicine—surgery—pulled in a variety of other fields of meaning and became reconfigured as something else, such as an experience of a deeply religious kind. Rather than an insulated site for the "pure" exercise of scientific rationale, hospitals such as the Bahir Dar Fistula Center are places of entanglement and encounter where relationships to various human and nonhuman actors are constantly kept up and regenerated. An analysis of these dynamics makes plain that biomedicine will never eclipse religion as an epistemic system because both fulfill profoundly complementary roles.

CHAPTER 3

The Cosmopolitan Hospital

Cheryl Mattingly

IF YOU HAVE ever spent much time in hospital waiting rooms in the United States, especially ones where children are being treated, you will recognize this kind of space, or something like it. In the Los Angeles hospital that is the ethnographic site for this chapter, the main waiting room where children are treated is filled with furniture made of pale, unyielding wood or plastic. The toys, if you can call them that, are large wooden spheres or cones. They are child height but are too slippery to sit on. They have no corners, no nooks or crannies. There is nothing to get under or lean against, no place to curl up or hide. And then there are those fluorescent lights, as institutional as anywhere. The colors on the walls are bright enough—reds, yellows, and iridescent blues—but their cheeriness strikes a brash note. You can tell the designers tried, but this is a hospital, after all. It is traversed by clinicians in green or white with their purposeful badges, anxious parents hurrying wheelchairs down corridors, and the whimpering of frightened children, dreading another visit to the doctor, another shot.

This is very much a city hospital. It is in a poorer section of town, but it specializes in uncommon or hard-to-treat illnesses and serious traumas, bringing patients from many parts of Los Angeles. You can stand still for five minutes in any one spot and you are almost guaranteed to hear at least three different languages—English and Spanish, of course, but also potentially Korean, Cantonese, Vietnamese, Mandarin, Thai, Haitian Creole, Farsi, Russian, Arabic, Akan, and Hindi. This hospital is, in short, a border zone. It is a place of "hybrid cosmopolitan experiences" (Clifford 1997, 25). It might seem strange to speak of an urban hospital as cosmopolitan, a word that more readily calls to mind a Parisian street café, a beach in Rio de Janeiro, or some other locale frequented by the well-heeled, globetrotting elite. This hospital does not serve the rich and few of the middle class. Yet I find it a particularly apt trope for calling attention to several things. Obviously, there is the cultural and linguistic diversity of not only the patients but also, to a lesser degree, hospital staff. Less obviously, patients are clearly travelers here, though reluctant ones. This is not a land they want to visit.

If, in everyday parlance, cosmopolitanism is still associated with an aesthetic sensibility of the educated, multilingual, sophisticated (and European) traveler (Werbner 2008), becoming a patient in an urban hospital generates another kind of cosmopolitan experience, a "rooted" (Appiah 2006), "vernacular" (Bhabha 1994, 2017; Werbner 2008) cosmopolitanism, a "cosmopolitanism from below" (Clifford 1992; see also Robbins and Horta 2017). Vernacular cosmopolitanism, as it has been theorized, characterizes non-elite travelers: labor migrants, refugees, the dispossessed forced to flee their homes and take up residence in foreign lands. Analogously, patients are also forced to inhabit the foreign land of the hospital itself, challenged to master practices and languages that are not their own. This means much more than struggling with English for the non-native speaker. The hospital, after all, is marked by its own cultural dialects, the idioms of biomedicine, the rhythms and rituals of its arcane customs, its architectural labyrinths, and these can be notoriously hard to decipher and navigate for outsiders who come seeking care.

I offer a related trope: the hospital as a cultural borderland. The borderland is one of the central metaphors of the contemporary social imaginary. Across a whole range of academic disciplines and in popular discourse, the recognition that social worlds are porous, that boundaries are fluid and contested, that objects and people are bound together or travel in all manner of unexpected ways continues to inspire imagination and provoke attention. Anthropologists began to focus on concept of the border several decades ago as a way to rethink anthropology's older vocabulary of culture. This generated a new interest in forms of connection and relatedness that were better understood as global or as, at least, neither isolated nor purely local (Gupta and Ferguson 1997; Gupta 1997; Olwig and Hastrup 1997; Appadurai 1996; Marcus 1999).

This reframing of the anthropological scene has looked at connections, often political, often unexpected, among diverse communities and commodities (Abu-Lughod 1991; Appadurai 1991; Metcalf 2001). But it has been especially attentive to the work of social Othering in which "culture" shows its politically charged face. Cultures, Bhabha declared, "recognize themselves through their projections of 'otherness'" (1994, 12). Culture emerged as a "contested category and . . . site of ideological and political struggle" (Mahon 2000, 469–470).[1] Practices of "Othering"—that is, creating social difference as a border practice—has been a key consideration. Postcolonial, feminist, and race theorists have led the way in attending to this largely negative capacity, a pernicious cultural virus that turns others into Others. "Culture," Abu-Lughod writes, "is the essential tool for making other" (1991, 143).

If hospitals are cultural borderlands, if they are spaces of Othering, if they demand (at least of patients who travel there) the cosmopolitan capacity to communicate in foreign tongues, it is obvious that clinical encounters can read-ily produce (and reproduce) mistrust. In what follows I ask: how, concretely, is mistrust produced in this border place? But, perhaps more interesting, how is it challenged? That is, how do actors attempt to create bonds of social connection in the face of this resilient mistrust, to counter its production and create a space of mutuality? How do they attempt to create communities of care that span clinic and home worlds in the face of enormous class and race divides? Can a theoretical framing of border zones and an ethnographic insistence on looking at processes at a micro level have something to contribute here?

MISTRUST, HEALTH CARE, AND AFRICAN AMERICANS

I draw upon a fifteen-year ethnography I have carried out with colleagues where we have followed African American families, many of them poor, as they traverse clinical spaces seeking care for their children who have serious, chronic, and sometimes critical medical conditions (Mattingly 2010). We have also studied the clinicians caring for those children to get at their perspective. From the parents' point of view, these navigations are not only fraught with worry over their children's medical difficulties but also menaced by the uncertainties and dangers marginalized minorities routinely face in trying to get clinical care. Balibar (2012) considers the proliferation of catego-ries of the "inhuman human" that have arisen in the name of global humani-tarian efforts to provide care to those in need. Urban hospitals are precisely those spaces where African American parents I have studied risk being classed as some version of the "inhuman human" and thereby unworthy of receiving care for their children. Clinicians, too, often find themselves confused and uncertain about how to provide care or connect with families far removed from their own class and cultural background.

From a social justice perspective, African Americans stand out in a very significant way. The racial history of the United States means that when interpersonal difficulties arise, the specter of race is always present. For decades, dramatic health disparities between African Americans and whites across a whole range of diseases have been documented; in most cases this gap is consistently wider than for other minority groups. These disparities have been linked to two overarching factors. One factor is the political economy of health care, that is, the persistence of poverty for a large sector of the Black population and the structural connection between race, class, and quality of care. A second major factor concerns what is often called the "communication barrier" problem. Or, in a word, *trust*. A wealth of research underscores the persistence of *mistrust* that haunts relationships between health providers and African American patients.

African Americans are far more likely than other ethnic racial groups to believe that race is a problem in health care and, unsurprisingly, there is tremendous evidence that such discrimination does occur. Black Americans are routinely subjected to the greatest racial stereotyping and to the least access to health services. They are more likely than whites to be seen by physicians as "at risk" for noncompliance, lacking adequate social support, being less educated and less intelligent than white patients.

The structural and the communicative are intertwined. Poverty plays an enormous role. Although the current socioeconomic situation for African Americans as a whole is by no means homogeneous and roughly one-third of African Americans are now middle class, those who fall below the poverty line—the extremely poor—continue to grow as well. For those on public aid or without their own physician, emergency rooms are more often used for routine health problems. This means that patients are receiving care from clinicians who do not know them and in clinical situations where clinicians are likely to be harried and exhausted. Emergency room waits are infamous; patients and families are also frustrated by the time they actually get to see someone. Not, all in all, a promising circumstance for trust-building.

THE CLINIC AS COSMOPOLITAN BORDERLAND

When things are desperately at stake, as they often are in hospital settings, border politics plays itself out in a particularly heightened way. In the world of clinical encounters, the patients or families are most obviously travelers through the cultural land of biomedicine, replete with unfamiliar languages, rituals, and moral expectations about how to act one's part as a proper patient. But, patient and family travelers also confront the problem that *they* may appear unfamiliar or exotic to health professionals. Worse still, they may appear as "familiar strangers," prejudged and slotted in categories where they are dismissed, invisible (Mattingly 2008, 2010). Parents may emerge as "won't step up to the plate" fathers or "not too educated" mothers, characterizations that challenge everyone's ability to create partnerships necessary for effective care.

It is not difficult to see that such a border space will be rife with misunderstanding. Interpretive trouble is particularly pernicious in clinical spaces, where life itself may be on the line. But so too—and for just this reason—is the need to create connection, to find paths that bring strangers together. Parents, especially, voice this as a central concern. They, more than the clinicians, have much to lose if they cannot develop bonds with clinicians to whom they must entrust the welfare of their children. For them, border crossing is a necessary, if treacherous, business. But it can also be a generative one. Border zones are not only spaces of Othering but also of what Anna Tsing has called "friction," a creative force that can ignite "interconnection across difference" (2005, 4). I will offer some examples here, considering how both parents and clinicians struggle to create moments of connection in the inhospitable confines of the clinical encounter, to make companions out of strangers.

I stress this creative possibility not in order to voice some naïve optimism about creating community out of pluralism but because these efforts at interconnection can easily go unnoticed, unappreciated, undertheorized. In attending to the discursive or categorical features of Othering, one runs into the danger of treating social processes in a preordained way. Indeed, while there is overwhelming evidence of racial Othering and its contribution to health disparities for African Americans, the very weight of this evidence can overshadow the means by which people, on the ground, use their frictive encounters to create interconnections across structural divides. So, rather than presume an overdetermined reality, I suggest we approach *both* processes of difference making and interconnection with a lighter touch and a more puzzled gaze. That we wonder, in other words, about the processes that lead even actors who share such significant common goals to mis-recognize the commonality of their purposes and their concerns. Why do things so often go so wrong? Why is there such *low* trust even in the face of highly valued common goals, like the care of sick children? An opposite puzzle also appears. If mistrust is so resilient, under what conditions can it be successfully contested and nascent bridging communities be created?

NARRATIVE PHENOMENOLOGY AND THE CLINICAL BORDER ZONE

To think through such matters as questions rather than foreordained conclusions, I will call upon what I have termed elsewhere "narrative phenomenology," a framework I have been developing for some years that highlights the dramatic, experiential, and dialogical qualities of social life, especially the social dramas that play out in the clinical world (Mattingly 2010, 2014). This framework has noticeable roots in Gadamer's (1975) philosophy of phenomenological hermeneutics, although my concern is not the hermeneutic problem of encounters with historical texts, as he primarily is, but with face-to-face human encounters. I look at the centrality of preunderstanding and the inevitability of misunderstanding in clinical encounters as unavoidable aspects of everyday interpretive efforts.

In the urban hospital, the practice of trust becomes politically charged as people find themselves trying to discern one another as motivated actors and locate themselves as participants in various dramas surrounding clinical interventions. Actors carry out what we might call "narrative mindreading"—an interpretive pre-understanding of their situation informed by culturally available stories that serve as resources for ascertaining the motives of their interlocutors, stories that situate any present moment within a projected past and anticipated future. Obviously, apprehensions of what will unfold, as guided by these cultural scenarios, can generate narrative anticipations of the social story they are in that produce misapprehensions of others and their intentions.

So, for example, African American parents in our study find themselves trying to "read the minds" of health professionals to discern whether they are being discriminated against. Take the emergency waiting room, a place many of them frequent with regularity. As one frustrated father put it about his many trips to the emergency room with his very ill daughter: "Sometimes you going through emergency, you . . . been there two, three, four hours. Then you see Hispanic kids come through or white kids come through. You notice they done went through fast but *we* still sitting. 'What the hell is going on?'" In the face of this worry, parents may conduct their own tests to see if their suspicions of waiting room prejudice are accurate. One mother, convinced she was made to wait longer because she was Black, decided to study her situation. As she sat with her son on one visit, she carefully noted when others were called and what their racial and class backgrounds were. When she ascertained that several white families were waiting as long as she was (including a Jewish one that she presumed to be of high economic status), she concluded with relief that she was not being singled out after all.

Producing Mistrust in Navigating the Clinical Border Zone: Learning How to "Shuffle and Jive"

Such interpretive puzzling is not merely passive. Parents also need to present themselves to clinicians as a certain sort of Black person in order to get care. It is dangerous to act "loud" or "go ghetto" even when they must protest. However, if they are merely compliant, if they simply follow the instructions of clinicians, they also risk not getting good care. This places them in the tricky situation where they must both be prepared to *mistrust* clinicians while at the same time projecting that they are trustworthy to these same clinicians. If they do find themselves disagreeing with a clinician's opinion, repair work can involve a re-creation of the subservient "Negro," one who knows how to "shuffle and jive," as one mother puts it. One skill many parents in our study have learned is how to appear *less* medically competent to clinicians than they actually are. Parents speak about their need to hide their own expertise when they believe this will threaten clinicians. This is a surprisingly common task in the case of children with chronic conditions as parents are increasingly asked to take on home care that was once the province of clinicians. Family caregivers need to gain medical competence (such as how to administer a shot at home) while, at times, taking care to disguise their competencies. On certain occasions, their very expertise may lead them to be categorized as "noncompliant" by clinical staff. I offer an example.

One mother, Dotty, whose daughter, Betsy, suffers from severe sickle cell anemia, is well versed in her daughter's medical condition. She is fluent in the clinical discourses of this disease. But such knowledge is not sufficient to ensure good care for her child. The cosmopolitan capacity to traverse clinical spaces adeptly requires something more. She describes how she has learned to "shuffle through and play this politicking thing"; that is, *appear* compliant even in situations where she knows more about her child's disease than the professional and may privately disregard what the clinician tells her to do. But this strategy does not always work. If her child's health is at risk, she must fight directly. Even when she is proved medically correct, she is then faced with yet more "shuffling" and "playing" the "politicking thing" to reestablish good relationships with estranged clinicians.

> A lot of times you, as parents you kind of specialize in a disease. You know a lot more than the doctor knows and it's scary when you have doctors that say, "Oh, I'm Dr. So and So," and . . . then they say something off the wall and you know that they are completely wrong. And how do you deal with a doctor and his ego?

She illustrates this dilemma by telling a story of one incident concerning a growing confrontation that occurs when she and health professionals disagree over what is causing her daughter's sudden fever:

> I had a nurse, with Betsy. She put in a PICC line. [This is a catheter that allows for intravenous access for a prolonged period of time.] And the PICC line, there was a problem with it. My gut told me something was wrong. [Betsy spiked a fever at home.] We took her into the ER and they said, "Oh yeah, she has a temperature, there might be something wrong with the PICC. Let's run all these standard tests." And then the tests came back that there was no sign of infection in the blood, but she's got this fever. I said, "It's gotta be the PICC line, we just put it in.

The clinicians disagree, believing her daughter has a bacterial illness. She replies, "Well, that's fine you think it's a bacterial illness, you can start her on antibiotics, but don't you think that a doctor should come up and look at the PICC line?" Though the nurses promise that a doctor will come in to check the line, no doctor appears. Dotty watches her daughter's arm swell, and she becomes increasingly anxious. With growing intensity, she asks the nurses where the doctor is. They phone him and he promises to drop by in the morning. At this, Dotty snaps:

> Finally, by that time I hadn't had any sleep. I'm anxious, you know. I just look at the nurse and I yell, "Look I'm not listening to anything you have to say! Get out! Go get the doctor, and I want him now!" So she runs out of the room. The doctor comes up twenty minutes later. They check and, sure enough, it's got a blood clot in it.

She recognizes the danger this could have posed to her child and confronts the nurses:

So I said, "So what would happen if I take my child home and I'm flushing it myself and there's a clot in there and I accidentally push that clot in? What happens?" [They tell her] "Oh, it could go to her lungs, it could go to her brain, um, you know, the body might absorb it but we don't know. We are going to pull that line.

She might have saved her daughter's life by demanding that the PICC line be checked, but she recognizes that she also has set up a situation in which she may appear as a "loud parent" (hence, performing a stereotyped "ghetto mom") and thus, worries about how to repair her own image and her relationships to the nurses and physicians whose good will she desperately needs:

And by that time, I'm all stressed out, anxious, I feel bad now because I've yelled at the nurse. Now they think, "Oh my God, she's just a really loud parent." And now I go in there, I wonder what these people think of me. I wonder and this is a constant thing—it's just this juggling thing of, "Well you be nice to the nurses so they'll take care of your daughter," but when you assert yourself and say, "Look, I want this and I want this now," what damage have you caused between the relationship that you have with the nurses, the doctors and everything else? And how are you gonna fix that?

Her solution is to bring in fruit baskets to the hospital staff along with profuse thanks and compliments on their excellent care.

Despite Dotty's strategic skills, over the years a number of the clinical staff grew increasingly hostile to her "interference," as they called it, and there was even a period where she began taking her daughter to another hospital for treatment because relations with some key staff had become so strained. And yet, even in this inhabitable climate, she and her daughter's primary physician, a hematologist, have cultivated a strong partnership, one which can even withstand their sharp disagreements over best care for her child that sometimes erupt between them. Dotty sometimes laughingly describes this physician as her "second husband." (The joke here—she has no first husband.) At other times, she has called him her "dad." (He is considerably older than she is.)

How does this social possibility of partnership get created? To think about this, I offer another example—a mother, Andrena, whose daughter was diagnosed with a brain tumor.

TRANSFORMING MISTRUST INTO TRUST: ANDRENA'S TRAVEL ADVENTURES

In my very first interview with Andrena, she launched almost immediately and with very little prompting into a harrowing story about her long journey for a diagnosis, an entire year in which she took her very sick daughter repeatedly to emergency rooms in hospitals all over the city, only to hear that there was nothing seriously wrong with Belinda. Her mounting fear and frustration as she witnessed her daughter become increasingly ill, with violent vomiting and headaches. Health professionals offered a wide range of advice and possible diagnoses. Improper diet or allergies were frequent suspects. Andrena followed these suggestions but nothing helped.

Andrena was at her wits end. One night, her daughter had a particularly violent spate of vomiting, "It was like in the *Exorcist!*" Andrena recalled with a shudder. She rushed Belinda to the emergency room, only to be turned away yet again by a physician who accuses her of abusing her child. Finally, the next morning, she took her daughter back, picking her up and carrying her through the hospital's administrative offices (off limits to patients) where she declared to the startled secretaries that she would not leave until someone saw her sick daughter. This act of trespassing finally results in a doctor ordering a CAT scan and the discovery of a cancerous brain tumor the size of an egg, one that had grown unchecked for at least a year. (Although I first heard this story from Andrena, I confirmed it by my review of her daughter's medical records.)

And yet, even with this inauspicious beginning, trust and community are created between Andrena and some of her daughter's clinicians, from X-ray technicians to the primary oncologist. Their success at doing so illustrates the hermeneutic proposition that misunderstanding is not the end point of dialogue but its necessary beginning. The following encounter between Andrena, her daughter, and the daughter's oncologist reveals how this dialogical possibility is produced through face-to-face interaction.

PRODUCING TRUST: THE YES I CAN/ NO YOU CAN'T GAME

Andrena and Belinda arrive at the hospital for an appointment with the oncologist. They are primarily there to find out the latest results of an MRI scan which will tell them whether or not the latest round of chemotherapy has been successful in shrinking Belinda's tumor. They are taken into one of the treatment rooms. There is the customary exam table covered with a white sheet and two chairs. Andrena helps Belinda hop up on the table and sits in one of the chairs. Belinda, as usual, pulls the otoscope and ophthalmoscope off the wall and begins nervously playing with them while they wait for Dr Hansen. Andrena waits painfully while trying to be calm for her daughter, fearing what he will tell them. Has the tumor spread? Or, she hardly dares to hope, has it shrunk or even disappeared altogether since the last bout of chemotherapy?

Finally, Dr. Hansen enters. He smiles a greeting to Andrena but goes immediately to sit beside Belinda. She instinctively puts her hand over her chest where her port is, fearing that he will give her a shot. She says nothing.

He notices her protective move and smiles, "No, no, I don't do shots. That's those other guys down the hall. I'm just going to check you out a little, use my stethoscope. You remember this, don't you?" Belinda visibly relaxes, letting her hand drop to her side.

"Hey," Dr. Hansen jokes, noticing the instruments still clutched in her right hand, "You can't have those! Give them back!" He playfully moves to take them from Belinda. She snatches her hand away, grinning. "No! I can have them!" she shouts. "No, you can't!" he says, raising his voice. "Yes, I can!" she repeats even more loudly, laughing now. "OK," he sighs in mock defeat. "I guess I'll just have to listen to your chest." Belinda hugs him and he puts his arm around her.

She leans against him and he strokes her head and back absently while talking to Andrena about the results from the MRI taken a few days earlier. A moment later he jumps down, telling Belinda that he wants to show her mother the X-ray films. He holds them up to the light as Andrena walks over to him. Together they look at the X-rays as he points out just where the tumor is. He compares it to the last scan. "It's holding stable," he says. "It's not shrinking, but at least it's not growing. This chemo might yet work." Andrena sits down again, relieved of her worst fears.

Dr. Hansen returns to Belinda's side, telling her he is just going to check out a few things. He gently prods her, which she now submits to without protest. The room is silent. A few minutes later, he looks up and asks of Belinda and then Andrena, "How was your Thanksgiving?" Andrena replies, "Okay, just my daughter and grandson came over this year. Very small." "Yeah," he says laughing ruefully. "My wife and I planned this big family dinner and then at the last minute, first my parents couldn't come and then my brother and his family couldn't make it. Then my two kids canceled out. So, it was just us and a huge table of food. We're still eating that turkey!" Andrena and Dr. Hansen laugh as he turns his attention back to Belinda for a goodbye hug. Shortly after, he leaves the room.

This visit lasts fourteen minutes. It may be routine for the doctor, but it is momentous for Andrena and Belinda. The oncologist is privy to secrets about Belinda's body, thanks to exotic tools like MRIs, that Andrena, who knows her child so intimately, cannot guess. This privileged knowledge is not trivial; it concerns life and death. For Belinda too, as for many children, though she may not know exactly what is at stake, doctors are frightening people. The hospital is a place she dreads, especially on days when she receives any shots. It is not a casual place. It demands vigilance. She instinctively places her hand over her port to ward off potential shots when Dr. Hansen arrives.

Andrena too is vigilant, and her vigilance concerns more than the medical news. She simultaneously attends to an equally subtle text, a text she reads in his body and in what clinicians might consider the "informal" or "nonclinical" aspects of his communication. She is assessing whether Dr. Hansen is doing all he can medically for her child. Race and class play a key role in the unstated content of their exchange. Will her child, though Black and poor, or the child of a single mother, be given good care? Will the doctors try hard to keep her alive? She tries to ascertain this through a number of common means, by trying to get second opinions, by scouring the Internet, by talking to other families she meets in the waiting room about their experiences at this hospital and with this physician. Although she relies upon all these avenues to assess quality of care, one of the most important means of assessment is the interaction itself. Does this doctor treat her and her daughter with respect? Does he go beyond being a "mere professional," a distant scientist, to engage with her in a personal way? Does he know and like Belinda? Does he indicate that it would matter to him if Belinda died? Medical encounters are not places in which such conversations take place in any explicit manner. These are not questions that she—or any of the other families—can put to clinicians and have answered. Rather, her questioning must be indirect, a reading of signs in the clinical encounter itself.

And so, Andrena reads the signs of Dr. Hansen's actions. She, in effect, reads his mind and this mind-reading is very much embedded in a narrative she has constructed about who Dr. Hansen is and what kind of relationship she has been able to cultivate with him. Andrena once mentioned after her child had died that she had heard some negative gossip about him. Other African American parents she met in the oncology ward had accused him of being prejudiced against Blacks. "I don't know if it's true but I don't care," she told me. This was a startling statement. What could she possibly mean? She went on: "He was good to me. He was good to Belinda. He really took care of her. He liked her. And not just like a doctor to a patient. But like a person, like a, like a . . ." and here Andrena hesitated in her choice of words, "almost like a father to a child."

How was this message communicated to Andrena, that he would not withhold treatment because of prejudice even if he had gotten this reputation? There is probably nothing Dr. Hansen could have directly said to assuage this fear. Rather, he spoke through his playful manner with Belinda, his fatherly warmth, and his relaxed confessional storytelling about a Thanksgiving fiasco. These small exchanges indicate to her a very real sense of partnership. His actions seem to say, *We are in this together.* His genuine and affectionate concern for her daughter is also evidence that together they hold Belinda's life dear.

Of all actions that Dr. Hansen takes, what Andrena remembers best is his capacity to play with Belinda. For this is not just any play. In some fashion or another, the "yes, I can/no, you can't" scenario becomes a familiar routine that transpires between Dr. Hansen and Belinda in nearly every visit. What I discovered in spending time with Andrena and Belinda at home is that it was an echo of a game (a reversal of a game) played commonly between mother and child. As Belinda grew weaker, Andrena often got a reluctant, frail

Belinda to do things by telling her that she could not do them. Andrena used this strategy to cajole Belinda into doing physical and occupational therapy exercises that Belinda shied away from. Andrena had cleverly incorporated exercises into play at home. But it was the "no, you can't/yes, I can" game that so often motivated Belinda to take on these difficult tasks. "You can't do that!" Andrena would exclaim, having asked her to climb some stairs or perform some other task that had become challenging post-surgery, radiation, and heavy doses of chemotherapy. "What?" Belinda would respond indignantly, but with a playfulness that indicated she recognized this as a pretend insult. "Yes, I can!" "Oh no you can't," Andrena would reply. "Oh yes I can," Belinda always continued to protest until they both dissolved into laughter. And so it went as Belinda, giggling and mock defiant, climbed the stairs or threw the heavy ball to her cousin.

Dr. Hansen had mysteriously acquired knowledge of the "no, you can't/yes, I can" game and used it for his own purposes, to put this frightened child at ease, a child who cried and pleaded every week when she realized that her mother was taking her to the hospital again. The apparent carelessness of this play between doctor and child belied its utter seriousness in terms of what it communicates to this mother. Andrena fondly remembered this several years later. For her, it offered some of the strongest evidence that she found a doctor who has come to care for her daughter as a "little girl, not just another cancer kid," as she put it.

The level of connection that is forged between doctor, child, and mother is deep in another way. In this hospital setting, where a frightened little girl has no power but must surrender her body week after week for poking and prodding, Dr. Hansen plays a game not only as an equal but, in fact, inverts their power relation. She does something that would ordinarily be forbidden—after all, otoscopes and ophthalmoscopes are not the toys of a child and Belinda clearly knows this. Furthermore, when he (all pretend sternness) forbids it and she tells him no, he concedes. Her no, unlike the many nos Belinda futilely voices on her trips to the hospital, wins the day. In fact, she can say no over and over and over with increasing delight. And, in the end, she keeps her stash of clinical tools clutched tightly in her hands while he moves into his examination or into conversations with her mother. Thus, in the middle of the grimmest scene, comes the possibility of humor, a momentary forgetting of the terrible reasons that bring these three together. It is precisely the embedding of the strictly clinical within a kind of family drama, the three of them together, that carries tremendous weight. Andrena encourages this with her appreciative laughter. Belinda encourages it with her delight and her affection. Andrena's whole body relaxes as she watches Belinda, who emerges as a delightful girl, a little charmer, leaning against Dr. Hansen.

Dr. Hansen's storytelling also reinforces the sensuous, embodied messages communicated by the play between doctor and child. Dr. Hansen points toward a family scene and briefly crosses professional/patient boundaries when he recounts Thanksgiving mishaps at his house. He and Andrena exchange knowing glances about the family dramas so likely to accompany traditional holidays. By referring to a common holiday, one celebrated across many gender, race, class, and ethnic barriers, he also initiates a common identification. Notably, he has told a confessional Thanksgiving story. He does not triumph in his little tale but is the unwitting victim of more powerful family members who fail to show up to dinner as promised. He may be the expert in his role as doctor, but as family member who has a hard time with his relatives, he and Andrena seem to share a similar space. Here again, the prevailing power structure of the clinic is quietly and fleetingly overturned.

The Fragility of Cosmopolitan Connections

This small moment, a single routine visit between an oncologist and his patient, takes on its profound meaning as part of a complex healing drama that involves Andrena's ability to cross this cultural border space successfully. As we already know, this border drama began long before Dr. Hansen was on the scene, in the year of Belinda's increasing illness and her fruitless attempts to get an accurate diagnosis from doctors. In this terrible place, Andrena felt she had come upon a doctor she could trust. Finding a good doctor is a measure of her own goodness and worth as a parent. The moral responsibility she still bears for somehow not managing to get her child diagnosed earlier is palpable. *Why did I listen to all those other doctors?*, she still asks herself. *Should I have fought harder? Why was I so compliant when doctors diagnosed Belinda with the flu or allergies? Why did I let myself trust them?*

Her own sense that she had done everything possible for her daughter, that she had given Belinda the best possible life despite her illness, hinged significantly on her relationship with Dr. Hansen. For if she felt she had allowed her daughter to be treated by someone who would not do everything, who was prejudiced or incompetent, and who therefore denied or was ignorant of experimental medical trials or the latest treatment techniques, how could she live with herself? A best possible life for Belinda is one in which Andrena is assured that she, and those she has allowed to treat her daughter, have done everything they could, have acted not only as professionals but with a kind of personal commitment that will transcend the obstacles of race, class, or clinical detachment. This is why, even when she later hears that Dr. Hansen is prejudiced, she does not waver in her opinion that she did the best for her daughter. How can this be? She prides herself and her daughter for their capacity to break through color barriers, to pull this doctor into a common humanity. Moments such as the "yes, I can" games, the casual exchange of a Thanksgiving story, serve as assuring indicators that she and her daughter have forged a trustworthy relationship. She does not, in other words, simply trust this doctor. Andrena and the clinician *actively* created and cultivated this trust. She trusts her own skills and those of her affectionate daughter to forge bonds of compassion. His playfulness, the gentleness of his hand on Belinda's back as he talks to Andrena, are the signs she reads to assess her own ability to bring this doctor into a genuine connection with her and her child.

CONCLUSION

City hospitals in metropoles like Los Angeles, Chicago, and Boston, where I have carried out fieldwork, are cosmopolitan spaces par excellence, dizzying scenes of border life. In such borderlands, there is ample opportunity for misunderstanding, for stigmatizing, and for fixing the other as Other. Race, class, and ethnic diversity play crucial roles in producing these negative effects, and a great deal of scholarly and educational effort has been directed to ameliorating it. Notable examples are the courses on cultural and structural competence offered in medical schools as part of clinical training. While such training may indeed be useful, what is less visible to the clinical world is the immense expertise that patients (or family members) must acquire. They are the ones who must develop competence in the culture(s) of biomedicine. Their task to become adept cosmopolitan travelers requires much more than simply acquiring specialized medical expertise or learning the proper patient role to win the trust of clinicians. Simple compliance will not do. Too often, trespassing and transgression are demanded if there is any hope to access decent care for their children.

What might attention to their efforts teach the clinical world? I return to Dr. Hansen. If I had asked about this clinical encounter, he would very likely have said that he was just "being pleasant" to Belinda and her mother, or that he was "calming Belinda down," or some other small and modest assessment of his friendly and respectful attitude to mother and child. In interviews with him, he spoke of the medical condition of Belinda, which concerned him greatly, but he would never think to recount something so "trivial" as his little "yes, I can" games with her or his chitchat with Andrena about Thanksgiving dinner.

His misunderstanding of his own role in building trust with Andrena and her daughter had a very direct impact. When it was clear that treatment was not working and Belinda was terminal, it was not Dr. Hansen who delivered this terrible news. He seemed to believe that since the "medical story" was over (the battle against cancer had been lost), his own part in it was also completed. In his last visit with Andrena, he simply announced that they were discontinuing the chemotherapy. In the hall afterward, it was the case nurse who said quietly to Andrena that she should "prepare." "You've probably got about three more months with her," she told Andrena. I remember standing there listening to these words in shock, uncertain I had heard correctly. Andrena was similarly stunned. She subsequently tried to reach Dr. Hansen on several occasions but he had "gone on vacation," she was told. "I thought he'd be with me through the death part," she remarked to me, anguished. "I thought he'd be the one to tell me." His sudden disappearance created new doubts, new mistrust. She thought Belinda was special to him. But perhaps she'd been wrong. Had she misjudged his level of commitment? Or her own skill as border traveler? Had she not, after all, found a doctor who would do everything he could for her child? In the months and years that followed her daughter's death, she struggled with this, at some point musing that perhaps she needed to extend empathy to him. Maybe the doctors need therapy, she offered, since they see death so much.

A great deal of work in medical anthropology has been directed to the inhumane inequities that permeate health care across the globe. I have also been concerned to expose social injustices. These become visible not only at the scale of large social structures or the global circulation of neoliberal practices, but also in the most ordinary and mundane clinical interactions. In this chapter, as elsewhere in my work, I have taken up the question of relationality across racial difference through the figure of the border traveler. In doing so, it has always been important to me to document not only the injustices so prominently on display but connections as well. In light of the formidable structural and racial barriers that undergird the hospital encounter, how and when do connections get created, even if these are fleeting and fragile? As I have followed African American families over the years, I have seen that when this happens, it is primarily due to the long, hard, and virtually invisible efforts parents make to forge partnerships where they can. They have the most at stake. It is their children's lives that are on the line.

ACKNOWLEDGMENTS

Earlier versions of some of the ethnographic examples in this chapter have appeared elsewhere, especially in Mattingly 2010. I particularly want to thank Mary Lawlor, a partner in the studies that informed this chapter. It was in our conversations and grant proposals to NIH that we proposed to study parental competencies in clinical encounters. We followed families and their clinicians from 1997 to 2011 in multiple clinical sites in the Los Angeles area. A team of researchers, including, for some periods, Carolyn Rouse and Lanita Jacobs, as well as a host of doctoral students, were involved over the years. Funding came from Maternal and Child Health in the Department of Health and Human Services and the National Institute of Child Health and Human Development at NIH: RO1-HD38878.

CHAPTER 4

"Dangerous Disease"

EPILEPSY IN ASANTE

William C. Olsen

THIS CHAPTER SHOWS how Asante households—part of the Akan ethnic group who are native to central Ghana—utilize hospital-based biomedical regimens as they treat epilepsy. Examples counter arguments in public health literature claiming hospital care is disregarded as vital due to local perspectives of disease causation.

According to the World Health Organization's (WHO) 2015 *Information Kit on Epilepsy*, more than a quarter-million people in Ghana live with some variation of the disease; it is regarded as one of the top medical and public health problems in the country. The study continues by reviewing Ghana's *Fight Against Epilepsy Initiative* (FAEI), which began in 2012 and rendered its findings in 2015. Challenges presented in the *Initiative* include "inadequate supplies of antiepileptic medication and distribution obstacles at regional and district levels, lack of health system resources, and social stigma and misinformation" regarding the nature and treatment of epilepsy (Ghana Ministry of Health 2015, 3). The WHO study confirms issues from the Ghana *Initiative*, saying, "In Ghana, stigma and discrimination are major obstacles for the early identification, treatment and social integration of people with epilepsy: a large majority of the population believes epilepsy is caused by evil spirits" (WHO 2015, 22). This finding has led WHO to incorporate pastors and diviners into its routine of health providers for epilepsy patients.

WHO's claims of avoidance of biomedicine by the Asante resemble those of Adjei et al., who claim that stigma presents social barriers, including limitations for expanded medical and public health treatment of epilepsy in all areas of Ghana. Stigma is characterized by "exclusion, rejection, blame, or devaluation that results from experience or reasonable anticipation of adverse social judgment identified with a particular health problem" (Adjei et al. 2013, 316). Their report contends that non-biomedical (non-hospital) modes of treating epilepsy are "widely accepted, and faith and psychic healers thrive."

Because of the widely accepted traditional medical systems, unrealistic perceptions of causes and treatments for diseases such as epilepsy can be extremely high and tend to fuel the perceptions of stigma" (Adjei et al., 316). Adjei and colleagues claim "stigma associated with some chronic diseases is recognized as one of the greatest challenges to the treatment of those diseases" (Adjei et al., 316). It is estimated there are 10.2 cases of epilepsy per 1,000 people in Ghana. Adjei et al. argue that because of public exposure, epilepsy patients in the north decline direct treatment in hospitals. Most epilepsy cases are reported to be the result of witchcraft or punishments from spirits, causing patients to be "stupid, mad, or cursed" (Adjei et al., 320). Patients with epilepsy "may fail to attend regular follow ups" with doctors (Adjei et al., 320), which lead to "treatment failures." Notwithstanding such predictions, Quansah and Karikari (2016, 18) assert that estimates of Ghanaian prevalence of epilepsy among non-hospital-based patients were lacking and sparse.

Hospital treatment is also circumvented in Benin, where mystical causes are suspected. Only 12.7 percent of patients turn to hospitals. Cultural beliefs have great impact and "*stigmatization et de recourse en premier lieu au traitement traditionnel*" (Adoukonou 2015, 138). A veteran surgeon at Malawi's *Embangweni* Hospital has reached a similar conclusion, saying it is "rare for a patient to come to hospital to be treated for epilepsy" (Watts 1989, 805). In Uganda, "stigma would need to be overcome in order for quality of life to improve with treatment of epilepsy in the developing world" (Fletcher 2015, 129).

In this chapter, I explore the Asante response to the medical problem of epilepsy. I reject public health analyses prima facie regarding stigma and African health reactions toward epilepsy. Epilepsy fosters a broad social stigma in the Asante, which creates avoidance and rejection. My argument refutes claims of public health researchers concerning hospital use by patients with epilepsy. Public health programs have been criticized for refusing to account for the impact of local culture on health planning. I argue that public health literature on epilepsy in Africa incorrectly describes alternative therapies as detrimental to hospital medicine as individuals seek to control witchcraft, which is suspected as a cause of epilepsy. I also contend this literature misunderstands the culture of stigma. Options for treatment of epilepsy may involve alternative medicine, but they rarely exclude biomedicine and hospital care. First, I argue stigma, noted by health intervention programs, is not an obstacle for hospital care. Using a premise of medical pluralism, I show how social stigma does not counteract patient use nor hospital care for epilepsy. In addition, hospital care works contrary to the notion that clinics exhibit "core values" of society (Van der Geest and Finkler 2004). Caring thus becomes a tool for healing. Second, stigma in regard to epilepsy is manifest at times of betrothal and marriage. Third, hospital access is fee based. Yet, epilepsy patients encounter assessments of their health conditions that accommodate for income and personal experiences. Fourth, diagnosis and dosage of prescriptions are administered by individuals who are not neurologists and may not be medical doctors. Drug effectiveness and precision remain a challenge.

Data for this research were gathered while interviewing forty-six epilepsy patients and their families, along with hospital staff, in 2005, 2009, 2012, 2014, and 2017 while living in Ashanti-Mampong in central Ghana. Conversations took place in hospitals in Mampong and in Kumasi; at divination sites in Penteng, Kofiase, and Apiakrom; at a prayer camp; and in the town of Mampong.

Writing on medical pluralism, Carolyn Sargent and I state, "How and why people can and do make health-care choices may have broad social consequences and reveal critical social relations that shape strategies for healing, whether biomedical or other modalities" (Olsen and Sargent 2017, 5). We also stress that human communities utilize multiple medical options, thus illustrating that "biomedicine alone is not sufficient to meet the needs of vast numbers of people" (Lock and Nguyen 2010, 62). Choosing primary options of hospital biomedicine in events of epilepsy presents a test case of this premise. Nearly all serious cases in Asante requiring medical care involve biomedicine. Even in cases where the cause of disease is linked closely with mystical agents, biomedical care is never excluded from the realm of possible health options (Olsen 2017). It has been stated that "even when health-education efforts are successful in helping people recognize that a vector or 'germs' are a cause of illness, pre-existing representations of causality are not necessarily replaced or superseded." Also, rather than becoming arcane, "indigenous notions of causality often interact with biomedical explanatory models, producing hybrid ideas" (Nichter 2008, 44). Janzen (2017, 90) makes a similar claim for the lower Democratic Republic of the Congo (DRC): "Clearly science-based medicine and technology have become the most prominent modes of seeking healthcare, but they do not *ipso facto* replace the older, yet ever-evolving, understandings of disease, threat, and misfortune."

As peoples' health choices utilize both hospitals and alternative medicines, it is possible to speak of a therapeutic continuum. "Generally, pragmatism, social relations, explanatory models, and perceptions of efficacy are among the factors that influence selection of particular practitioners along the therapeutic continuum" (Olsen and Sargent: 2017, p. 5). As with other West African mental health clinics, the Mampong psychiatric unit is "a border zone of sorts" (Kilroy-Marac 2019, 140). In it, medical pluralism is a foundation for how diseases are experienced in Asante. Two examples illustrate treatment of epilepsy along this medical continuum.

Case 1: Mary is a forty-five-year-old married mother of six children. She has epilepsy and has been symptomatic for five years. She feels an aura and then stays quiet and still for several minutes. Saliva and sputum protrude from her mouth. Mary says she obtained the epilepsy when someone gave her tainted food that included a contagious substance. She suspected harmful intent and thus ate only a portion. The rest was given to a neighbor. The mixture was passed from a co-wife to Mary after she and Mary had a row regarding one another's workload. Symptoms began soon after eating. Some friends recommended an herbalist; but many others told her to go to the hospital, which she did right away. Mary is prescribed carbamazepine (*Tegretol*). Mary has come to the hospital once each month for five years.

Case 2: Three-year-old Grace developed the tension and stiffness in her body one year ago. Grace also showed no ability to walk and speak; *sunsum yareε*, or spiritual sickness, was suspected. However, other family members suggested she go to the hospital. Since the Mampong Government Hospital's (MGH) medical staff diagnosed the problems as related to epilepsy, her parents are confident in following a course of action prescribed by the doctor.

These cases show the likelihood of hospital use by epilepsy sufferers even as witchcraft suspicions are prevalent. This context of disease demonstrates African patients as actors seeking to form understandings of their circumstances. They negotiate meanings of disease and reshape its parameters, rather than being constrained by limitations of culture or by imposed public health models.

The body—as viewed by the Asante—is a composite of material, social, and mystical. Medical ailments are biological realities as well as social facts. Dynamics of diseases require scientific responses. But the human body may be at odds with social relations and with mystical powers. Epilepsy symptoms, like stroke (Olsen 2017), are reasons for hospital care. Symptoms may require pursuing alternative modes of treatment. They are known as spiritually caused, or *sunsum yareε*, and are considered beyond the scope of science. Because of education and the hospital, Asante health care perspectives utilize science and Western modes of treatment. Professional convergence of science and alternative health care has dismantled the "facile contrast" between one single mode of therapy to the exclusion of another. Applications of knowledge, and proof of power, integrate differing kinds of medicines for patients (Last 1986, 8). Asante also experience "health/communicative inequities" (Briggs and Mantini-Briggs 2016, 8), such that Western modes of treatment for diseases like epilepsy remain largely inaccessible because of cost; patients are given only limited medical explanation due to the restricted numbers of specialist care found anywhere in the country.

In Europe and the United States, doctors determine how long someone may be regarded as symptomatic, thus requiring wider recognition, which often extends beyond a patient's desire to make such things public (Trostle 2005, 14). Much greater attention has been given in anthropology and in public health literature to exotic remedies and healing than to the more prevalent use of hospital modes of treatment and recovery (Whyte 1995).

STIGMA

Diseases associated with stigma have received a fair amount of attention. Cecilia Obeng argues that understanding epilepsy in Akan must certainly account for the "cultural basis of disease" (2007, 97). Notoriety of epilepsy within families carries its own forms of public scrutiny. Ugandan school children with epilepsy participate in classroom routine though concern is expressed for the safety of children who make contact with the body of epileptic sufferers (Reynolds Whyte 1995, 238).

Stigmas for body abnormalities in Asante reveal barriers to living that are not experienced by those whose bodies are free from involuntary or restricted movement. An afflicted body is indeed a "creative source of experience" (Good 1994, 118). Family and neighborhood stigma arise in Mampong when they see "themselves being endangered by the actions" of patients with disease-related body impairment or dysfunction, such as tuberculosis (TB). In another compound, some spoke of stigma regarding a resident TB patient. They claimed stigma to be irrationally composed of "archaic fears," which existed only among women (Ence 2006, 22).

Asante perceptions of epilepsy include adversarial stigmas. It is identified as ɛfam yareɛ, or a "falling down" disease. This is because the "body cannot do anything at that time" while under seizure. There is the presumption that the person will "lose control of the body," which may result in "cuts and marks" on the face and hands. Patients and the elderly often fall. But children playing or elders stumbling are not seen as out of control. Convulsions, stiffness, and thrashing or foaming at the mouth and falling uncontrollably are indications of epilepsy. Epilepsy is also known as ɛtwa yareɛ, or a "disgraced disease." This is identified with the public loss of restraint and control, especially in adults. They may urinate or even defecate on themselves, thus bringing disgrace to their family. Public displays contribute to the spectacle of ɛtwa yareɛ. Random movements of epilepsy "make that disease very scary." Epilepsy is also experienced as yareɛ a ɛhu, a "dangerous disease," meaning symptoms are themselves quite serious and may cause bodily impairment and harm or even death. There is believed to be no real cure for yareɛ a ɛhu; often "people with these diseases lose all hope that they will recover." Epilepsy is thought to be spread by eating the same food as the one with epilepsy. It can also be transmitted by sleeping in the same room as someone with epilepsy. Persons with epilepsy are avoided. "People stay away from you. That person is considered not part of society." Epilepsy results in individuals losing "legitimation as social persons" (Allotey and Reidpath 2007; Jilek-Aall 1997). Such individuals in Africa may be identified at the pinnacle of social "destitution risk" for social disengagement (de-Graft Aikins 2015). Most extreme cases of yareɛ a ɛhu in West Africa include HIV/AIDS and TB.

The Asante Twi word for epilepsy is ɛtwerɛ. ɛtwerɛ is known to produce fluids from a body stricken with the disease; these fluids are regarded as unclean and dangerous. Dangerous bodily fluids, as well as unnerving body spasms, in Asante provide a platform for presenting what has become in much of Africa and elsewhere as an unnecessary obstacle between medical practices within a hospital and those found through local modes of healing. Two examples demonstrate the loss of control. They also demonstrate social stigma associated with epilepsy.

> Case 3: In 2015, Adoma was roasting hide for food when the fur on the hide "all caught fire and greatly flamed up." At that same moment, Adoma suffered an epileptic seizure; the grip of the seizure caused her to fall into the fire. Finally, a family member pushed her out of the fire. Adoma was initially taken to MGH, and then to *Komfo Anokye* Hospital. The family said they could not pay the cost of ICU treatment. Her infection went undetected, and she died one month later.

The second scenario is quite different from the first, yet it contains some similarities:

> Case 4: Comfort is twenty-three years old and the only one in her family with an advanced education. She became symptomatic of ɛtwerɛ as a teen. Comfort's symptoms became manifest only when she declared her desire for advanced schooling. Comfort believed the epilepsy was the result of sent sickness, or ɔma yareɛ, in the form of witchcraft, or bayeɛ, sent by a relative who was jealous of her education achievements. Beginning at the age of fourteen, she would fall down, experience twitching, bite her tongue, and feel a seizure aura that lasted about two minutes. Her family took her to an herbalist, but Comfort and her family were still not completely sure of the cause. After six months, Comfort sought the assistance of a doctor at the hospital.

Both cases demonstrate modes of treating epilepsy consistent with the severity of disease symptoms. In Case 3, no prior narratives were given regarding how Adoma and her kin addressed the extreme manifestations of epilepsy. It is likely these were "breakthrough" seizures since Adoma had been receiving medication for regular episodes of epilepsy at the local hospital. Second- and third-degree burns became the emergency concern, and this required the attention of a hospital. Case 2 demonstrates common Asante assumptions. Even though symptoms were mild, suspicions arose concerning witchcraft. Facts of the case yield little doubt about such suspicions; these were confirmed by the clergy.

Cases concerning Adoma, Comfort, and Mary involve body fluids. In Adoma's case, the flailing body was left untouched because of fear of the disease being contagious, or *nsaayareɛ*. It is thought that direct contact with body fluids of an epilepsy victim may transmit the disease. "So they let here lay in the fire where she developed severe burns over most of her body. Fears of contact make the body something that must not be given assistance. Contact resistance is common; however, most family members show little hesitation to administer to a son or daughter or spouse even in moments of seizures. Susan Reynolds Whyte (1995) argues that the correct African perspective of body emissions with epilepsy involves notions of contamination rather than contagion. Following the work of Mary Douglas, she notes that emissions during seizure transgress social boundaries between the body and the wider public. These fluids offend an order of bodily control and public space. Discharge is thus seen as threatening. As a local healer in Penteng claims, "in the case of epilepsy, the person with the disease may be thrashing around or other strange movements. It will appear almost as if that person is not human. The movements make that disease very scary. It is so frightening when you witness this in public."

In the story regarding Comfort, educational skills and advancement fit well into narratives of witch attacks in Africa. As a leveling device, witchcraft debases those whose financial and professional abilities exceed others within their kin network (Geschiere 1997, 2013). Nevertheless, such suspicions were never viewed as social barriers to Comfort and her family as she reached out for serious help on several fronts of medical pluralism, including normalized hospital remedies.

Epilepsy cases in Asante in the town of Mampong demonstrate stigma and fear. However, investigation into stigma indicates that declarative results by public health researchers are wide-ranging and vague, and they are given little support from narratives by those living with the affliction. On the contrary, the stigma of epilepsy in Asante is unlikely to prevent the use of biomedical options. We will now see how people construct an understanding of living with epilepsy within a framework of treatment that involves the hospital.

MAMPONG HOSPITAL

Mampong Government Hospital (MGH) was built in 1973 in response to a national initiative that attempted to address fundamental health and medical concerns of a growing rural population. MGH is a level C district hospital, meaning health personnel administer, evaluate, and supervise health concerns for the entire Sekyere West District. MGH maintains several medical wards: maternity, physical therapy, men, women and children, outpatient department, pharmacy, laboratory, surgery theater, mental health/psychiatric, X-ray room, and administration. The facility was widely praised and broadly used from its beginning. Long-term residents speak of the celebrations surrounding the opening, and locals have made heavy use of hospital care, especially after the country adopted the National Health Insurance Scheme. MGH is a

167-bed facility, serving a regional population of nearly 500,000. Staff includes six MDs, four of whom are Cubans and two are Ghanaians. Patients have varied levels of education. When Kofi (1996) wrote a thesis on MGH in 1996, one-quarter had only limited education, 30 percent were educated up to middle school, 24 percent had gone to secondary school, while 19 percent had finished secondary school (Kofi 1996). Hospital patients were farmers, traders, teachers, mechanics, government workers, and unemployed. Ninety-four percent were consistent to moderate users of hospital facilities. Reasons for hospital use included proximity (38%) and "better treatment" (54%). Some patients expressed problems with the hospital. These dealt mostly with cost of drugs and with the unavailability of necessary medications. Currently, the MGH medical doctor to population ratio is 1:66,214, a rate that has decreased in recent years. The number of visits to the Psychiatric Unit, which includes review of cases of epilepsy, was 1,757 in 2016.

A mental health diagnosis at MGH is made by outpatient doctors who are Cuban trained and are Spanish-speakers and also doctors who are Ghanaians. Drugs are dispensed mostly based upon affordability. Drugs may be issued after a single consultation of symptoms, thereby providing hit-or-miss effectiveness according to patient symptoms. At MGH, a majority of the mental health patients seek therapy from herbalists, pastors, and diviners before seeking hospital care. Patients also use alternative sources after a hospital prognosis and Western pharmaceuticals, since the hospital "did not make the patient better" (Case 2014, 56). The Mental Health/Psychiatric Unit at MGH consists of three full-time psychiatric nurses and a support staff. The three practitioners, Sally, Clement, and Aziz, received additional medical education and training. They diagnose low-level disorders and dispense psychotropic medications to epilepsy patients. They also contextualize symptoms. For example, one epilepsy patient seeks a regimen of pharmaceuticals in the mid-price range. Her family accepts the diagnosis. But the boyfriend did not agree, and he talked of ending the engagement. He believed the popular idea that epilepsy is contagious and felt uncomfortable about marriage. Clement explained to the boyfriend of the unlikely possibility of such contagion, and that "he would not get this disease simply by touching or having sex with the girl." The boyfriend accepted the explanation and the couple later married. Clement also related the story of a former patient who had visited a diviner subsequently to accessing help at the hospital. The diviner was able to "transfer the epilepsy from the body of the client to the body of a dove." Ritual action "freed the client from any further symptoms of epilepsy." The bird then developed spasms and fell to the ground "almost as if it had lost consciousness." Due to repeated telling and variations of the story, it had strong credibility in the mind of hospital workers.

Epilepsy is a neurologic disorder occurring in about 3 percent of the population in low- and middle-income countries throughout the world. Epilepsy encompasses an assortment of diverse syndromes whose predominant symptoms are manifest in unprovoked seizures. Seizure manifestations are often indicative of the kind of epilepsy within the patient. Genetic factors are associated with general modes, and symptoms originate in both sides of the brain. Partial epilepsy includes localized neurologic activity that may spread to various parts of the brain. Seizures are the result of one or more "central nervous system insults, but in many cases the nature of the insult is never identified" (Chang and Lowenstein 2003, 1258). In tropical Africa, seizures are also likely associated with malnutrition due to impoverished circumstances. Other proximate causes in Africa include perinatal activity such as restricted breathing, head injury, sickle cell disease, and cardiovascular complications (Kariuki et al. 2014, 79). Common African causes of epilepsy, according to public health models (Ngugi 2013), include DNA, maternal seizures, abnormal delivery, home delivery, head injury, malnourishment, hypertension, stroke, and diabetes. Alcohol and acute malaria have also been noted as proximate causal agents. Other secondary modes of epilepsy are brought on by brain tumor, brain lesions, infection, and parasites (Preux 2005, 26–27). Most Asante consider the disease to be chronic. Treatment may address symptoms, but it cannot be cured. Through active community outreach, hospital staff listen to patients' circumstances. They educate through pharmaceutical applications.

Recognizing limits of medical care in Ghana due to finances and proximity for specific cases of epilepsy is also noted, yet neither WHO's *Information Kit on Epilepsy* nor the *Fight Against Epilepsy Initiative* analyze the tremendous impact of household income on health care. "Neuroscience attracts relatively low interest from Ghanaian students and scientists, leading to a disparity in research output" (Quansah 2016, 21). These limitations challenge research funding, training, and the medical infrastructure. Restricted access to hospitals is a common experience throughout rural Africa, and yet this important hurdle is not reviewed in the WHO and FAEI reports. For example, Coleman and colleagues report that 74 percent of those in her study in Gambia had attempted to find treatment from more than one source. Half of those with active epilepsy cases utilized biomedical remedies via a clinic. However, "attempts to obtain preventive treatment from a clinic were intermittently thwarted either by lack of personal finances or by inadequate drug supplies" (Coleman 2002, 380). In Mampong, those who suffer from epilepsy and schizophrenia are sometimes abandoned at prayer camps for care because the family cannot afford hospital medications.

Perspectives of science in public health programs often assume the qualities of bureaucratic rationalization as described by Max Weber (1980). Such models of reality, he said, work like an "iron cage" in which rules and laws are so greatly taken as evidence of reality that creative imagination and other cultural attributes of moral systems like value or metaphor appear as superfluous or incredible. At the margins of science, the meaning of "stigma" seems unnecessary. Stories of stigma are seen as a threat or contrary to science. In the literature of science and medicine, public health agendas identify cultural narratives as barriers. Hanna and Kleinman note that understanding the limitations of bureaucratic rationalization will serve public health policymakers by enhancing the realities of nonscientific (cultural and social) dimensions to outbreaks of diseases. Identifying social relationships that shape behavior will "help us design better programs, guide practical solutions to health challenges, and develop habits of critical self-reflection among practitioners" (2013, 32).

Within a public health model, African responses to epilepsy may appear irrational or as obstacles to real, working resolutions. This approach is evident in the work of six neurologists from Nigerian medical schools (Nwani et al. 2013). These researchers argue the primary modes of treatment for epilepsy in Nigerian populations include herbal medicines, divination, pastors, and homeopathy. "That these beliefs are erroneous is obvious because these remedies do not produce cure but that they still influence the treatment-seeking behavior of people living with epilepsy" (Nwani et al. 2013, 27). Further, "these superstitious and cultural beliefs strongly . . . influence the treatment seeking behavior of the people with epilepsy and their care-givers" (27).

A study focusing on urban and rural approaches to epilepsy in Zambia concludes that "stigma towards people with epilepsy in developing countries is mainly due to lower levels of education and to the more disadvantaged setting" (Pupillo et al. 2014, 44). Similar levels of social stigma to epilepsy are seen as limited medical access in Cameroon (Nijaminshi 2009), Benin (Rafael et al. 2010), and Tanzania (Winkler 2010). Conclusions drawn from these studies demonstrate that as a public health model is utilized, countervailing premises to disease causation theories appear to function as inhibitors to a population's reliance on hospital medicines for treatment. Public health literature thus reiterates its own dualities between traditional and orthodox medicine. Its claims indicate a frailty of the former in producing results in effective health recovery.

Nevertheless, my own inquiries into epilepsy in Mampong failed to produce such therapeutic dichotomies. Rarely, if ever, did patients pursue a course of medical action involving one mode of treatment that was exclusionary of other forms of therapy. Patients seeking help through MGH embrace science. They recognize the neurological conditions of epilepsy. Yet, many also sought other medical assistance, mostly through herbalists and divination. They did not consider the various options as mutually exclusive. This reality was continuously affirmed within MGH by patients and hospital staff. As noted by Sally in the Psych Unit, "Education and medicine have prevailed more; and people now understand epilepsy is hereditary or due to trauma." The quest for therapy commonly involves multiple remedies. Disease trajectories change as patients and their management groups engage in varying levels of therapeutic negotiation. Because herbal or spiritual treatments are so readily available and affordable, they are often the first resort for addressing complicated symptoms. Two case studies illustrate this process.

> Case 5: Kwame became symptomatic in 2015 at the age of fifteen, with headaches, blurred speech, and his eyes rolling back into his head. The family restricted the boy to being mostly inside the home. Kwame's parents were concerned about his mother's work. She is a baker. Many people believe epilepsy is contagious, so they were concerned about telling anyone for fear that through her some substance—even saliva from the boy—would be passed along to the customers. The family took Kwame to an herbalist. After five months, the family began bringing the boy to MGH. He was diagnosed by an MD. Now Kwame comes to the hospital for all medications, including phenobarbital. The drug has reduced the frequency and intensity of Kwame's seizures.
>
> Case 6: Now forty-six years old, Joel's symptoms began as an infant: aura, rigid body, "heavy" heartbeat, eyes rolling back. His family visited a diviner, who confirmed the *sunsum yareɛ*. Joel's father died, and his mother took on the landlord as a lover to help pay the rent. Because of her faith, the mother ended the relationship after two years. The man became enraged and began a course of vengeance by putting "witch-substance" in a pot hidden in the apartment. A diviner discovered the substance in the pot. Joel and his mother relocated to another town. As a youth, Joel was seen by "many, many *ɔkɔmfɔ* and a pastor." Joel's devotion to Christianity blossomed. He eventually married. Seizures prohibited him from obtaining an advanced education. He worked as an unskilled farmer while he and his wife had two children. His seizures increased, and his wife became enraged and frightened. She took the children and left Joel. In his early forties, Joel had enough money to seek medical help at MGH. Joel was prescribed *carbamazepine* (Tegretol). Joel now lives mostly free of seizures.

These examples demonstrate biomedical and alternative options. Hospital medications are a consistent choice. Hospital regimens were pursued after other options, and this often is the result of restricted finances. Medical choices offered and taken are not singular with Asante medicine. Obeng's (2007, 101) argument includes age in this equation, where Akan individuals under age fifty, or 66 percent in her survey, were more likely than not to utilize hospitals for epilepsy treatment. Robert was a young man in Mampong and was eighteen when he told me he had been symptomatic of epilepsy for ten years. At age eight, his parents took the boy to an herbalist; but after having a seizure in school at age sixteen, a teacher suggested the family go to the hospital. His parents first took him to Tafo Hospital and then to MGH. Both hospitals diagnosed epilepsy and the boy received phenobarbital for his nighttime seizures. Narratives such as these indicate initial responses of confusion about symptoms, uncertainty about a course of treatment, and cost concerns. Moving forward may involve choices beyond biomedicine. But alternative options are rarely definitive of a conclusive scope on health care. They are almost never final. Public health models identify such options as contrary to good health or even harmful.

Asante, by and large, seek alternative options of medical care provided in hospitals. In Mampong, herbal remedies are offered on the two main streets in town. For decades, Alex Mensah (Dr. One Man) has made a living processing and distributing forest herbs for administering a wide range of illness symptoms involving pain, congestion, heart problems, hypertension, dizziness, fatigue, malaria, and convulsions. Easily accessible is another herbal merchant who sells processed medicines in bottled, tablet, and ointment forms. Some of these regionally produced medicines are labeled in Arabic, thus appealing to residents of Mampong's Zongo, where several hundred migrants from northern Ghana, Burkina Faso, and Niger reside. Many senior patients travel a few kilometers to Ninting seeking herbal remedies for stroke and hypertension (Olsen 2017). Most people in Mampong self-medicate with herbs and with Western pharmaceuticals purchased at one of the three pharmacies and five chemical stores in town. More serious symptoms, such as epilepsy, are taken to the hospital. These symptoms are also brought to the attention of a dozen spiritualist healers who are pastors and local prophets in independent Christian churches. Divination healing is readily available to the sick. Diviner shrines are found just north of Mampong. Patients will also travel by vans to Kofiasi, Daho, Apiakrom, Krobo, and to the renown shrine in Penteng where they consult with deities via a diviner who goes into a trance to decipher messages from the gods (*abosom*). This transaction involves disclosure of medical problems to the diviner, payment for services, offerings of a chicken or larger item to *abosom*, and acknowledgment to adhere to the divine admonitions of medical and moral instruction. Rendering of mystical powers in medical procedures is legitimized in Asante ethos. This structure dates to the founding of the state in 1701, when Okomfo Anokye, the great high priest, legitimized the founding of the kingdom and became a paradigm for state power and for divine intervention in human society (McCaskie: 1995).

CARING

Clement, one of the three practitioners at MGH, reflects on years of treating epilepsy at the hospital. "Most patients believe epilepsy has no cure. Others believe it can be healed only with herbs or through divination." Others, he explained, are certain that residual problems, such as poor memory or lack of ability to create good human relations and social skills, are products of seizures. Poor work habits make it hard to find and keep employment.

Seizures decrease the likelihood marriage. Seizures sometimes begin in child-hood. Others experience their first seizures as teens. Some are adults when they notice symptoms. Adults with epilepsy are claimed to be shape-shifters, changing at night into horses carrying witches through the air. This explains their exhaustion the next morning. Epilepsy is chronic. It is ɛtwa yareɛ because the body is not in control. The person may see flashes of light; or they may scream; or they may lose consciousness. Some fall. Others lose sight for "many minutes." Even though other chronic illnesses, like cancer or diabetes, do not carry this stigma, epileptic seizures imply a curse or sent sickness. sunsum yareɛ is present. Seizures are manifestations of neurological disruptions caused by witchcraft. Patients are never discouraged from being treated by local healers while also coming to the hospital. Asante experience epilepsy as a kind of mental illness that forms in the head and then engages the whole body. A hos-pital goal is to build bridges between science and Asante medicine. "In most cases, a family will bring the person to the hospital or doctor first. They will be in search of drugs or some kind of hospital remedy." Clement claims that numbers of hospital patients are increasing who meanwhile seek other modes of therapy. Seizures make living a normal life nearly impossible. Seizures also perpetuate notions of instability and vulnerability. Clement and I listened to Elizabeth.

> Case 7: Elizabeth's husband opposes the use of household funds for Eliza-beth's symptoms. He believes the expense of the hospital drugs do not warrant taking the funds which would otherwise go to other household expenditures. In her protest to her husband, Elizabeth declared an embargo on sex as long as he refuses to pay for the medication. He remained steadfast in his refusal to provide funds. Because her occasional seizures are quite severe, she cannot entirely control her body during the episodes—which sometimes last for up to thirty minutes. During those minutes, Elizabeth says her husband takes advantage of her vulnerability and forces her to have sex during the epileptic seizures, which render her body mostly uncontrollable and incapable of resistance.

ɛtwerɛ impacts family relations and public mobility. Epilepsy impedes mar-riage choices and family planning. Within families, however, adjustments are generally made to accommodate access to education, employment, and social functions. Sally, Clement, and Aziz respond to personal tragedies with tre-mendous empathy. They legitimize the plurality of medical practices. Patients seeking assistance for epilepsy in the psychiatric unit at MGH also often believe that the disease is sunsum yareɛ. "This is true even among the enlight-ened ones. These are educated people who read a lot and who are informed of the medical and chemical realities of ɛtwerɛ." They will take drugs and visit a pastor. "Nearly all patients who come into this unit for pharmaceuticals for ɛtwerɛ will also seek therapy among traditional healers such as a prayer camps, pastors, or a diviner—the *ɔkɔmfɔ*." Sally reiterated that some try self-medication. However, "that will not be enough. Instead you must go to the hospital. They are the people qualified to make a diagnosis. You must see them for their understanding of the disease. With epilepsy, the doctor's diagnosis would be better because their medical knowledge is deeper."

For many Asante, *ɛtwerɛ* is the result of *ɔma yareɛ*, or sent sickness—which is a kind of evil, or *bɔne*. Moreover, for "any population to classify evil is to establish a mode of power, the power to bring about suffering. Associating expressions of evil with a medical system is similar to that of any other sectors of life that form people's being, their identities, and their futures" (Olsen 2019, 264). Sally, Clement, and Aziz do not resist or deny this reality. Neither do they confront it nor ridicule those who accept it. They also participate in the suffering of patients and the community. Asante recognize suffering and body control to be associated with mystical forces, which themselves take shape within global economies and forms of power. Hospital settings provide ample space for stories of occult beings and their victims. MGH staff work with patients within these spaces. Working within professional and legal parameters, the hospital offers the comfort of healing via pharmaceuticals, advice, and attentive listening. Clement, Aziz, and Sally also legitimize patient narratives by listening to epileptics and other psych patients describe their afflictions, and by acknowledging the realities of both spiritual and biomedical healing. MGH and Tafo hospitals pursue the reality of science. They do not condescend.

Hospital staff at MGH are not deterred by this spectrum of pluralism. No patient seeking medicines in the hospital is ever discouraged from also pursuing treatment within the spiritual realm or through herbal remedies. Moreover, the staff regularly visit local prayer camps. Their objective is to teach both pastors and patients about the healing capacities of biomedicine. The MGH psych staff educate pastors of prayer camps in the use of medications that decrease seizure rates and intensity. Larger numbers of patients from the camps now receive Western pharmaceuticals in addition to seeking the healing powers found at the camps. Drugs are dispersed to such patients in three ways: the patient lives close and may come to MGH; the patient lives closer to another hospital and is referred there; or staff take the medications and dispense them at the camps. Clement and Aziz visit the camps and confirm prescribed and regular use of medicines. They determine if patients need any additional or alternative drugs. Patients continue also with fasting, prayer, and faith healing, as overseen by the camp pastor. Drugs taken to the camps are broad-spectrum and are of low cost. MGH staff comprehend how the lives of epilepsy patients continue interactions with family and other social networks. Their goal is to not disrupt medical options beyond the hospital if pharmaceutical regimens are maintained by the patient. Nor does the staff deny the efficacy of alternative medicines. "We try to help in any way possible. We can help people at the hospital."

MARRIAGE

Asante marriages often do not endure for a lifetime. Marriage residence is often neolocal, although bride and groom may live separately for a time at the homes of their natal families. Contemporary marriage choices, such as that of Robert, are based on romantic love.

> Case 8: Robert (34) was a young man in secondary school when he and Yaa (28) fell in love. A courtship was unusual because of Robert's epilepsy. Under no circumstances would anyone want to marry somebody who has epilepsy. The couple announced their affections to their parents, but Yaa's mother stridently objected to the relationship due to Robert's condition. She refused to permit her daughter to marry, but the two were determined to wed. When their plans were announced, Yaa's mother threatened the relationship with a curse upon the couple from river deities. She promised both Robert and Yaa if they did not break up that they would both suffer great harm. The couple kept their liaison secret. Robert lived and worked in Kumasi while Yaa lived in the town of Kofiasi; they would visit each other on weekends. They began "acting like a couple." That is when "the curse" took effect. Robert contracted malaria, which worsened into paralysis due to a stroke. Within weeks, Robert died. Yaa developed a blood disorder and died within three weeks.

A prominent diviner in Penteng elaborated on this story. "In Asante, we have ideas of physical imperfections, or *asikman*." Beyond distorted physicality, *asikman* also implies "put a stop to the marriage." The word is derived from circumstances of betrothal. Marriage will be prohibited to someone who is disabled or who has committed a crime or who is a witch. Upon engagement, family attempts to discover unacceptable social and physical disqualifying features. These include thievery, murder, suicide in the family, laziness, prostitution, or witchcraft. Medical conditions include "madness," epilepsy, infertility, blindness, disability, and mental illness. If such things are discovered, it is "expected that the family making the discovery will end the engagement." In Robert's case, the bride's family wished to avoid "dread and embarrassment" of such a marriage. The diviner elaborated further: "In many cases, ɛtwerɛ is the result of inheritance. The person has the disease because of the mother or father. ɛtwerɛ is sometimes sent to an individual to impact their future life. It disrupts their present life, but also their future: their income and their progeny." Witches are aware of such things. A witch has "no moral regard for their damage in peoples' lives. Symptoms of *asikman* may be seen as witchcraft desires to confound and destroy lives of their victims and his family," the diviner explained.

At Tafo Hospital (Kumasi), Wanda described how she showed signs of epilepsy at age eighteen. Symptoms included dizziness, falling down, and unconsciousness. Relatives identified this as ɛtwerɛ; and noted the cause as *sunsum yareɛ*, the result of a curse. Because she was not married or unemployed, Wanda agreed and sought a cure from an herbalist. Around the same time, Wanda's mother separated from her husband, claiming there is no ɛtwerɛ in her family; the ɛtwerɛ of Wanda and her younger brother must be inherited from the father. When family members suggested Tafo Hospital, Wanda began treatment within the psych unit. The Tafo Hospital regime of medications has kept Wanda asymptomatic for three years.

Avoidance of epilepsy is more a social restriction for fear of contamination, as noted by Whyte (1995). Spousal selection is restricted to individuals who show no physical or social imperfections. Epileptic individuals are the restricted ones. Like other Africans, Asante place boundaries upon individuals believed to have impaired brains. In Asante, the nature of impairment shapes networking. But what is true for marriage does not apply in a quest for medical therapy. Care and efficacy of drugs bring patients to MGH. Medications and professional nurturing improve lives for persons who have a plurality of options for epilepsy, yet they return for the tools that work in their lives.

Marriage restrictions based upon social character or biological and physical disability are part of the corpus of anthropological literature. What limits marriage arrangements between two households may be symptoms of epilepsy, as it is in Asante. It may be also historical and ethnic exclusions based on differences in identity, language, and moral disqualification. Such is the case in much of the Mediterranean: Italy (J. Davis 1973), Spain (Lison-Tolosano 1966, Collier 1997), Greece (Campbell 1964, du Boulay 1974), second marriage in Egypt (Inhorn 1996), Turkey (Benedict 1976), Portugal (O'Neill 1987; Cutileiro 1971), Morocco (Rosen 1984), Libya (Peters 1990), Israel (Rabinowitz 1997), Bosnia (Bringa 1995), and Lebanon (Khuri 1975). Shakespeare's Jessica elopes with Shylock due to marriage prohibition between a Christian and a Jew.

CONCLUSION

Claire is a nurse in Mampong. She claims epilepsy is believed by all patients to be *sunsum yareɛ*. Patients may come to the hospital to obtain drugs. But they also return to their town where they visit a pastor or an ɔkɔmfɔ. Some use the hospital for years. Some cannot pay for the medications in part or full. "At that point, they will default"; symptoms will relapse, which is sometimes thought to be *sunsum yareɛ*. When symptoms do not begin in childhood, *sunsum yareɛ* is suspected. People then consult with doctors and go to the hospital for drugs to address the symptoms. Hannah, also a nurse at MGH, has seen hundreds of epilepsy patients. "In most cases, a family will bring the person to the hospital or doctor first. They will be in search of drugs or some kind of hospital remedy." Grace has been a nurse at MGH for over ten years. She claims epilepsy patients are "outcasts" and are avoided by the public. "That person is considered not part of society. Some even believe those with epilepsy should all live separate somewhere amongst themselves." Grace also knows people in her Kumasi community with epilepsy who are not treated poorly and whose neighbors and family never suspect *sunsum yarɛ* in cases of *ɛtwerɛ*.

Dr. Jectey, the medical chief of staff at MGH, says,

> There used to be a huge void between biomedicine and traditional healing. But we are doing much more here in the hospital to change that and to diminish that void. We reach out to especially psychiatric patients to let them know what we do: our pharmaceutical resources and our medical skill. For some, the hospital is a frightening place. But we are expanding our medical profile by showing people how we read an X-ray, how to take blood pressure, and how to diagnose basic illnesses. The division between biomedicine and traditional healing is like a room with a sheet down the middle. We want to reach through that barrier, and then bring the person through it.

Research reiterates this reality as MGH psych staff seek feedback from local healers as they extend biomedical services to patients whose modes of treatment have only marginally included hospital care. Very few Asante deny the realities of *sunsum yarɛ*; and yet hospital care is never outside the realm of health options. Few approach a quest for therapy as restricted to a singular path of treatment, especially when serious symptoms such as epilepsy are the purpose of medical care. Wider public health literature has yet to embrace such engagement of medical pluralism.

Epilepsy is a medical reality in Asante. Asante see difficulties mostly in areas of family identity, biological inheritance and genetics, and public embarrassment. Epilepsy is especially problematic in men or women in their late teens through mid-thirties who wish to marry and have children. Like most African populations, Asante see much of their personhood connected to bearing children and perpetuating the lineage. Epilepsy presents an impairment to the human person and for progeny. Epilepsy creates firm barriers to family consent and marriage-partner choice. Robert's case illustrates the severity of such family resistance. Epilepsy is also considered dangerous. Its victims lose control and become public spectacles while in seizure. It is thus associated with *sunsum yareɛ*. Yet like other forms of physical, mental, and neurological diseases, epilepsy is rarely regarded by Asante as being beyond the realm of treatment by hospitals. Ghanaian hospitals are sought out for medical attention at different stages of treatment just as they are throughout the world. Identifying medical problems as *sunsum yareɛ* does not prohibit recourse to hospitals in Asante. Cases in this study show that Asante pursue medical treatment beyond a basic etiological cause, of which there may sometimes be more than one. Hospital care for epilepsy patients at the Mampong Government

Hospital accommodates alternative notions of how a patient may have become sick. That care is also counteractive to how patients are often treated or regarded beyond the hospital, in the core values of the population at large. Epilepsy patients carry a range of economic, social, and existential problems when they seek assistance in MGH. Regardless of these issues, assurance of professional medical care is well provided within the hospital and sometimes beyond its clinical parameter.

CHAPTER 5

The Salience of the State
in Biomedicine

CONGO AND UGANDA CASES COMPARED

John M. Janzen

THIS CHAPTER EXAMINES the role of the state—at various levels—in the shaping of biomedical institutions—hospitals, clinics, and public health units—and their approaches to dealing with endemic and epidemic diseases. Two Central African settings of this state–biomedical institution relationship, each in a distinct time period, will be compared: the Lower Congo of the Democratic Republic of Congo (DRC) during the "collapse" of the Zairian state from the mid-1980s to mid-1990s and Northern Uganda in 2000 during the Ebola outbreak in Gulu's Lacor Hospital, in the midst of a sustained assault by Joseph Kony's Lord's Resistance Army. Following a sketch of the two settings, and ethnographic accounts of the biomedical institutions involved, the chapter brings an anthropological perspective to the analysis of state and biomedicine.

Although the focus of this chapter is Central Africa, I find it necessary, as I write these lines in the year 2020 from the "shelter-at-home" quarantine, to compare these cases to the novel coronavirus (COVID-19) pandemic raging in 200 countries around the world. This global crisis has laid bare the interdependence of states, hospitals, and disease control. As the media reports daily statistics of new cases, deaths, and the progression of countries through the trajectory of infections, "hot spots," hospitalizations, deaths, and survivals, a massive global comparative experience unfolds. Here in the United States daily White House briefings cast in vivid relief the lines of federal state power, control, and policy testing, in relation to states and local communities, and the hospitals that are the front lines of an epic struggle between humans and a new virus for which there was no vaccine. As hospitals scrambled to find enough bed space for the critically ill, and demanded protective gowns and masks and ventilators, political authorities alternatively tried to provide these materials and protections or blamed "others" for the shortages and bungled warnings and preparations. Suddenly, in a matter of weeks, the pandemic had become a great leveler, as the same questions about the "salience of the state" in hospital and public health responses to diseases faced leaders and citizens around the globe. State policy and governance, at whatever level—whether leading effectively or failing by errors in judgment or by simply not engaging with the issues—make a difference in the work of medical institutions.

How does the state—whether national, regional, or local—marshal its financial, legal, scientific, moral, and material resources to deal with a disease outbreak? How does it identify or establish policies for routine or emergency action? How is scientific or other knowledge marshaled, and the keepers of such knowledge involved in analysis and decisions? Which agencies can step up quickly? How do the leaders act, and what strategies or policies do they invoke? What powers do they claim? How do particular hospitals or clinics, or public health measures, engage with these powers, resources, and strategies? What outside, international agencies or nongovernmental organizations (NGOs) are called on to lend financial, medical, personnel, and logistical assistance? The COVID-19 pandemic, like other viral outbreaks before, casts in complementary and co-dependent relief the relationship of public health to hospitals, as diverse strategies of containment, quarantining, lockdowns, testing and tracking cases, determining when to "open up" society while "keeping safe." On a global scale, the range of policy alternatives set in motion by governments has been dramatic. Some countries have succeeded in imposing or evoking popular measures of lockdown for weeks or months, while others have been unable to achieve a unified response. Time will tell which trajectories, guided by states or by popular reaction, and which medical measures, will be most effective in curtailing the virus. These emergency experiments are sure to be studied in great detail and written about as the human community figures out how to rein in this latest new disease.

EPIDEMIOLOGY, ECONOMY, AND "STATE SALIENCY" IN LOWER CONGO AND NORTHERN UGANDA

Meanwhile, the more measured, and historically closed, Central African case studies may provide insights into varying state postures toward biomedical institutions. My original interest in this comparative study was whetted by an opportunity to visit Northern Uganda shortly after my 2013 fieldwork in the Lower Congo (Janzen 2019). I was struck by the sharp divergence in state involvement in public health and health care in the two settings: in the Lower Congo case, an example of a "fragile" state; in the Uganda case, a more "resilient" state. In the first case, the lines of authority and distribution of resources that had been expected—at least normatively—to flow from the state, dissipated while, at the same time, a revised structure of the decentralized "health zone" inspired by the World Health Organization's (WHO)

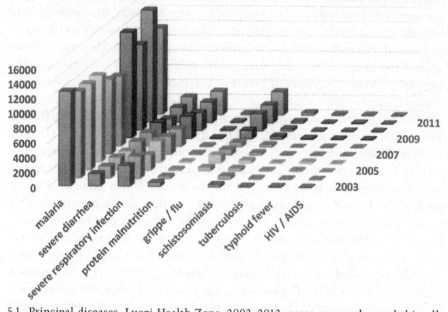

5.1. Principal diseases, Luozi Health Zone, 2003–2012; cases seen and recorded in all health posts, health centers, and the referral hospital.

primary health care plan was being put in place. Preexisting church-related, private, and state institutions were incorporated into this new decentralized structure that featured many local health posts, a number of health centers, and one referral hospital for each zone. The implications on patient care, where to go with which problems, and how to navigate individual or family health crises became a significant issue for many people. In the Northern Uganda case, rigorous state intervention and control in general, but especially dramatically so during the Ebola outbreak of 2000, lent the hospital in question significant authority to take decisive action. This case study illustrates how biomedicine may be shaped by authority structures and oversight, access to resources, control of information, and management of patient cases and their kinsfolk.

A view of the "principal diseases" tracked by one health zone in the Lower Congo from 2003 through 2012 (see figure 5.1) provides a clear picture of the major health challenges during the period being analyzed. These are major infectious diseases reflective of the early stages of the "health transition," that is vector-borne diseases such as malaria, and among riverside dwellers, schistosomiasis; water-borne and sewage-related diseases such as severe diarrhea; and respiratory diseases having to do with problematic housing. Malaria is by far the most serious of the endemic diseases reported and dealt with in the entire region. Severe diarrhea (mostly in children) and severe respiratory diseases (related to dusty, smoky cool dry-season conditions and inadequate housing) are the next most common. The disease rising in frequency over the decade was the seasonal flu (*la grippe*). Diseases that remained steady, at a relatively low level, were tuberculosis, HIV/AIDS, and typhoid fever. Protein malnutrition showed a significant decline, thanks to WHO and other agencies' interventions. Conspicuous by their absence were smallpox and polio, both diseases earlier eliminated by WHO and agency campaigns, and trypanosomiasis (sleeping sickness), a major disease at the turn of the twentieth century that only occurs in sporadic outbreaks that are quickly treated, although still much feared.

Although the Uganda hospital comparative case in this chapter will focus on the Lacor Catholic Hospital in Gulu in 2000, in connection with the Ebola outbreak there that year, a brief contextualizing picture of overall diseases in Northern Uganda highlights the war footing of the region during the time of the outbreak. Attacks by the Lord's Resistance Army (LRA) led by Joseph Kony upon villages and towns created major camps of displaced people near the larger cities like Gulu. The conditions of war and displacement produced outbreaks of water- and sewage-related diseases, food shortages, and physical trauma. The kidnapping of children to serve as child soldiers was a common LRA strategy that created a generation of traumatized youth who if they escaped or managed to return home were often rejected by their families, or found rehabilitation extremely difficult. This was especially true of young women who returned with children fathered by LRA soldiers.

HOSPITAL ETHNOGRAPHY, LOWER CONGO 2013

In my 2013 fieldwork I visited two referral hospitals, three health centers, and a number of private clinics and health posts in several cities of the Lower Congo. I regularly stopped by the health zone headquarters to follow up on the staff's work with the rural health posts and the distribution of medicines. Then, too, with the generous help of assistants,[1] 105 households were interviewed to create an "intensive sample." I also read regional government reports and scanned student theses from the several medical institutes and the local university in the territorial capital of Luozi, where I was based. Finally, I had many formal and informal conversations with a variety of people both health related and at large.

The activity around the three levels of health care institutions—post, center, hospital—differed. The health posts received mainly walk-in cases with typical conditions—infections, injuries, children with diarrhea, and episodes of malaria. Theoretically, any cases that were too serious to handle by the health posts were referred to health centers or referral hospitals. The majority of serious cases, resulting in hospitalization, were handled at the health centers that had a resident physician and nurses, and had the reputation of dependable care. Here is where the maternity units were organized, where some surgeries were performed, lab tests conducted, and medications distributed. The referral hospitals were often less crowded than the health centers.

The most common cases seen in health centers or referral hospitals were cases of malaria in children who had experienced several bouts of fever and were as a result seriously anemic. In my months of fieldwork, every one of the households with whom I was in contact experienced serious malaria attacks requiring a visit to a clinic or hospital. The second most frequent type of case resulting in hospitalization was a serious bout of flu.

Medical professionals complained that the populace avoided available health care services but rather resorted to less-able practitioners, even charlatan healers. All DRC hospitals, health centers, and health posts charged fee-for-service, sometimes on the official scale, sometimes more. An analysis I conducted of a typical household's income suggested that a family could afford one major medical episode per year while still paying school fees for children and paying other costs. But by and large the households in my intensive sample demonstrated that they needed to economize on medical expenses. Fewer than half of sickness episodes (table 5.1) even reached the health care hierarchy, with the medical centers receiving most of those clients. Nearly half of sickness episodes were taken care of through self-medication, mostly with medicines purchased from independent pharmacies or plants picked from the environment or gotten from a healer. This was particularly true of the cases of schistosomiasis, of which only one was hospitalized; the rest, from riverside dwellers who fished for a living, treated themselves with drugs purchased mainly in pharmacies. Many of my informants complained about the high cost of health care (along with school fees and other necessities) and their difficulty making a living.

The economy of hardship had a strong grip on people's ability to access adequate medical care. And yet the culture of care in these institutions is a powerful one, based on a strong professional ethos, a sense of community, and in some a staunch religious faith. The sense of care and the identification with the community is evident in the views shown below of one of the health centers in Lower Congo. The surgery as well as the laboratory are functioning without electricity (see figures 5.2 and 5.3).

As already noted, the background context of this ethnography is the simultaneous collapse of the Zairian/Congolese state and the introduction of the World Health Organization's primary health care infrastructure. State "collapse" is a complex phenomenon that analysts have tried to detail with economic, political, civil society, and military/security dimensions. The Fund for Peace maintains a global ranked list of states on a continuum from "fragile" to "resilient," the former reflecting loss of state functions—security, prosperity, population stability, political cohesiveness, and so on. During the years from 2012 through 2018, the Democratic Republic of Congo varied from second most fragile to sixth most fragile, of 170 states worldwide. Relevance

TABLE 5.1

Disease episodes and treatment venues reported in Janzen intensive sample, 2013, with 579 individuals in 104 households

Diseases and conditions/venues	Referral hospital	Health center	Health post	Self-pharmaceutical	Self-herbal	Healer-prophet-diviner	Episodes not treated	Total episodes/disease
Malaria	15	37	12	47	6	3	17	137
Grippe (seasonal flu)	6	10	1	31	3			51
Schistosomiasis		1		21	9		11	42
Stomach pain	5	6	2	4	3	3		23
Pain in joints "rheumatism"	3	2	1	3	4	5		18
Appendicitis (operated)	1	16						17
Hypertension "excess de sang"	2	5	3	1	1	3		15
Fever	3	5	1	7	2			15
Hernia	3	7			2	1		13
Ovarian cyst (removed)	1	6						7
Filaria			2		2	1		5
Hemorrhoids				2	1	2		5
Tuberculosis	2	3						5
Varicella (chicken pox)				2		2		4
Earache		3						3
"Miome" (adenomyosis)		3						3
Other conditions (2 or less)		20		3	1	2		26

(continued)

TABLE 5.1

Disease episodes and treatment venues reported in Janzen intensive sample, 2013, with 579 individuals in 104 households (continued)

Diseases and conditions/ venues	Referral hospital	Health center	Health post	Self-pharmaceutical	Self-herbal	Healer-prophet-diviner	Episodes not treated	Total episodes/ disease
Total episodes in intensive sample	38	124	22	121	34	22	28	377
Episodes treated in clinics		174						
Episodes self-treated					177			
Episodes not treated							28	

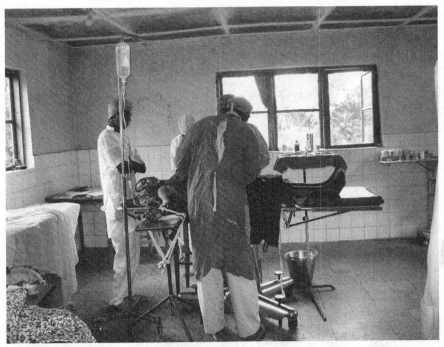

5.2. Surgery without electricity, Sundi-Lutete medical center, April 2013.

to the current topic of biomedical institutional functioning, collapse of the state meant complete cessation of state funds for regional hospitals and health care infrastructure.

The simultaneous ending of central government support and the introduction of the health zone system of decentralized health care and public health created ambiguous lines of authority, or at least a shifting, a realignment, of existing authority structures. The health zones were administered by either church bodies that had been created uniquely for this new work or by midlevel governmental authorities. In the region where I did my field study, a church directorate had been created in 1992 to administer two adjacent health zones and several urban clinics in Kinshasa and Matadi. A neighboring health zone was administered by a Catholic directorate. Up to two-thirds of the health zones in the DRC were thus headed by newly created church hierarchies, leaving the rest to what coordination could be mustered by government officials. The directorate I witnessed most closely was headed by an MD/MPH physician who operated from the old headquarters of the Swedish Protestant Mission. In some senses his role and the organization he headed was a recreation of the colonial-era Protestant medical mission.

Early in the postcolonial era, even before the 1974 Alma Ata WHO meeting that spawned the Primary Health Care movement "health for all by the

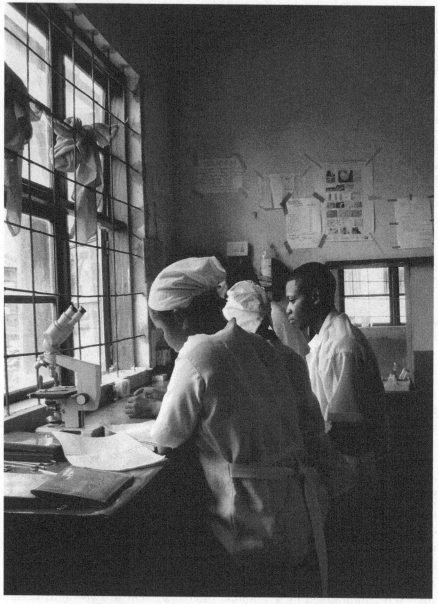

5.3. Lab technicians, Sundi-Lutete medical center, April 2013.

year 2000," mission medical innovators in the Congo had created model
health zones, pilot projects in public health administration. This creative
innovation served DRC planners well when WHO introduced its program. A
series of initiatives by these independent public health actors brought into
being a middle-man agency called Santé Rurale (SANRU) that brokered

funds for infrastructure development, vaccines, and medicine acquisitioning to supply the new health zones across the country. Because SANRU existed outside of the national Ministry of Health, it was to some extent insulated from the chaotic forces that affected the federal government. In due course, SANRU became an independent Congolese NGO, still independent of the Ministry of Health, able to raise significant funds for the purpose of mass inoculations, creating or re-creating health zone infrastructure, and supplying the hospitals and clinics with necessary funds and supplies. Thus, at the height of state collapse and beyond, an independent agency was bringing in funds and supplies for both public health and curative medicine. This is a largely untold story of amazing work in the midst of state paralysis and civil war.[2]

Despite the successes of this independent agency to compensate for a failed state ministry, local institutions still struggled with the transition. The newly dubbed "referral hospitals" still had to maintain their buildings, pay their staffs, and deliver services and medicines. Yet with the emphasis on local lower-level service, these referral hospitals had fewer patients, thus less income from fee-for-service billing. The health centers, most of which had been semi-independent hospitals, struggled with what amounted to a status demotion that curtailed what they could perform, and restricted the funds that they might have gotten from patients and other sources. Health posts functioned well, performing the basic services expected of a nurse-aid and a lay committee, assuming that they had the medicines and materials they required. Some of SANRU's grants did go to upgrade hospitals and health centers.

HOSPITAL ETHNOGRAPHY, NORTHERN
UGANDA 2014

This hospital ethnography was conducted in November 2014, while offering a two-week course on medical anthropology at the University of Gulu.[3] Ezra Anyala, one of the students in the class, worked at Lacor Catholic Hospital in Gulu and joined me to visit the hospital and conduct an interview with the director, Dr. Martin Opira. The Ebola outbreak of 2000 had been carefully followed and well documented. Quick action by the staff, in particular Dr. Matthew Lukwiya, director, to implement the WHO protocol for steps to take in an Ebola outbreak, undoubtedly saved many lives. Action taken included sending blood samples to a lab in South Africa (which took three weeks for results to return), notifying the Ministry of Health immediately when Ebola was suspected, the creation of an isolation ward where all suspected cases were placed and cared for, and the organization of a burial unit to dispose of bodies quickly without family or public ceremony. Of the 425 people infected, about 50 percent survived, which is one of the highest survival rates of African Ebola outbreaks at the time of this writing. This high survival rate is attributed to the quality of care in the isolation ward. But that came with a cost: among the dead were twelve hospital staff and Dr. Lukwiya.

A somewhat different picture of the epidemic emerges in an interview of Dr. Martin Opira, in 2014, through the connections of an intermediary, graduate student Ezra Anyala. It was common knowledge that the Ebola Case #1 of the 2000 epidemic was a prominent military figure in the Ugandan army who came home infected from Zaire, where he was fighting alongside Kabila's army against Mobutu's forces. Museveni's—the Ugandan state's—imposition of a media ban on this information, and subsequent control of information about the epidemic, indicates the first of the state's interventions in hospital care at Gulu. When asked about this, Opira and Anyala emphasized that the country was on a war footing with the Lord's Resistance Army, raging in Acholi country in Northern Uganda, so the army and Museveni's government were used to emergencies, and this included controlling the media. In this case that meant suppressing public knowledge of the infection and death of Case #1, the high-ranking army officer or general in the Ugandan Armed Forces. Official Ugandan government policy maintained that Uganda was not involved in the struggle between opposing militias, exiled armies, and rebellions of neighboring countries. The office of the president was thus directly involved in managing the Ebola outbreak in Lacor Hospital in Gulu. All of the 425 cases that came to be infected in Gulu spread from this original case. The fact that Case #1 was not publicly known or ever revealed—until much later, and then not really publicized—reflects the state's close control of the media and messaging about the outbreak.

The Ugandan state also intervened in the Gulu Ebola outbreak early on when the hospital staff realized that they would not be able to control the disease in the hospital and beyond without more rapid lab results than the three weeks it had taken to ship material to a South African lab and await the results. The national Ministry of Health, and the president's office, allocated funds to establish a lab right at Gulu hospital. This permitted the hospital to act quickly to adhere to the WHO protocols by now well-known by African medical authorities.

In addition to interviews with hospital staff and director Opira, my ethnography of St. Mary's Lacor Hospital included a guided tour of the hospital complex and a lengthy interview with the hospital director and some of his medical staff. As we walked slowly through the halls and into the courtyard, we could see the various wards and departments in action and could easily visualize what it must have been like during the Ebola epidemic. The west building, now a ward like several others, had been designated as the isolation ward early in the epidemic. Access was carefully guarded; entrances became sites of dressing into and undressing out of those white suits that were supposed to protect the medical caretakers. It was the ward into which most of the four hundred infected individuals were forcefully if lovingly moved after their lab tests confirmed their status.

The basis of the commitment to care for Ebola patients was a topic of questioning by me and further conversation by Director Opira and the staff. What accounted for the dedication of Dr. Lukwiya and his staff in the face of grave risk, even when staff began to display signs of Ebola infection and died within days? Was it perhaps the ethic of Catholic Christian dedication? Dr. Opira was quite firm in his rejection of this explanation. Rather, it was the bravery of Dr. Lukwiya, the dedication he displayed to care for the sick and dying, that inspired the staff. Dr. Opira emphasized that the death rate had been kept low, for Ebola, by the excellent quality of care—assuring sufficient bodily fluid, nutrition, and comfort.

Yet the firm resolve to quality care also included an equally firm approach to the burial of the dead. Early on the hospital, with the backing of state authorities, resolved to disallow family of the deceased to participate in common African burial rituals. The danger of spreading the infection was simply too great. Thus, a special team handled all burials with dispatch following death, with no family permitted close to the body. Similarly, sheets and clothing of the deceased were burned by another team. The isolation ward was routinely cleansed with strong disinfectant.

By 2000, health experts had accumulated some degree of experience with the epidemic. Specific procedures and protocols were the expected norm for control and treatment. Tracking networks of infection was a high priority and was carried out in this case by teams intent on quarantining those who had been exposed by those whose lab tests proved positive. Quarantine was maintained for the predictable time of incubation. If no signs of infection appeared, the quarantined subjects were released but kept under watchful eye. There was a well-recalled precedent in the protocols that had been developed and used in Uganda's earlier, remarkably successful, intervention in the HIV/AIDS epidemic. The creators of memory and monuments were able to claim ultimate victory, despite the martyrdom of staff, over these two terrible disease scourges.

Yet the state of knowledge about Ebola, and the means of effective treatment, were considerably limited in 2000 compared to what it would become after the massive 2015 outbreak in West Africa, and the subsequent rapid development of vaccines by pharmaceutical companies in the face of threatened global outbreaks. In 2000, best practices included the knowledge that some patients—especially those with a strong constitution, otherwise healthy—could survive Ebola with good care. Caregivers could safely treat the sick with appropriate protective clothing and its careful maintenance. Already at this time, African medical specialists were the vanguard of treatment protocols for Ebola.

The grim memories of 2000 seemed surreal as we walked through the grounds of the obstetrics ward of Lacor Hospital. Expectant mothers were

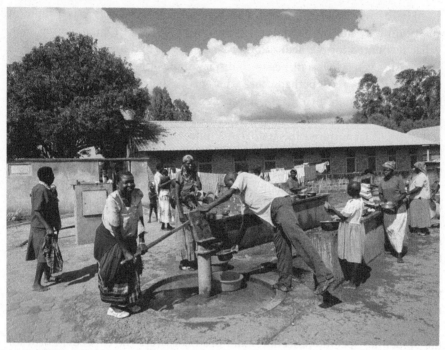

5.4. Water pump, Lacor Catholic Hospital, Gulu, Northern Uganda, November 2014.

lounging on mats or cots, often with women relatives nearby to attend to them. Or they were in the yard where cooking and meal preparation was being done, or they were at the water pump filling their containers, or they were washing dishes after meals. In the maternity ward mothers were caring for their newly born babies, again with kinfolk attending them. Generally, Lacor Hospital had the feeling of a busy market (figure 5.4). The medical departments, like a variety of vendors, were at work in their specialties.

Yet the memories of individuals, the mementos on walls and in large photographs, were very fresh. Prominently displayed at the entrance to the hospital were photo murals of the hospital's long-time directors Piero Corti and Matthew Lukwiya, and long-time surgeon Lucille Corti (see figure 5.5).

Dr. Piero Corti, an Italian pediatrician who arrived in Lacor in 1961 with his wife Lucille, had developed this hospital, founded by the Comboni Missionaries in 1959. Many Ugandan doctors and nurses gained excellent skills and a deep sense of dedication to their patients from the Corti couple.

Dr. Lucille Teasdale Corti, a Canadian surgeon, arrived in 1961. She treated four generations of Ugandans and operated on thousands, before contracting HIV while working in the surgery theater. Dr. Matthew Lukwiya began practicing medicine at Lacor in 1983. His outstanding qualities led him

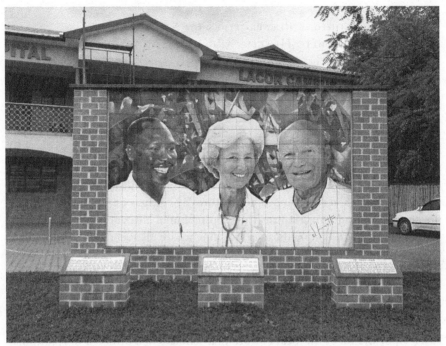

5.5. Portraits at entrance to Lacor Catholic Hospital, Gulu, Uganda (left to right): former director Dr. Matthew Lukwiya, Dr. Lucille Teasdale Corti, and Dr. Piero Corti.

to become medical superintendent and designated successor to the Corti team. In 2000, while directing the fight against Ebola, his leadership inspired one hundred hospital staff members to risk their lives assisting the patients. He and twelve staff members died in that fight.

By 2014, peace had come to the Acholi region of Northern Uganda. The Lord's Resistance Army had been quiet for a while, its leader Joseph Kony was reported to be hiding in the dense forests of Central African Republic, or had been killed. Many of the surviving child soldiers had emerged from the bush and were either reunited with their families or were struggling with unwelcomed status in shelters that ministered to them. Girls who had been kidnapped had often become the "wives" of the male soldiers, and came out with children from these unions. Such women, and their offspring, were often rejected, or shunned, by their families. They represented a new class of marginalized, liminal, community members. My seminar students and others who worked with them, or had such individuals in their families, said these were the most difficult trauma cases to deal with and saw little hope of resolving their situation. Gulu and Northern Uganda were rebuilding, reorganizing, celebrating. We attended a festival of women's emancipation sponsored by a national ministry.

Anthropological Perspectives on States, Hospitals, Public Health, and Biomedicine

A theoretical pillar in anthropology is that states and biomedical institutions are socially constructed, historically situated, rather than sui generis entities that possess intrinsic characteristics. Scholarship on just what those historically situated, socially constructed features may be has varied significantly. Foucault's influential work on the nineteenth-century Western hospital as a focus of social control (biopower), and of the penetrating "medical gaze," has influenced anthropological scholarship on hospitals and biomedicine. Some recent writing on biomedical hospitals outside of the Western world has identified these and other features as vestiges of colonialism and of the agenda of modernization to which postcolonial elites are beholden (Street 2014). Hospitals and biomedical establishments are also seen as providing sites for the exploitation of local blood, genes, and research subjects for northern scholars and biomedical developers (Geissler, Rottenburg, and Zenker 2012). Yet other scholars have held up the distinctive culture and morality of care, of responsibility to the patients in practitioners' communities, as a defining feature of non-Western biomedical institutions (Wendland 2010, 2014). In this latter view, the focus on local culture that scholars had directed to traditional healers now includes the distinctiveness of biomedicine (Lock and Nguyen 2010; Wendland 2014).

In all of these perspectives, an overriding feature, sometimes hidden from view, is state power and the way it is (or is not) extended to, or into, biomedical institutions. In any case, these specialized institutions—hospitals, clinics, and public health networks—are never autonomous bodies of experts and knowledge, floating freely in the clouds of social structure, power relations, and cultural sentiments. They are always embedded in a context of corporate structures, legal codes, and supporting or controlling conventions and actors. Hospitals are corporate institutions with organizational hierarchies, staffs, budgets, rules, and procedures. They are not autonomous entities; rather, they are embedded within public or governmental structures that give them their authority, their right to operate for the common good. All of the weighty writings on corporation theory (M. G. Smith 1974; Weber 1980) are relevant to the study of medical institutions.

The state's shaping of biomedicine in its particularities and variations—hospitals, clinics, pharmacies, public health, medical research—is nowhere more pronounced than in Africa (Biershenk and Sardan 2014; Ferguson 2006; Chabal and Daloz 1999; Wendland 2014) and as analysts like the Fund for Peace (2020) monitor, the fifty African states include a continuum from effective states to failed states, and many in between. State robustness, as defined by the multiple criteria of the Fund for Peace "failed state index" (2018) includes economic, populational, institutional, and educational criteria, many of which shape institutional biomedicine. This is in sharp evidence in the findings of my fieldwork in Lower Congo (Democratic Republic of Congo) in 2013 and Northern Uganda in 2014. These cases in specific moments reveal the contours of power and legitimacy and the allocation of available resources to the institutions in question in response to the major diseases confronting them.

"The state" is a complex entity, made up of many parts and dimensions, whose regulations and behaviors are expressed by many individuals. Sometimes the state is likened to its president, king, or potentate, as when Louis XIV of France is to have said, "l'état c'est moi" (the state is me), or Donald Trump tweets "I have total authority." In Congolese "art populaire" paintings, the state is sometimes depicted as a beautiful woman, lying on a bed of diamonds, but who is ailing from schisms, armed conflicts, disease, and corruption. In these visually rich depictions, she is ministered to by a host of specialists, national as well as foreign. Analysts of state failure can cite statistics of declines in income, or numbers of internally displaced citizens, or falling gross domestic product. But what is often missing from political science or economics reports of failed states is the overwhelming feeling of absence, of a vacuum, where there should be something—for example, the postal service, universities, good roads—there is nothing. Furthermore, there is usually no one to blame, for there is no "there" there. Ferguson's (2006) notion of the "shadow" state captures the image of the shell of officials present in their offices without the substance of financial means to carry out their responsibilities, or even receive their salaries, as a consequence of which they must perform "moonlight" work to make a living.

The impact of state failure on biomedicine is therefore similar to the shadow image. Institutions are there, but their functions are curtailed, their capacities crimped. There may be doctors and nurses about, but they are often elsewhere tending to private practice, personal needs, or emergencies. Their dedication is not in doubt, but their means to carry out their responsibilities is often limited by very tight or no budgets. The creation of decentralized public health "zones" is an important measure against various diseases that continue to plague the Congolese populace. But the health zones are not a solution to the absent or very weak state support for medical care. The health zone with hierarchies of institutions—from local health posts, health centers, and one referral hospital—may well be a most efficient arrangement combining both public preventative health and curative health care. But if the resources are spread too thin, both types of programs are shortchanged. In an economic environment that is neoliberal, the most significant source of funds for institutional operations is the fee-for-service arrangement. This results in those who are least secure, the poor, to have the highest disease rates. They cannot afford medical care.

Are hospitals as institutions ever able to operate autonomously? I think not. They are embedded within broader corporate or public institutions that give their personnel and knowledge the legitimacy and resources they need to operate. In the case of the Lower Congo, this larger, legitimacy-granting corporate authority was ambiguous, or "divergent," at best, embedded in local government, ad hoc political alliances, churches, or foreign NGOs (Janzen 2015, 2019). Not only was the transition to a new hierarchy fraught with confusion, a certain desperation was evident in the realization that there was no superior authority who could find financial means to keep the institutions going. Fee-for-service surgeries and prolonged hospitalizations became the means to extract operating funds from patients; yet patient numbers were scanty—people resorted to self-medication for many conditions that would have been cases for hospital or clinic care.

The case for public health and for something like "health zones" is clear without by default approving a failed state scenario. In the DRC case, the public health infrastructure, and the resource brokering operation of SANRU, have made a difficult situation more livable. The DRC may have one of the best and most flexible public health setups in developing countries. But public health by itself is not a substitute for hospitals.

State resilience, on the other hand, makes more likely a robust response to medical emergencies like the 2000 Ebola outbreak in Gulu. It must be emphasized that Dr. Lukwiya's and his staff's quick and thorough diagnosis and response played an important role in limiting the outbreak, regardless of whether it was due to an ethic of Christian charity or to professional calling. But if he would have had no quick response from the Ministry of Health it is unlikely that the additional support he needed would have been forthcoming. Thus, in all likelihood the state's presence and intervention played a decisive role in the quick ending of the epidemic, in just over four months, from October 2000 to January 2001.

Although this chapter has some of the qualities of an apples and oranges comparison, it comes as close as we can get to a controlled experiment concerning the variable of state salience in biomedical institutions.

CONCLUSION

The point that is most important for this chapter's account and argument is that corporate organizations are usually embedded in other, more encompassing corporations that give them their legality, their professional legitimacy, their power, their access to resources, their very life. Of primary interest in the Lower Congo case is what happens to hospitals when the state weakens or withers. Does some other institution or network move in to give medical institutions their legality, power, resources, and professional legitimacy? In the case of the Lacor Hospital during the Ebola epidemic, what is of interest is how the state took over emergency powers to move Lacor in a certain direction, with great speed and authority. The two cases, the first case(s), loss of overarching authority, in the second, enhancement of such authority, taken together, illustrate the state's salience in medical institutions and disease control.

The issues raised in this chapter are very much in play in the successes and failures by states to deal with the novel coronavirus of 2020 and beyond. Although, at the time of this final writing in early 2021, new vaccines offer hope of eventual control while the virus continues to spike and spread. The salience of the state in COVID-19 control has become evident in the looming gap between countries that have kept infections and deaths low (e.g., China, Vietnam, Taiwan, Rwanda, New Zealand) and those where they have burgeoned (the United States, India, the United Kingdom, South Africa) (World Health Organization 2020). Although the final outcome of these patterns of response to the pandemic is uncertain, several factors are anecdotally evident in the role of the state in shaping health, including leadership rhetoric and role modeling, decisive action plans, public health infrastructure, and the enablement of the scientific community. Although it is not possible to elaborate on these issues here, a microcosm from the United States illustrates both state salience in public health and scientific work in monitoring effective intervention. In summer, 2020, the U.S. Centers for Disease Control and Prevention (CDC), in the course of tracking COVID-19–related mortality and morbidity, identified a natural-occurring experiment underway in the state of Kansas that clearly demonstrated the efficacy of a mask mandate issued by the governor in June. In the twenty-four municipalities that re-issued the mandate, infection rates dropped significantly over the course of two months, compared to the eighty-one where authorities did nothing or rejected the mandate (Van Dyke et. al. 2020). Still, the CDC's research and publication, and the national media's attention to this bit of evidence of the effectiveness of masking, did not persuade the county commissioners who justified their recalcitrance with the assertion that there is no evidence masking makes a difference, and besides, it is a curtailment of our "freedom." As a result of such sentiments in the populace, shared by then U.S. president Donald Trump, the United States had the largest number of COVID-19 cases and deaths of any country worldwide.

ACKNOWLEDGMENTS

An earlier version of this chapter was presented in the panel "In and Out of Biomedicine: Hospital Ethnography" at the 2017 American Anthropological Association meetings in Washington, D.C.

NOTES

1. Luheha Luyobisa Jackson skillfully administered most of the interviews.
2. Individuals to whom I am greatly indebted for this information on the origin of the health zones and the subsequent development of SANRU, are Drs. Malonga

Miatudila, its current head, Ngoyi Bukonda, Pakisa Tshimika, and Franklin Baer.

3. This course was part of a master's program in medical anthropology organized jointly by Professor Ruth Kutalek of the Medical University of Vienna, Austria, and Professor Grace Akello, senior lecturer in anthropology at the University of Gulu.

PART TWO

 Care Giving and
Hospital Labor

CHAPTER 6

Creating a Therapeutic Community

LESSONS FROM ALLADA HOSPITAL BENIN

*Mark Nichter, Ghislain Emmanuel Sopoh,
and Roch Christian Johnson*

PROVIDING INPATIENT CARE for people afflicted with diseases
requiring long-term hospitalization is a major challenge in low-income countries. In these countries, health staff must manage patients with limited
resources. At the same time, patients struggle to maintain a positive attitude
while far from their families and burdened by concerns about both the progress
of their treatment and the welfare of their households during their absence.
Patients and hospital staff live and work in close quarters, yet they are often
socially distant, their interactions cordial yet primarily focused on disease
management tasks. While considerable literature exists in developed countries
on the hospital as a social system and on formation of therapeutic communities
to care for long-term patients (primarily mental health and substance abuse
patients) (Hautefeuille 2011), hospital-based research on other types of therapeutic communities is sparse, and virtually nonexistent for Africa.

This chapter describes a pioneering attempt to establish a therapeutic
community for patients suffering from the neglected tropical skin disease
Buruli ulcer (BU) and other chronic ulcers requiring long-term care in Benin,
West Africa. The hallmark of a hospital-based therapeutic community, as we
define it in this chapter, is a communication process that invites open and
respectful dialogue between patients and health care staff, patient participation in problem-solving associated with everyday living, ways and means of
resolving conflicts that arise, and information exchange that fosters adherence, as distinct from one-sided directives demanding compliance. Our definition of therapeutic community is based on the principle of mutual respect
and recognition that respect is only forthcoming when patients and staff better understand the works, responsibilities, challenges, and constraints each
faces. Respect, dignity, and communalism, an ideology know as *ubuntu*, is the
cornerstone of problem-solving in much of Africa (Kamwangamalu 1999).

Buruli ulcer (BU) is the third most common mycobacterial disease in the world. A majority of cases are found in rural West Africa (Pluschke and Rölt-gen 2019). Cases diagnosed early can be cured with fifty-six doses of a combined regimen of intramuscular streptomycin and oral rifampicin. Treatment of advanced cases of BU often requires surgery and long-term residential treatment. During their stay in hospital, a patient's dressings must be changed daily or at least three times a week, and the patient must undergo physical therapy to prevent disabilities and joint contractures (World Health Organization 2012).

The Allada Buruli Ulcer Treatment Center (CDTUB) is one of the four primary reference centers for BU care in Benin and a recognized center of excellence for clinician training in BU management. The hospital also treats patients suffering from other types of chronic ulcers of various etiologies, such as sickle-cell disease, necrotizing fasciitis, and phagedenic or vascular ulcers. Patients with advanced BUs residing at the hospital require extensive postoperative care. BU patients receive subsidized treatment thanks to the government and international nongovernmental organizations (NGOs). Other chronic ulcer patients have to pay for much of their therapy out of pocket.

When patients suffering from more advanced stages of BU and other chronic ulcers come to hospitals like Allada, they have to adapt to a new way of life in unfamiliar surroundings. They have to learn to get along with other patients who are members of groups they have had little contact with in the past. They then have to cope with the uncertainty of their illness trajectory, the demands of treatment, and the physical discomfort associated with the frequent changing of bandages and physical therapy sessions. For more advanced cases requiring skin grafts, the duration of treatment is uncertain and difficult to predict due to individual variability in wound healing.

Given that the duration of BU treatment is long, and patients are unable to care for themselves, family caretakers are asked to accompany patients and attend to their daily needs such as cooking, washing clothes, and daily assistance. One of the main conditions for being admitted to the hospital is identifying a suitable caretaker from one's extended kin network. This is often difficult, as removing household members responsible for agricultural operations or child care at home can place the well-being of an entire household in peril (Agbo et al. 2019). In some cases, caretakers come and go, and in other cases they are not able to remain at the hospital and the patient is abandoned (Aujoulat et al. 2003). Food is partly provided free of charge for BU patients, but not for their caretakers, and not for patients suffering from other types of chronic ulcers. Although treatment is subsidized for BU patients, there are indirect costs related to hospitalization that can prove burdensome.

METHODS

Study Setting

The CDTUB is located in Allada, a small city of 127, 493 inhabitants. It is staffed by four doctors, eighteen nurses, laboratory technicians, and support staff. The director of the hospital is a doctor actively engaged in both the care of BU patients and BU-related research. The hospital receives approximately two hundred new patients a year, out of which around forty are BU cases. BU patients typically remain in the hospital for eight to eighteen months, but some remain much longer. Patients in the hospital range from two to seventy years of age, with 60 percent being children. There is an even split between male and female residents in the hospital, with residents divided into nine wards segregated by gender. Caretakers range in age from nine to fifty years of age, and an overwhelming majority (over 90%) are female. At the CDTUB, all patients are required to obey rules put in place by the hospital administration to assure a sense of order as well as quality of care. Compliance with hospital policies is mandatory.

Study Design

HOSPITAL ETHNOGRAPHY. A hospital ethnography was conducted followed by the development and pilot testing of two complementary interventions. A hospital ethnography encompasses a social systems analysis that investigates the ways in which the social organization, administration, therapeutic practices, and interactions among hospital patients, staff, and administrators reflect and conflict with social norms, cultural values, and economic contingencies. It begins with a study of the day-to-day routines, division of labor, and patterned forms of behavior one encounters within hospitals as well as perceptions of quality of care that go beyond clinical guidelines. It then identifies areas of stakeholder concern, tension, and conflict, and assesses existing as well as potential processes of problem solving. Hospital ethnographies are a social science contribution to health service research.

In 2013, a three-person local social science research team trained by an experienced medical anthropologist (MN) observed patient–staff interactions in Allada Hospital for two months and interviewed forty-two BU and non-BU patients (Amoussouhoui et al. 2016) to identify treatment concerns and social relational issues. Illness narratives were first collected to ascertain patients' health care seeking history, treatment expectations, and understanding of their illness and current treatment. Patients were then asked how they were being treated at the hospital, their interactions with staff, and if they were encountering any problems in everyday living. They were also asked about their level of social and economic support while in the hospital. Interviews were also carried out with five staff members to determine what they saw as their scope of work and common patient compliance problems. Assessment of baseline data by the social science team lead to the generation of intervention options and a SWOT (strengths, weaknesses, opportunities, and threats) analysis to assess the feasibility of each option.

The two complementary interventions designed to transform the hospital into a therapeutic community were supported by the medical director after conferring with his administrative and medical staff. The interventions were introduced simultaneously. The combined impact of these interventions on patient–practitioner relations was then assessed through interviews with both patients and hospital staff.

The first intervention was designed to provide a space and time for open dialogue about issues causing discontent in the hospital. Considerable research in Africa has pointed to the importance of collective problem-solving in community settings. An open forum was designed to facilitate this process in the hospital. Weekly meetings were held at the hospital in the evening and attended by both patients and hospital staff. These meetings were designed for two purposes: for continuing education and information exchange, and to provide a collective space for the articulation of grievances. Educational themes selected for weekly meetings included facts about BU and other chronic ulcers, wound and scar care, and health promotion topics related to diet and hygiene. Most of these interactive sessions followed a question-and-answer format modeled after a successful community outreach education program designed by the social science team following a year of qualitative research (Nichter et al. 2015). Health staff conducted the educational sessions using PowerPoint presentations containing evocative photographs and key messages pretested by the social science team for comprehension. Patients were encouraged to ask questions of health staff in attendance. Educational sessions informed patients about health issues so that they could return to their communities as "go to" resource persons for information about BU and wound care.

Following education sessions, participants were encouraged to voice concerns about life in the hospital, medical treatment, and conflicts that were brewing. The aims of this open dialogue were not just problem identification and conflict resolution but also rapport and trust building. A social scientist moderated each open forum. Over a seven-month period from March to September 2014, twenty-two meetings were held, with an average of sixty attendees per meeting, including patients, caregivers, and staff. Issues raised at open forum meetings were then referred to a patient committee composed of elected representatives from each of the hospital's nine wards. Meetings of this committee were held every two weeks. Working together with health staff, the group would try to find solutions to the issues raised in the open forum. The issues and proposed resolutions were then reported to the director of the hospital, who attended some meetings in support of the process. In some cases, conflicts raised led to a review of hospital policy. One or more social scientists attended each meeting and took notes on both the process of communication and attempts at resolution.

The second intervention provided patients with an opportunity for an individual consultation with a social scientist as a means of facilitating patient-centered care (Laine and Davidoff 1996). There are economic, psychosocial, and treatment-related issues patients prefer to discuss in private. Social scientists served as therapy facilitators, a cultural broker role established in other hospital settings (Nichter, Trockman, and Grippen 1985). The social science team built on the rapport they had developed with patients while conducting illness narrative interviews (Kleinman 1988) and discussing patients' level of social and economic support while in the hospital. Therapy facilitation entailed being attentive to the many "works of illness" patients face during their hospitalization (table 6.1). The male and female social science team members maintained an office with an open-door policy in the hospital. Patients and caretakers were encouraged to drop in and discuss emergent problems. Hospital staff occasionally asked a social scientist to talk to a patient who appeared despondent or who was having trouble securing medications necessary for treatment, in the case of non-BU patients.

The overall effectiveness of the two complementary interventions was assessed through in-depth, open-ended interviews with hospital residents carried out by two of the social scientists who did not play an active role in the implementation of the open-forum intervention. Forty-four informants were interviewed about changes in the quality of their care as a result of open-forum meetings and drop-in patient counseling: Fifteen long-term adult BU patients and their caregivers and twenty-nine non-BU chronic ulcer patients and their caregivers were interviewed (Amoussouhoui et al. 2016). Key questions focused on changes in lines of communication, changes in levels of knowledge about one's health condition, shifts in social relations with staff, and problem-solving in the hospital. Participants were specifically asked about the impact of biweekly meetings attended by representatives from the nine patient wards. Questions asked included: Did patients and caretakers have a better understanding of hospital rules and regulations as a result of discussions at meetings, and were any issues/problems raised resolved in a way that improved the quality of their life? Staff were interviewed about their impressions of the impact of open forum and follow-up meetings on patient–staff relations as well as their use of the forum to express their own discontent about issues in the hospital. During these interviews, social scientists were attentive to staff works of illness (table 6.1) and changes in how they view the scope of their work following the interventions.

All interviews were recorded, transcribed, and coded to facilitate content analysis. Codes were generated from project objectives as well as emergent themes identified from transcript reviews. Data from interviews were triangulated with observational data recorded at weekly meetings. Grounded theory (Pope, Ziebland, and Mays 2000; Strauss and Corbin 1994) guided data collection and analysis, which focused on both problem recognition and processes of problem-solving. Ethical approval was obtained from Benin's National Ethical

TABLE 6.1

Key works of illness and treatment for ulcer patients and health staff (adapted from Corbin and Strauss 1985; Nichter 2005)

Works of illness: Patients	Brief explanation	Comment: Each kind of work entails different types of effort, consultation, information gathering, accommodation, and adaptation
Pre-hospital illness recognition and self-treatment work	Symptom recognition as warranting treatment; self-medication	Consultation with others
Health care–seeking work	Where in pluralistic health care arena should one seek treatment? For how long to evaluate effectiveness?	Decision-making—taking into account predisposing and enabling factors, as well as reputation of healer, clinic, and more
Illness comprehension and treatment work	What does one know about their disease? ■ *Were they or their family ever told diagnosis by practitioner? ■ *Do they have any idea of how long they will be taking treatment at hospital?	From whom have they gotten information—health staff, other patients? Do they feel comfortable asking staff questions?
Preparing to go to the hospital work	How did household prepare? (e.g., ramifications of hospitalization on household and livelihood)	What support do members of larger social network offer, and what kinds of support are requested?
Monitoring healing progress work	How do they feel healing progress is going? Is it what they expected?	Informing family members who inquire
Pain and sensation management work	How do patients manage pain and uncomfortable sensations?	Request staff, for medication, self-medication using herbals or medicines bought in market; also work of bearing pain and being stoic
Compliance/adherence work	Doing what is requested by staff, managing wound hygiene, physical therapy	Finding resources to do the work expected, following correct procedure
Subsistence work while in hospital	Caretaker work, hygiene, food acquisition, and the like	Resources a concern, uncertainty for many; direct and indirect costs

TABLE 6.1

Key works of illness and treatment for ulcer patients and health staff
(adapted from Corbin and Strauss 1985; Nichter 2005) (continued)

Works of illness: Patients	Brief explanation	Comment: Each kind of work entails different types of effort, consultation, information gathering, accommodation, and adaptation
Social relational work	Getting along with other patients in the ward and with health staff	Interacting with unfamiliar ethnic groups
Emotional work	Maintaining morale during long hospitalization, fighting boredom, fear of abandonment	Managing own emotions plus emotions of household members, managing despondency and depression
Spiritual work	Dealing with fears associated with possible etiology, protection from sources of evil	Reduction of fear

Works of treatment: Health staff	Brief explanation:	Comments:
Treatment management work	Adhering to best practices, tailoring treatment to patient	Disease management is primary goal, time pressure due to heavy patient load
Health education and conceptual translation work	Explaining to patients how treatment is progressing in terms they can understand	Poor resources exist for this task, often not seen as falling in scope of practice
Compliance work	Convincing patient to follow treatment protocol	Patients typically treated as passive
Trust-building work	Reassuring patient they are receiving quality care	Favoritism can undermine trust
Collaboration work	Collaborating with all stakeholders in hospital, from patients to staff to hospital administration	Teamwork essential, social tensions need to be defused
Making do work	Making do with resources at hand	Creative problem-solving
Motivation work	Fostering and sustaining motivation	Management needs to foster strong work ethic and provide incentives that reward teamwork

Committee of Health Research, and informed consent procedures already in place at Allada hospital were strictly adhered to over the course of the project.

RESULTS

Interviews conducted at baseline revealed that patients were poorly informed about their disease by health staff. Information was rarely provided to the patient about the type of affliction from which they suffered. At the time of admission to the center, they were told they had a serious health problem that required hospital care and wound dressing. They were then informed that they needed to secure the services of a caretaker to reside with them at the hospital and were told what treatment-related products they would have to pay for out of pocket. Caretakers were required to assist the patient with washing their wounds and changing dressing on a bi-daily basis. Patients were asked to reside in the hospital compound as a clean environment to hasten the healing process and to reduce contact with the world outside the gates of the compound. Notably, twenty-six of forty-two interviewees (61%) were unaware of the type of ulcer for which they were being treated. Levels of awareness did not differ among BU and non-BU cases. When patients and caretakers were asked where they received most of their information about their disease, twenty-six of forty-two (61%) cited more experienced patients in residence at the hospital, not hospital staff.

Notably, twenty-eight of forty-two (67%) interviewees complained that they were given little idea of how the treatment was progressing and how much longer they might have to remain at the hospital. Following admission to the hospital and an initial conversation with staff in which staff sometimes mentioned probable length of stay, these patients and caretakers stated that they received little information about how many more months of hospitalization they were likely to require before being discharged. Patients lived in a liminal state, with great uncertainty about the duration of treatment. They described this as highly stress-provoking. For example, one nineteen-year-old patient expressed his frustration and anger in the following manner:

> It has been over three months since I've been here (in the center) with my mother. I was told that after six weeks I should be healed. But I do not know exactly when we will be able to return to my village. . . . The last time my dressing was changed, the nurse examined the wound and reported to me that there was no improvement. But the nurse did not say what this means in terms of my recovery, and the nurse did not tell me what I should do differently. If there is a product to buy, the nurse should tell me.

All patients interviewed at baseline reported that they did not feel comfortable asking hospital staff questions or voicing concerns during routine interactions. Forty-two percent of patients interviewed stated that the only time they would express concern is when they experienced severe pain, and that even then staff were typically unsympathetic. Patients described being rendered docile by busy staff who did not invite questions and referred their complaints to busy doctors who were seen as even more unapproachable than staff. As noted by one patient, a thirty-seven-year-old woman who had been in treatment in the center for nine months and was increasingly frustrated by the quality of care:

> Health workers do not allow patients to bother them with our concerns. They are difficult to talk to and they shout at us when we complain about pain. . . . There is always pain, it is our main suffering.

Another patient, a twenty-two-year-old BU patient, complained: "I do not approach hospital staff with my problems, because they will just refer you to the doctor. And seeing a doctor is very difficult."

Follow-up research with health staff identified the pervasive perception that poorly educated and illiterate patients and their caretakers were unable to understand both basic information about their disease and its treatment, and reasons why they were being asked to follow hospital rules about sanitation and the like. Staff were busy and did not see education or conceptual translation (translation of science into lay terms) as their responsibility. Staff generally defined their role in the hospital as treatment goal oriented. Further, they did not see eliciting or responding to patient concerns as part of their charge. In short, they expected blind compliance on the part of patients and their caretakers.

Patients perceived staff lack of sensitivity as a sign staff cared more about their disease than them as a person and complained about being treated in a disrespectful manner. One example of this lack of regard related to maintaining ward hygiene. In order to maintain basic levels of hygiene in the wards, hospital staff would pour water over the floors, even when caretakers and patients had left their possessions on the floor, an act that greatly angered ward residents. Health workers justified their behavior, saying that this was the only way they could communicate the importance of hygiene.

These findings greatly surprised the director of the CDTUB, who has been instrumental in initiating community-based BU outreach education efforts in the endemic catchment areas covered by the center. As a result of these findings, interventions were developed and piloted in the hospital.

The Effectiveness of Interventions

Forty-four informants were interviewed about changes in the quality of their care as a result of open-forum meetings and drop-in patient counseling: Fifteen long-term adult BU patients and their caregivers and twenty-nine non-BU chronic ulcer patients and their caregivers were interviewed.

Open Forums: Effectiveness of the Education Sessions

Hospital education sessions were modeled after community-based BU outreach programs developed by social scientists from the Stop Buruli

Consortium following a year of qualitative research in Benin, Cameroon, and Ghana (Nichter et al. 2015). These sessions followed a question-and-answer format that was iterative and covered all aspects of BU, wound care, hygiene, and nutrition. All patients and caretakers found these weekly meetings quite informative. Patients felt at ease to ask staff questions during educational sessions, and staff did the best they could to answer questions in ways patients could understand. They were assisted by anthropologists attending the meetings, who had become skilled in conceptual translation after having participated in community outreach programs for several months. During hospital-based outreach sessions, many of the same issues surfaced: Why were so many days of medication required for some kinds of wounds but not others? Why do some ulcers spread to different parts of the body? Why are ulcers so commonly found on the extremities of the body? Other questions were more specific and related to current illness experience. For example, patients asked questions about pain management, foods to avoid during treatment, the difference between BU and other chronic ulcers that patients were being treated for at the hospital, and whether medicine for BU was good for other kinds of ulcers.

An assessment at the conclusion of the intervention found that patients had far better knowledge about BU and other ulcers than at baseline. Ninety-two percent of interviewees (N = 44) were able to respond correctly to questions about the signs of BU and could name at least two key clinical signs. Ninety-seven percent now had adequate knowledge about what kinds of factors did not cause BU as well as possible risk factors. All informants now recognized that BU was caused by a pathogen "worm" (*wevi* in the local language) that required at least fifty-six days of medication to treat and guarantee that all remaining worms had been eliminated from the body. All now recognized that if BU were treated at an early stage, surgery could be avoided. Patients were also better able to distinguish BU from other ulcers, and they could identify differences in treatment. There was also increased knowledge about disease progression for BU versus non-BU ulcers, particularly slow-healing and difficult chronic ulcers arising from diabetes or sickle-cell anemia. All patients had also learned the basic principles of wound care, which focused on wound hygiene. Importantly, staff now recognized that patients were able to grasp basic ideas about their disease when presented in culturally appropriate ways.

Weekly Open Forum and Biweekly Follow-Up Ward Meetings

Following education sessions, an open forum invited discussion of social tensions influencing life in the hospital and issues fostering discontent. For example, complaints surfaced that staff treat patients better when they provide them gifts. As noted by one forty-five-year-old patient: "If you want hospital staff to respond to a request, then gifts are the way to do it . . . only then will they give you special attention."

Giving gifts to reinforce social relationships is a common practice in Benin, not limited to hospital contexts. It is used to develop personal relationships and resolve problems within the bureaucracies of the educational, judicial, and legal systems. The problem with giving gifts is that a number of very poor patients living in the hospital are unable to do so. In practice, this creates two tiers of patients in the hospital, which results in discontent. For the poorest patients, giving voice and acknowledgment to their frustration helped diffuse tension around the issue.

The administration quickly came to see patient forums as a useful mechanism for effective exchange and communication that had not been previously available. Health staff would attend the meetings and explain hospital policies and their medical rationale. The real value of the forums lay in the possibility of not merely conveying rules to the patients, but in patient–staff negotiation that led to protocols that at once protected patients and were responsive to their social and psychological needs. Negotiations took place during biweekly ward representative meetings. Requests raised at these meetings were then forwarded on to the hospital director, who examined them and introduced new policies when they appeared reasonable.

One example of a productive exchange concerned patient mobility. Hospital staff had become increasingly frustrated with patients who were leaving the hospital without permission to travel over the weekends, visit local markets, or establish relationships in the larger community. For patients this was a chance to engage in petty entrepreneurial activities to earn much-needed resources as well as visit with relatives or take a break from the rather monotonous life in the hospital. Although these activities were an important part of the social and economic life of patients, they were also a threat to their healing process and increased the risk of secondary infections. As a result, the hospital had imposed a stringent system of constraints on patient mobility. Patients were confined to the hospital premises and had to request permission to leave hospital grounds. Open-forum discussion identified the issue as a major source of discontent.

Hospital policies were altered through a process of negotiation. The hospital agreed to relax its policy on patient mobility outside the hospital but made it clear that patients had a responsibility to the community to keep the hospital clean and to participate in their own healing process. Patients were allowed to leave the hospital but they were made aware of the risks of engaging in different types of activities that exposed their bandages to sources of contamination. Following a change in rules, social scientists observed that patients have not abused their newfound freedom. Indeed, as a result of increased education, they have limited their movement outside the hospital, preferring to give errands to their caretakers whenever possible.

Not all types of discontent aired during open forum were able to be resolved. The most difficult issue that emerged was a systemic problem generic to all linear disease control programs funded by foreign sources of philanthropy that privilege one health problem over others. It was very difficult for patients who have non-BU-related chronic ulcers to understand why preferential treatment is offered to cases of BU as distinct from other ulcers. As noted, the care of patients with BU is subsidized through external support offered to the hospital by international NGOs and partners. BU patients do not have to pay for treatment costs and receive a monthly food ration, while other ulcer patients have to pay for treatment and do not receive free food. Non-BU patients, many of whom were unaware of their diagnosis, did not understand this policy and saw existing practices as discriminatory and a display of favoritism. Even when patient diagnosis was clarified, there were patients who felt that preferential treatment by diagnosis was unjust particularly since BU was noncontagious. For example, one male patient aged thirty-two noted at an open forum: "We do not understand why patients with BU receive free care . . . and we have to pay for our care . . . but we all suffer from ulcers, we share the same rooms, and we get the same dressings." As a systemic problem reported by other horizontal programs (diabetes patients complaining about preferential treatment for patients with HIV, for example (Men et al. 2012; England 2007), there was little that the CDTUB could do given existing funding streams and MOH policy. While the grievance could not be resolved, at least the reasons for the policy were rendered transparent. Greater understanding of the issue was an impetus for an integrated wound care program presently being introduced in Benin.

One positive outcome of open forum health education sessions was increased staff–patient communication about a key patient concern: pain. In the past, when patients experienced pain or sensations such as itching or burning, they did not report this to staff because such complaints were typically brushed aside. Many patients engaged in self-medication, obtaining medicines from shops, other patients, or healers. Staff complained that this practice often impeded the process of healing, and it became a source of tension. Following education sessions that addressed pain, the need to keep wound dressing moist to reduce itching, and how certain sensations constituted a sign of wound closing, patients were more willing to report these symptoms to staff. Patient practices of self-medication also decreased. One informant, a twenty-two-year-old male, commented on how increased staff accessibility and the ability to ask questions altered the way he attempted to manage pain:

> Before, I had a fear of approaching hospital staff and would not think of knocking on their door. . . . Now it's easier to approach them and tell them our problems. If, for instance, you experienced pain and did not sleep all night, you can go and tell them and they will assist you. Before these meetings, we did not do that and went and purchased street drugs suggested by friends or other patients. . . . The weekly discussion sessions also helped me understand many things. When the hospital staff is interested in teaching us, this is very good.

Another positive outcome of educational sessions and open forum discussion was increased patient and caretaker participation in improving hygiene and sanitation in the center. As one nurse noted:

> Before the intervention, it was necessary to put pressure on patients and caregivers to involve them in the cleaning of the hospital rooms. Now there is a big improvement. We can say that they have understood the need for good hygiene in the improvement of their health.

PATIENT COUNSELING AND THERAPY FACILITATION

One of the most significant contributions of individual therapy facilitation meetings was enhanced communication between staff and patients about how treatment was progressing. A decrease in uncertainty was greatly appreciated by patients and their families. For example, one young man, aged twenty-one, with a chronic ulcer had been growing increasingly frustrated and despondent after having to spend his third Christmas away from his family as an inpatient. He had little idea why his wounds had not healed while those of other patients in the ward had healed. During counseling he was informed that his wound was different than the wounds of these other patients, although they looked alike. They were caused by a vascular problem that was explained to him in terms he could understand. He was also told that further tests might provide additional insight into why his wound was not healing as expected. The tests were not particularly expensive, but there were well beyond his means. Seeing his anguish, health staff contributed to the costs of the tests. Following an explanation of the underlying cause of his wound, the reason why this kind of wound is difficult to heal, and attention from the staff, his spirits lifted and he felt reassured that he was getting good care.

Therapy facilitation led to many other examples of greater compassion shown to patients by staff. For example, in one case a nurse became so frustrated with a patient's noncompliant behavior (by failing to follow a bandaging procedure in a particular sequence) that he refused to continue with his treatment, referring him to other staff. After the nurse was made aware of psychosocial problems facing the patient, he not only cared for the patient, but he did so with genuine empathy. Social scientists documented multiple instances in which patients who had previously been snubbed or summarily dismissed by staff were better treated following therapy facilitation sessions, where the patient had the opportunity to provide an illness narrative and voice their concerns.

Therapy facilitation also entailed dealing with emergent problems that might jeopardize treatment. The hospital has limited funds available to assist the poorest of patients with food and medicine. However, staff do not have the time to make careful assessments about who qualifies, and patients whose financial circumstance worsens during their stay often reveal the gravity of their situation to health staff. Patients in dire need felt comfortable approaching social scientists, who carefully assessed whether the problem was short or long term. When appropriate, they referred the case to the hospital administration to see if they qualified for support.

Another contribution of therapy facilitation was resolving interpersonal conflicts that were too delicate to air in open forums or be dealt with by ward meetings. In one instance, long-term patients complained of the smell of new patients in the ward, since the necrotization of fresh ulcers produces an unpleasant smell that becomes particularly strong in close quarters. In this case, the problem was presented to the staff member in charge of assigning patients to their beds. An arrangement was made to keep separate wards for new patients and for those whose wounds had largely healed over.

DISCUSSION

Challenges to Implementing and Sustaining a Therapeutic Community

Three core challenges to establishing a therapeutic community were identified during the pilot project. The first challenge is how to establish an open forum where patients and staff feel comfortable enough to speak their minds without fear of reprisal. If staff feels they are being criticized and that this will have negative impact on their job performance, they will assume a defensive posture. This challenge requires the active support of the hospital director and hospital administration. In the present case, the hospital director let it be known that he viewed the airing of discontent as the first step of a problem-solving process that was valued at the hospital. Establishing trust in this process took time and required change on the part of all members of the therapeutic community. By the end of the seven-month pilot project, all stakeholders interviewed had enough trust in the process to feel they could communicate their problems without compromising their position or the quality of care they received.

The second challenge faces social scientists attempting to establish a therapy facilitator/cultural broker role. It is important that they not be seen as the handmaiden of the hospital administration or an advocate for either health staff or patients. Trust demands a neutral position, where the charge of the social scientist is to identify, investigate, and present all sides of a dispute and to provide in-depth understanding of issues affecting administration–staff–patient relations. During the project, there were times when various parties attempted to gain the support of a social scientist in opposition to another. It became important for the social scientist to be clear about what they can and cannot do as part of a process of problem-solving. For example, when a patient became destitute because they lost a caretaker or the resources needed for treatment, the social scientists assisted the patient in presenting a case to the administration but could not be seen as directly solving the resource problem themselves. During the community outreach program that preceded the therapeutic community intervention, the social science team created a resource assessment screening tool to facilitate patient referral to the hospital. The same assessment tool was used in the hospital when an economic crisis was revealed to a social scientist. The screener enabled the case to be systematically presented to the administration after all data necessary to make a decision had been acquired.

A third challenge is sustainability and cost-effectiveness of the social scientist role. The therapeutic community model presented in the study requires the presence of a social scientist and justification for the resources needed to support the position. Based on the results of the pilot study, the Allada hospital administration has decided to employ a social scientist to assist in therapy facilitation and community-based outreach activities, and to secure the services of a psychologist in cases where patients need to be treated for mental health problems requiring medication.

CONCLUSION

In this chapter, we have described a pioneering attempt to transform an African hospital serving long-term residential patients into a therapeutic community. Although the focus of this case study is chronic wound and BU patients, the model and experience presented here are relevant for many other types of patients. It requires a rethinking of hospital staff–patient relations in concert with the tenets of patient-centered and humanized patient care (Bardes 2009; Epstein and Street 2011; Fujita et al. 2012; Laine and Davidoff 1996) and people-centered health policy (Sheikh, Ranson, and Gilson 2014; Sheikh, George, and Gilson, 2014). For patients, it addresses their concerns, enhances their sense of well-being, and provides a feeling of support and compassion during their long hospital experience. For staff, it leads to greater patient adherence and the resolution of conflicts that can compromise care. In addition, it provides staff as well as patients a forum to articulate their grievances. And for administrators, it provides them with a finger on the pulse of everyday life in the hospital such that tensions can be identified and resolved, policies revisited, and greater transparency provided when necessary.

The pilot project proved to be highly successful as assessed by patients, staff, and administrators. Communication patterns improved, patient uncertainty about the status of wound healing decreased, and patients became far more knowledgeable about their illness. Socially, petty disputes were resolved in a far more amicable fashion, and both patients and staff felt vindicated by expressing discontentment and being heard by others, who could then better understand their position.

The pilot project made use of two distinct but complementary forms of problem-solving as a means to establish a therapeutic community in keeping with culturally meaningful modes of conflict resolution in Africa. Much has been written in the anthropological literature about the value of both collective and individual forms of conflict resolution in settings ranging from the settling of social disputes between factions in villages, to processes of divination used to air grievances both past and present (Chuwa 2014; Geschiere and Roitman 1997; Sambala, Cooper, and Manderson 2020). An open forum both facilitated collective problem-solving and enrolled public support for one's position, serving to establish their moral identity (Price 1987). Individual counseling provided the patient a complementary opportunity to speak to an empathetic witness (Kleinman and Benson 2006) about difficulties that one would not like to share in public, for reasons ranging from embarrassment to spiritual danger.

Is it feasible to transform African hospitals serving long-term patients into therapeutic communities? We would argue that it is practical given two conditions. First, hospital administrators need to recognize the utility of building a therapeutic community and be willing to engage in the problem-solving processes outlined in this chapter. Second, health social scientists need to receive basic training in health systems analysis and conflict resolution as well as hospital ethnography (Van der Geest and Finkler 2004; Long, Hunter, and van der Geest 2008) and an anthropological approach to patients' illness experience attentive to their many "works of illness." Treating patients as active agents in the hospital will serve as a corrective to paternalistic approaches to patient care that treat them as passive recipients of treatment whose only work is compliance with medical advice (Emanuel and Emanuel 1992). Life is far more complicated, and when both patient and staff needs are not met, discontent undermines quality of care.

We end with one last observation: There is another important way establishing a therapeutic community benefits the hospital. Former satisfied patents are positive sources of information about both the hospital and the community-based outreach program it has promoted to identify early stages of BU. As the adage goes, the best advertisement is a satisfied customer. This is particularly important in a disease like BU, where the reputation of the hospital is essential to the success of community outreach and the entire BU program. Patients educated in wound care as well as BU re-enter the community as a valuable resource and "go to" person for information about the disease and wound management. In Benin, former patients already play an active role in identifying cases of BU in some communities (Barogui et al. 2014). Increased patient education and a more positive experience in the hospital increases the likelihood that they will refer chronic ulcer patients to health staff they know and trust.

ACKNOWLEDGMENTS

This chapter was adapted from : Amoussouhoui, Arnaud Setondji, Roch Christian Johnson, Ghislain Emmanuel Sopoh, Ines Elvire Agbo, Paulin Aoulou, Jean-Gabin Houezo, Albert Tingbe-Azalou, Micah Boyer, and Mark Nichter. "Steps toward Creating a Therapeutic Community for Inpatients Suffering from Chronic Ulcers: Lessons from Allada Buruli Ulcer Treatment Hospital in Benin." *PLoS Neglected Tropical Diseases* 10, no. 7 (2016). The study was funded by a UBS Optimus Foundation "Stop Buruli" grant.

Chapter 7

Medical "Errands" among Women with Cervical Cancer in Guatemala

Anita Chary and Peter Rohloff

It's been a long day. Dominga, Miguel and I arrived at the oncology hospital (the Instituto de Cancerología [INCAN]) at 5:30 A.M., after a two-hour journey from Tecpán. It was still dark outside, but the city traffic had already begun. Dominga is getting her third cycle of chemotherapy today. She was diagnosed with cervical cancer three years ago, but after a few visits trying to make it through INCAN by herself, she gave up and never started treatment. She's a subsistence farmer from a mountaintop village, never went to school, and speaks Kaqchikel Maya and very little Spanish. When she first came to Guatemala City by herself to get tests for a staging workup, she could barely understand the doctors and couldn't communicate with anyone, since services are only available in Spanish. She didn't know how to get the imaging done, since the scanner at the hospital was broken and she didn't have money to go to a private clinic for it. She told me in an interview that she had initially "resigned herself to die." When her vaginal bleeding became worse, she visited our non-governmental organization clinic this year looking for help. We enrolled her in our patient navigation program. Miguel, one of our staff members, coordinated her appointments at the hospital, accompanied her to each appointment, and interpreted between Kaqchikel and Spanish for Dominga and the medical teams throughout a new staging workup. She started chemotherapy two weeks ago and is in the salon now. Miguel and I are waiting outside, and feeling exhausted now at 4 P.M. I can only imagine Dominga feels even more tired. Yesterday, she walked an hour from her village to the bottom of the mountain to catch a bus to town, so that Miguel could help her get bloodwork done as a prerequisite for the

chemotherapy appointment. She stayed at a hotel overnight
so that she could travel with us to the capital early in the
morning. Despite getting to INCAN early, we waited in the
chemo queue for two hours, and then the chemo team told
us we needed to repeat her labs today because they wanted
to trend her blood counts. Miguel, who speaks Kaqchikel
and Spanish, helped Dominga get to the cashier to pay for
the labs, go to the lab downstairs for the new bloodwork,
brought the paperwork back to the chemo floor, and got a
written prescription for the drugs she needed. Next, Miguel
went to the social worker to apply for a discount on the
drugs, left the hospital to get to an affiliated pharmacy to
buy the drugs, delivered Dominga back to the salon with the
medications, got her paperwork stamped, and got her a
number to enter the salon. The process took hours, and
there's no way she could have made it through each step
without Miguel. It will be a few more cycles of chemotherapy, followed by radiation, for Dominga. Thankfully, Miguel
will be at her side each time.

—*Excerpt from field notes (AC), Instituto
de Cancerología (INCAN), 2013*

THE *INSTITUTO DE CANCEROLOGÍA*, INCAN, is the only
oncology hospital serving impoverished public sector patients in Guatemala.
The hospital sits near the smoggy intersection of major highways of the bus-
tling metropolis of Guatemala City. Every morning, a line of patients and
family members snakes beyond INCAN's front gates along the building's
exterior walls, waiting to be seen.

While the Guatemalan constitution guarantees citizens free government-
sponsored health care, underfunding of the public health system severely limits access to medical care. Approximately one-fourth of the population of
sixteen million lacks access to basic primary care (USAID 2015). The majority (60%) of the country lives in poverty (World Bank 2019), making paying
out of pocket for services in the growing private health care sector an infea-
sible option for many (Chary and Rohloff 2015). The government of Guatemala has long struggled with chronic budget limitations, which have prevented
investment in cancer and chronic disease care (Palacios 2013). As such, impoverished Guatemalans with cancer have only one option: traveling to Guatemala City to seek care at INCAN.

INCAN was founded in the 1950s by a charitable organization created by
family members of cancer survivors. Technically a private hospital, INCAN partners with the Ministry of Health to offer discounts to patients referred from public health facilities. However, patient volumes are large, and government subsidies

to INCAN are unreliable, making INCAN a severely under-resourced hospital. It often lacks basic medications, laboratory and imaging exams, and personnel. The hospital is only open for outpatient consultations in the mornings, as it cannot pay its staff full-time living wages. Physicians work there part-time, largely as "social service," and spend the rest of their time in better-compensated private practice. The front windows of INCAN are plastered with nurses' protest posters about low wages. Patients often must buy their own chemotherapy drugs if government subsidy payments are late. Radiation therapy suffers from long downtimes due to the maintenance requirements of aging equipment. As such, the waiting list for radiation therapy is over 1,000 patients, and patients wait several months before beginning treatment. Like Dominga, one-third of patients never start treatment, and only one-third of patients complete treatment (Chary 2017).

As described in the field notes above, the process of seeking care at INCAN is tedious and exhausting for patients. Staging workups require multiple visits for lab work, imaging, and biopsies, some of which must be performed at outside facilities. As in Dominga's case, treatments require patience and perseverance over hours waiting in line, often without food, water, or access to restrooms. Given the multiple steps associated with care at INCAN, patients and their family members frequently described how tiring it was to "*dar tantas vueltas*" or to "*vueltear*." The phrase literally means "to turn around," or more colloquially, "to run an errand." *Vueltas* and *vueltear* refer to both running errand after errand within the hospital as well as traveling back and forth between the hospital and one's home multiple times. While the noun form of "vueltas" is common in Guatemalan Spanish, we have only ever encountered the verb form, *vueltear*, in conversations about seeking biomedical health care. Indigenous language speakers, like Dominga, use *vueltas* and *vueltear* as loan words when speaking about care-seeking.

Errands are common requirements for patients in low-resource hospital settings, who must make trips outside of the hospital to private pharmacies, labs, and other facilities to obtain medications, exams, and imaging that are otherwise unavailable within the hospital itself. As such, the anthropology of the hospital in low-resource settings necessarily involves study of the journeys into and out of the hospital. This chapter explores the meaning and function of *vueltas*, the many errands required for patients to obtain hospital care. We draw from six years of ethnographic and clinical interactions at INCAN with Maya women with cervical cancer, one of the leading causes of cancer deaths in Guatemala (Ferlay et al. 2012), to show that medical errands, which ostensibly serve the purpose of compensating for infrastructural gaps, also function to ration care and may be deployed by health care providers for profiteering. Following van der Geest and Finkler's (2004) suggestion that the hospital, as an institution, is "a domain where the core values and beliefs of a culture come into view," we argue that medical errands and tasks provide insights into how hospital staff deal with and conceptualize scarcity. Errands also reflect and reinforce the marketplace mentality characterizing Guatemala's fragmented health system (Chary and Rohloff 2015). We begin with context about Guatemala and cervical cancer, followed by a description of methodology, and then turn to cases that highlight our arguments about medical errands.

GUATEMALA AND CERVICAL CANCER

Guatemala is a Central American country with a large rural and indigenous population. Over half of the population lives in rural areas, and 45 percent of all Guatemalans identify as Maya (Ministerio de Salud Pública y Asistencia Social [MSPAS] 2015). Markers of indigenous culture traditionally recognized by scholars include practices of subsistence agriculture, wearing of woven indigenous clothing, and speaking of distinct Mayan languages (Adams 1994), though these markers are in transition (del Valle Escalante 2009; Metz 2006). Centuries of Spanish colonialism and more recent civil war and genocide of the Maya population (1960–1996) have resulted in enduring marginalization of Maya people. The majority of Maya people (79%) live in poverty (Central Intelligence Agency 2020), have limited access to biomedical services (USAID 2015), and face disparities in health outcomes (MSPAS 2015).

Like many low- and middle-income countries, Guatemala faces an increasing prevalence of chronic diseases, including cancer. In recent years, cervical cancer surpassed maternal mortality as the leading cause of death among women of reproductive age in Guatemala (Ferlay et al. 2012; USAID 2015). While cervical cancer is a preventable disease, Guatemala lacks public health infrastructure to systematically offer women cervical cancer screening exams or refer women with positive screening results to higher care. Prevention through vaccination against the human papillomavirus, the sexually transmitted infection that causes cervical cancer, is currently not available through public health facilities (Chary 2017). These issues are particularly salient for Maya women, who face numerous geographic, economic, and social barriers—specifically regarding gendered expectations of modesty and lack of family support—to cervical cancer screening and cancer care (Austad et al. 2018).

Nearly 40 percent of women diagnosed with malignancy at INCAN each year have cervical cancer (Waldheim and Villeda 2014). Due to high patient volumes and under-resourcing at INCAN as described above, most women wait months to start therapy. A recent clinical chart review-based study found that approximately 25 percent of women diagnosed with cervical cancer at INCAN do not complete treatment (Zamorano et al. 2017). While hospital registry data are not currently available to compare treatment rates and outcomes between indigenous and nonindigenous women, during interviews, administrators and providers at INCAN expressed that rural and indigenous women are more likely to drop out of treatment than those from urban areas or of mixed descent.

METHODS

This chapter draws from fourteen months of ethnographic fieldwork at INCAN. AC performed participant-observation in hospital inpatient wards and outpatient clinics as well as interviews with administrators and fifty women with cervical cancer from 2011–2014. Thirty of these women were recruited from INCAN during their treatment, and twenty of these women were recruited through nongovernmental organizations (NGOs). Like Dominga, seventeen of the twenty women recruited through NGOs had dropped out of treatment at INCAN and subsequently sought assistance from local charity health care projects.

This chapter also builds on the authors' experiences as physicians (AC, PR) involved with a care navigation program for rural Guatemalans with cancer, sponsored by the NGO Maya Health Alliance. In 2010, Maya Health Alliance began a Complex Care Program to facilitate referrals and support specialty care for impoverished patients from rural areas through cancer, surgical, and chronic disease treatments available in hospitals in Guatemala City, as described in detail elsewhere (Chary et al. 2016). Trained care navigators like Miguel coordinate the logistics of patients' appointment scheduling and transportation, interpret for patients and medical teams between indigenous languages and Spanish, and provide moral and emotional support while accompanying patients through clinical visits. Costs of therapy are subsidized by donations, online fundraising campaigns, and collaborating NGOs, such that patients pay very little if any costs toward treatment. To date, this program has supported over one thousand patients, approximately one-third of whom have cancer.

Research was conducted with approval of the Ethics Committee of INCAN and the Institutional Review Board of Washington University in St. Louis, Missouri. All names used herein are pseudonyms.

GRISELDA: RUNNING ERRANDS IN VAIN

Griselda and I (AC) sat inside of her bedroom with mugs of dilute instant coffee warming our hands. The bedroom was sparse, dotted with a humble collection of belongings: a thin mattress on a wooden plank, propped up by cement blocks as a bed; a cracked mirror; a small open chest of colorful hand-woven blouses and traditional women's skirts. Griselda's daughter emerged from inside with a plastic tub full of fresh bananas, harvested from their land nearby, and handed one to me. "*Kawa'*," Griselda told me, smiling, "Eat." She adjusted a pile of newspapers beneath her, spotted with blood.

Griselda had been diagnosed with cervical cancer four years prior. Like many other Kaqchikel Maya women of her generation, she had grown up caring for younger siblings and farming her family's land. She had married and had her first child in her early teens. Griselda's husband was murdered in the 1980s during the peak of Guatemala's civil war and genocide, and she raised their five children as a single mother.

In her mid-fifties, years after menopause, she developed vaginal bleeding. She made the journey to the nearest government health center, where she had the first Papanicolau smear of her life. The doctor there told her that he thought she had cancer, but that it might be curable, and referred her to INCAN in Guatemala City. Griselda had a strong will to get better, and she decided to sell off several traditional woven blouses and skirts—her most valuable personal possessions—for money to travel to INCAN for treatment. By public bus, her journey to Guatemala City took six hours.

When Griselda arrived at INCAN, she waited outside the hospital for several hours to get through security with her referral letter. She was seen by a triage doctor, sent to pay a cashier for her appointment, and then to various departments to fill out paperwork. She was finally seen by specialists who gave her recommendations for further tests. At each step, she waited in a long queue of people, and, unable to read and write or speak Spanish, she could not read the signs or ask others for help or directions. She had difficulty understanding what the doctors had told her during her first visit, but she took away a list of laboratory and imaging tests that she would need to get before her next appointment.

Some of the tests were not available at INCAN itself. Rather, Griselda would need to go to private labs and imaging centers and bring back the results. As a rural woman, Griselda was unfamiliar with the notoriously dangerous environment of Guatemala City. Concerned about being mugged or robbed, Griselda enlisted one of her sons to travel with her and help her figure out the city bus routes.

"They sent us to Zone 7, to another hospital where we had to go to get the radiology studies, the ultrasound. Just one exam there was 300, 400, 800 *quetzales* [40, 50, 105 USD]. They ask you for exams one day, and the next day you don't have any money for tortillas," she recalled. Her comment about not being able to afford corn tortillas, a staple food for rural Guatemalans, was a testament both to the impoverishing effects of seeking care and to enduring hunger throughout long waits at INCAN—a common complaint among patients.

Griselda made it through four more visits to INCAN, each of which brought more of the same: waiting in lines, hunger, confusion, demands for more errands, going between departments all day. She found it particularly difficult to manage her paperwork. The medical record system at INCAN is limited, and patients are left in charge of keeping their own exam and imaging results and bringing them to appointments. Griselda had trouble keeping track of what she was supposed to bring where, and as a result was scolded by secretaries and nurses multiple times. Recalling the numerous errands she had performed with emotional exhaustion, Griselda stated, "One day, I almost threw myself under a bus. You know, how the hospital is right next to the highway. But I stopped myself."

Gupta (2012), in an ethnographic account of poor people's interactions with Indian government programs, offers the term "uncaring" to describe the ways that state interventions designed to enact care toward the poor simultaneously enact violence through bureaucratic procedures. He characterizes "uncaring" as "not a psychological state of government employees but a constitutive modality of the state" (23). INCAN's constitutive modality can be similarly conceptualized: despite being a space of care, the hospital's bureaucratic procedures and errands demanded of patients comprise a form of violence against impoverished patients. This very violence is captured in Griselda's suicidality as a reaction to her experiences in the hospital.

The concept of "uncaring" also highlights an important tension between the essentiality of the errand and the violence that it enacts. Errands are a vital aspect of patient care and hospital function. In high-income settings, hospitals often employ personnel as well as communicative and electronic systems to perform many types of medical errands: transporting patients from one department to another, obtaining medications from central pharmacies and delivering them to specific patient care areas, and storing and releasing medical records to patients. However, in low-income settings, where underfunding, stockouts, and disrepair of equipment are the norm, the burden of these aspects of care devolves to patients, who must fill in for crumbling infrastructure. Indeed, INCAN would come to a complete standstill if patients did not perform errands. Errands are—despite being performed by patients—a form of patient care.

At the same time, errands constitute a form of violence. Patients find errands exhausting, and at times frightening. Patients complete one errand only to be assigned another, leading to feelings of futility and unpredictability, mirrored in other ethnographic accounts of welfare bureaucracies (Auyero 2012; Petryna 2002). Women interviewed at INCAN commonly used the language of performing errands "for nothing" or "in vain," expressing sentiments that their care did not seem to advance as expected. These feelings lead patients to give up on care, as Griselda related:

> Those exams, the papers, the tests—one day, out of desperation, I decided those papers weren't going to help me anymore. I gathered them all up, and I burned them. I got frustrated, because we couldn't do anything more. We didn't have money, and we had debts, and I was going on just the same, not getting any better. It was for nothing that we were fighting, and with me getting worse.

Rather than simply discarding her INCAN records, Griselda destroyed her paperwork in such a way that it would be unrecoverable. She intended to permanently sever her link with the hospital. This act of destruction was not simply Griselda's reaction to economic, geographic, or linguistic barriers to care. The paperwork symbolized the numerous errands and bureaucracy of the hospital.

For Griselda and many other women, the terms of *vueltas* and *vueltear* bear semantic resemblance to the English concept of "being given the run around." *Vueltear* was not simply about the physical mechanics of moving back and forth between different departments or between the hospital and the home but the experience of performing tasks that seemed twisted or convoluted, with no clear gain in sight.

Three years passed after Griselda's initial visits to INCAN. Her vaginal bleeding worsened to the point that she was nearly constantly oozing blood. Growing increasingly desperate, she reached out to a group of local health promoters in hopes of accessing care. The health promoters, familiar with Maya Health Alliance, referred Griselda to us. Through our care navigation program, Griselda made it back to INCAN for a new staging workup, and we arranged for her to have palliative radiation.

DELMI: THE ROLE OF ERRANDS IN RATIONING CARE

We diagnosed Delmi, a single mother in her forties, with advanced cervical cancer when she developed abnormal vaginal bleeding. Maya Health Alliance coordinated her staging workup at INCAN through our care navigation program and found that she would need radiation therapy. At that time, there were nearly 1,500 patients on INCAN's waiting list for radiation, and Delmi would not be able to initiate treatment for an estimated six months. Delmi understood her prognosis was guarded, and she hoped to maximize her time with her children, three of whom were under the age of ten. Our organization's clinical and administrative leadership, which meets weekly to review the care navigation program's patient caseload, agreed that delaying Delmi's radiation by six months could significantly reduce her overall life expectancy and remaining time with her children. Private oncology facilities in Guatemala City could offer immediate treatment, though typically at up to ten times the cost of treatment at INCAN. Osvaldo, one of our trained patient advocates, was able to negotiate a discount at a private hospital for Delmi to receive radiation therapy immediately, and the organization successfully raised money for Delmi's treatment through an online fundraising campaign.

Dr. Vargas, the physician at the private hospital in Guatemala City, required a referral letter from Delmi's oncologist at INCAN to offer us the discount. He arranged an appointment for her to obtain the letter at INCAN, as he also worked there part-time. As previously described, many physicians in Guatemala City split time between low-salaried positions in public institutions and more lucrative private practice. When Osvaldo brought Delmi to

INCAN for the appointment, much to their surprise, the physician responsible for writing the referral letter to Dr. Vargas was none other than Dr. Vargas! Dr. Vargas instructed Osvaldo to present the referral letter—written by him to himself—at the private hospital, where he would then be willing to begin administering Delmi's radiation therapy at the discounted price. We did not get to interview Dr. Vargas about this interaction and cannot comment on his specific motivations. However, his actions reflect a general sentiment we have observed among health care providers at public health institutions in Guatemala: that patients must show commitment to treatment by jumping through hoops in order to receive care.

INCAN providers practice within an environment dominated by the principle of triage. Simply put, there are too many patients and not enough resources, and providers must constantly make decisions to offer care to some patients preferentially over others—a common dilemma anthropologists have described in low-income and humanitarian settings (Fassin 2011; Nguyen 2010; Ticktin 2011). At INCAN and other under-resourced institutions in Guatemala, providers must consider who is the likeliest to comply and make it through treatment, or who is the likeliest to survive. The centrality of triage to daily interactions at INCAN greatly shape what is expected of patients there. Parsons (1951) theorized the "sick role" to describe the set of social expectations an individual enters when ill. These expectations include that a sick individual demonstrate desire to recover through seeking help and complying with suggested medical treatments. In Guatemala, performing medical errands is both an obligation of the sick role and a way to reflect one's interest in treatment.

During interviews and in informal conversations, health care providers often discussed the tension between high patient volumes at INCAN and the limited resources to treat patients. Several Guatemalan providers recognized numerous barriers that patients face to care but simultaneously made statements that "the patients have to collaborate" and "the patients have to do their part." Indeed, while hospital administrators and public health officials generally appreciate the ways that our care navigation program benefits patients and health care providers alike, a few have cautioned us against "coddling" or "doing everything" for patients, who might start to "take their care for granted." Social expectations of patient "collaboration" or "doing one's part" refer not only to help-seeking and following clinical recommendations but also to wading through institutional bureaucracy to show one's commitment to getting better.

At the same time, a patient's failure to perform medical errands becomes a way for providers to rationalize triage decisions and denials of care. Whether INCAN providers intend it to or not, triage occurs not only based on a patient's ability to pay but also their ability to perform and endure multiple rounds of medical errands. Providers sometimes described those who could not survive the bureaucracy as patients who did not "collaborate" or "do their part," and they described patients who discontinued care as "abandoning" their treatment. As we have described elsewhere, these patients tend to be the most marginalized of society—rural, indigenous, women (Chary et al. 2016)—and their deaths end up being written off as a normalized outcome of the practice environment. As one physician told us with a shrug, "What can you do? Some of them just never come back." Prince (2018) similarly describes how in an under-resourced Kenyan hospital, providers must make triage decisions based on their perceptions of patients' abilities to pay for treatment. While such triage is driven by practicality, over time, ethically fraught decision-making and poor patient outcomes, including death, lead to providers' detachment and rationalization of the status quo.

Mariel: Errands as Weapons

At age fifty-nine, Mariel heard about a woman in her village who had died of cervical cancer and decided to get her first Papanicolau smear. She arrived at a screening campaign sponsored by the Maya Health Alliance in a village nearby her own. When one of our staff nurses, Glenda, performed a pelvic exam, she discovered a tumor on Mariel's cervix. Mariel had not had any symptoms before that day.

Maya Health Alliance supported Mariel through initial visits to INCAN and confirmed a diagnosis of early cervical cancer. However, due to a combination of fear, denial, exhaustion, and lack of family support—Mariel's husband had been killed in the civil war, and she never had children—she ended up dropping out of treatment. She lived in a small coffee-farming village near the southwestern coast of Guatemala, about five hours away from INCAN by public bus. Despite accompaniment by one of our patient navigators, Mariel found the journeys to INCAN tiring. We performed home visits with her regularly, offering to re-enroll her in care, and she regularly declined.

About a year after we had facilitated her initial workup, however, Mariel's neighbor and closest friend showed up unannounced at Glenda's house in a panic. "Mariel is bleeding—but *a lot*," she told Glenda, earnestly. "Can you come see her?" Glenda and Anita paid Mariel a home visit later that day. Mariel's neighbor, now temporarily in charge of the store, was fanning herself under the corrugated tin roof. When she saw us, her eyes perked up, and she escorted us inside Mariel's home.

We found Mariel in tears, sitting on a wooden chair with a large swath of woven cloth tucked between her legs. Every so often, she would retrieve a clot from between her legs, toss it into a bucket, and shift the position of the cloth. The bleeding had begun months ago as sporadic spotting, but in the last two weeks it had become heavier and heavier, she told us. She found herself unable to leave the house and run errands to keep her small home-based store in business; going over bumps in the road and straining herself to carry packages made the bleeding worse.

Mariel was, for the moment, clinically stable with a normal range heart rate and blood pressure, but she would likely suffer significant blood loss and become dehydrated within days. She would then need to go to the regional hospital for fluids and likely a blood transfusion. If we had been in a higher-resource country or setting, she'd get admitted to an oncology service, where she'd get an immediate cancer grading and staging workup and begin treatment within a few days. In rural Guatemala, the regional hospital would do nothing but resuscitate her with fluids and blood and send her home with a referral to INCAN, if even that. It would take weeks to months of workup before she could start treatment at INCAN.

We knew that if we sent Mariel to the regional hospital without lab work, she would likely be turned away by the security guards at the front gate. The Maya Health Alliance clinic had just run out of phlebotomy equipment—everything was in short supply due to closure of the main road, which had been ravaged by rains—and we would need to travel to the nearest town to buy more. We told Mariel that we would return in several hours to draw a blood sample so we could send her to the hospital with paperwork. We also reassured Mariel that, if within her wishes, we would help her get a biopsy and the imaging she would need to get treatment at INCAN. However, shortly after we left to buy the equipment, Mariel fainted and her neighbor arranged for a friend with a pickup truck to emergently drive Mariel to the regional hospital.

Hours later, we received a desperate phone call from Mariel. Dr. Varon, who was taking care of Mariel at the public hospital, had told Mariel that she would need to perform a number of *vueltas*—a complete grading and staging workup—in order to get treatment at INCAN. Dr. Varon owned a private clinic near the regional hospital and offered to arrange all of the tests Mariel would need for the next day at a discounted price of approximately $10,000 USD. Mariel would be able to save time and headaches of traveling between multiple centers to get the tests and wonder if she was getting the right ones, Dr. Varon told her, because the private clinic had resources to do all of the testing at once, and Dr. Varon's staff would follow her orders without asking Mariel questions. Mariel declined, stating she didn't have that kind of money and would instead go through a local organization that had offered to help her. Dr. Varon told her that she would give her the night to reconsider and speak with her family. We reassured Mariel that we would indeed help her with the requisite testing for INCAN, and that she did not need to make her own arrangements to go to Dr. Varon's clinic.

The next morning, hearing that Mariel had not changed her mind, Dr. Varon threatened Mariel that if she did not do the *vueltas* at her clinic, she would kick Mariel out of the hospital. Mariel apologetically declined once more, reiterating that she did not have the money. Dr. Varon delivered on her promise; we received a call from Mariel when she arrived at home, asking if we could remove the IV in her arms. Mariel had been escorted off of the hospital premises so quickly that the nursing staff had not removed her IV there. "They told me not to come back," Mariel told us in tears.

As described earlier, on top of their private practices, many medical professionals work part-time in the public sector, due to social commitments to the impoverished patient population, opportunities to see a wider range of pathology present among those with poorer access to care, and benefits of tenure or social security available through government institutions. While at hospitals such as INCAN, codes of conduct forbid physicians from recruiting their public sector patients into their private clinics, it is common for physicians to do so (see also Chary 2015; Pezzia 2015). In our experiences through our care navigation program, providers at INCAN and other institutions have referred their public sector patients to their private clinics in order to provide therapies unavailable through the public health system—such as psychotherapy—or in order to accelerate treatments that might otherwise be delayed due to long waiting lists, such as radiation. We have also witnessed cancer patients experience public to private referrals for costly tumor debulking surgeries, with subsequent bankruptcy, unpayable debts, and continued illness, leading them to question their surgeons' motivations and seek out our organization's assistance.

While we were unable to interview Dr. Varon, it is possible that Dr. Varon felt she was doing Mariel a service by offering her an easier though more expensive option to obtain a grading and staging workup. However, Dr. Varon's economic incentive to do so cannot be overlooked, nor can the confrontational nature or outcome of her interaction with Mariel. Mariel felt betrayed by her experience at the regional hospital, which deepened her distrust of health care providers and the public health system. Regardless of any benevolent motivations, Dr. Varon ultimately used medical errands as a tool to recruit Mariel into her more lucrative private practice. Dr. Varon also wielded errands as a weapon by using Mariel's refusal to comply to deny her continued public sector care.

That errands can be capitalized on and deployed for profit reflects the marketplace mentality characterizing the health care landscape of Guatemala and many other low- and middle-income contexts (Ecks and Harper 2013; Prince and Marsland 2014). As public health infrastructure—limited to begin with—is continually retracted in the face of political scandals and budget shortfalls, individuals must increasingly access the expanding private health sector for care (Chary and Rohloff 2015). The privatization of care fundamentally shapes provider–patient relationships, as profit becomes more central to clinical interactions. The boundaries between the public and private health sectors are already blurred by medical errands, which are typically requested of patients in public health settings but carried out in private clinics and laboratories. These boundaries become even more nebulous as providers use errands as tactics to recruit patients into private practice and, regardless of providers' intentions, reinforce to patients the primacy of profit.

CONCLUSION

This chapter has explored the multiple functions of and meanings associated with medical errands in a low-resource hospital. Errands are crucial to hospital functioning in Guatemala and are indeed a common aspect of a low-resource practice, where patients must fill in for gaps in infrastructure. However, errands exact a severe toll on patients, who find them emotionally exhausting, frustrating, and at times futile when care does not appreciably advance. Errands also function to ration care, as providers expect patients to perform errands to show commitment to treatment. Within the framework of medical triage, providers can more easily rationalize poor outcomes among or denying care to those who do not successfully complete errands—a topic we are currently studying further at other specialty care centers in Guatemala that collaborate with our patient navigation program. Finally, errands can be deployed by providers to recruit patients into private practice, reflecting and further contributing to the increasingly privatized landscape of health care in Guatemala.

Medical errands are an important part of anthropology of the hospital in low-resource settings, where much of hospital care occurs outside of the hospital itself. Tracing these journeys ethnographically allows for a better understanding of hospitals as institutions with particular cultural milieus, of local social expectations of the sick role, and of the complex and fragmented ways that public and private health care fit together.

POSTSCRIPT

We offer a brief postscript given that at the time of publication, years have elapsed since the women featured in this chapter embarked on their hospital care-seeking journeys. Dominga remains cancer-free, five years after finishing treatment, and has returned to farming her land. Griselda passed away three years after receiving palliative radiation. She spent her last months of life at home, enjoying the company of her children and grandchildren. Delmi was able to spend nearly two years with her children after finishing radiation therapy. Her eldest daughter now cares for her youngest children. Mariel finished palliative radiation one year ago and is in bright spirits. She continues to operate a small shop out of her home.

CHAPTER 8

Routinized Caring or a "Call" to Nursing

SHIFTS IN HOSPITAL NURSING IN RUKWA, TANZANIA

Adrienne E. Strong

I SAT IN the office of the regional reproductive and child health coordinator, Rosemary, asking her questions about maternal health in the Rukwa region and the changes she had observed over her many years there. She was, at the time of our interview in 2015, just one year from retirement. Based on conversations I had had with, and comments I had overheard from, the older generation of nurses working in the regional hospital, I asked Rosemary if she noticed a difference between the young nurses just starting work and those of her generation. She told me, in her no-nonsense manner, "Me, the problems that I see a lot are just that people don't know their obligations, their responsibilities. They leave school, they don't know what they are coming to do." She continued, "But our people, like I've said, a lot, they enter this profession now not like how we were entering it, us in those days. I mean, you *feel*, you even see their appearance is different!" Intrigued, I asked her to continue, to explain more about what she meant by the younger nurses having a different appearance. She told me,

> A [nurse] she is sitting on the labor ward, she is using the phone, chatting while a mother is hurting over there. Then that same nurse, she will claim, "My rights aren't being respected!" What rights? Those that are studying these days, frequently they have just gone into this profession of nursing as though they lacked somewhere else to put themselves. They see maybe they can just sit there. Then a lot of them, their minds are just to think that, "If I go to study more . . . I should just be in a high position so that this patient, I don't have to touch her."

Rosemary explained how skilled personnel are the ones who should be close to the patients, physically caring for them. But, she lamented that these nurses nowadays sought to be removed from direct patient care, leaving physical contact to paramedical staff, such as medical attendants. She concluded, "They do this because they don't have a calling, *wito*, they don't know their responsibilities. A person, if she knows her responsibilities, she will do each thing that she should be doing. But, if a person doesn't know their responsibilities, yes, every time she will sit complaining, blaming [others]."

Shifts in broader society and in the health sector have deeply affected the institutional environment of hospitals. As a result, the older nurses often stated there had been a shift in nurse-caring from selfless, emotionally warm, and characterized by physical proximity and intimacy, to distanced, constrained by resource scarcity and increased workloads, and mitigated by technology in the form of social media escapism. Public media portrayals of nurses and the nursing field have also decreased respect for the field and increased public perception of nurses as corrupt, cruel, and uncaring. Institutional and societal changes, as well as those within the professional of nursing, sometimes resulted in conflicts between older and younger nurses or nurses and their patients and patients' families. Ethnography with this critically important group in the hospital setting sheds light on these transformations and their implications for community trust in, and satisfaction with, the health care available to them.

Generally, these comments from Rosemary were representative of the older generation's perceptions of their juniors. Many were concerned that the younger nurses were treating nursing like any other occupation, as opposed to going into the profession because they have a calling, or *wito*, to be a nurse. I suggest we read this difference, or perceived difference, as related to nursing's close ties to care, specifically a particular, historically feminine, form of caring that includes a positive emotional component. In teachings about Florence Nightingale, held up as the paragon of nurse caring in Tanzanian nursing education, nurses learn about how they should live up to ideals of selflessness, forbearance, and comforting care. Additionally, the different perceptions of the role of nurses and their duties or place in society can be interpreted in light of a shift from socialist collectivism to greater capitalist individualism.

In this chapter, I begin to explore the intergenerational differences between nurses as they understood their profession, the hospital as an institution, and how technology, specifically social media and smartphones, has transformed the nursing profession. I touch on nurses' reflexive accounts of their professional practices to analyze how nursing care has transformed since the last days of the Nyerere presidency. Uneven investment in health care infrastructure in the colonial and postcolonial period in Tanzania paved the way for health institutions that are necessarily flexible and adaptable but also partial and often characterized by scarcity. As more and more people utilize biomedical health services, as technology changes, and clinical advances march onward, different generations of nurses describe a profession that sounds as though it has become a sort of chimera—composed of vastly different goals to be accomplished by rather different means.

I argue that a shifting global health landscape and national developments, moving from socialism to capitalism, have transformed nurses from valued nation-builders, vital for the future of the Tanzanian nation-state, to objects of suspicion and mistrust, demonized in popular media for a perceived lack of caring with suspect motives for entering the field of nursing. These suspicions are present in the community, leading to loss of professional prestige, but also present in young nurses' own workplaces as their elders accuse them of working by rote, being uninterested in being close to patients, and only looking for money, as opposed to accomplishing the lofty ideals of Nightingale-esque caring demonstrated through a vocational calling to the nursing profession.

In my broader project, I was primarily interested in how pregnant women still come to die in a regional referral hospital and the sequences of events within the Mawingu regional hospital that precede their deaths there. Part of this investigation has included, from the time I first visited the Rukwa region in 2012, health care workers from the hospital repeatedly telling me of the low levels of morale and poor motivation among the health care personnel in the hospital. In seeking to understand what might underlie these low levels of motivation, or this discourse of poor provider motivation, one thread repeatedly arose—that of the difference between the new nursing school graduates and the older nurses. New nursing school graduates are a product of a globalized world and health landscape, and rapid advances in technology. On the other end of the professional spectrum are those nurses close to retirement who trained in the 1970s and 1980s, in the last several years of the Nyerere presidency and, by extension, the socialist era. These older nurses trained in an era imbued with strong nation-building rhetoric and socialist goals of community solidarity, national self-reliance, and health care for all as a product of the post–Alma Ata primary care push during this same period.

THE MAWINGU REGIONAL HOSPITAL AND THE RUKWA REGION

The Mawingu Regional Referral Hospital, located in Sumbawanga, the main town in the Rukwa region, is the highest level of care in the region. The Rukwa region is one of the most peripheral regions in Tanzania, and the central government neglected it for many years in terms of investment and infrastructure-building. In the 2010 national Demographic and Health Survey (DHS), the region ranked in the bottom five of the twenty-one mainland regions for nearly all indicators of maternal and reproductive health; for example, at that time, only 29.5 percent of births were taking place in health facilities, one of the lowest numbers in the country (National Bureau of Statistics and ICF Macro, 2011, 134). Given the poor performance of the region, the DHS provoked an influx of programs and investment in the region, including in the form of new, young doctors and nurses assigned to the regional hospital.

I spent approximately two years in the region, between 2012 and 2015, for my broader project on maternal death in government health facilities. During this time, I conducted more than 1,600 hours of participant observation on the hospital's maternity ward, largely working alongside the nurses and doctors. I attended meetings, spent time on the night shifts, took samples to the lab, helped wheel gurneys to the operating theater, changed bed sheets, and fetched supplies. I am also trained as a doula, a labor support person, and spent many hours alongside women in labor providing emotional, physical, and instrumental support for them. Through the many hours on the maternity ward, I often overheard complaints about the other generation of nurses, either by the older ones about the younger or vice versa. Based on my experience in another region of Tanzania, in which I had witnessed a stark difference between the conduct of older nurses and that of their younger counterparts, I began to purposefully pursue these questions as an integral component of understanding working conditions and how these differences in work attitudes might translate into different outcomes for women in obstetric crisis. The ethnography presented here is primarily derived from my observations and one-on-one interviews with maternity ward nurses and nurses working in the region who were nearing retirement age.

Body Work and Nursing

Returning to Rosemary's comment that nurses "these days" sought to physically distance themselves from hands-on patient care, this section explores the idea of body work in nursing. Nursing has historically been a profession that includes a demanding physical component, requiring close physical proximity with patients through the work of moving, bathing, and grooming patients. It was, at one point, this type of physical closeness to patients that set nurses apart from other hospital staff members, including physicians (Sandelowski 2000, 2). I draw on the sociological concept of "body work" to help analyze these comments and the importance of physical proximity or distance for nursing. In a review article, Gimlin (2007) explicates four types of body work. In the discussion here, I primarily draw on her second type: body work/labor. Gimlin (2007, 358) writes that body work/labor is that "labor performed on behalf of or directly on other peoples' bodies." In the health care setting, doctors are often distanced from direct interaction with bodies, engaging in relatively little body work and "confined to the high-status activity of diagnosis, or as mediated by high-tech machines" (Twigg 2000, 391). In the context of nursing, Twigg (2000, 391) notes, "Though bodywork is at the heart of nursing, it has an uncertain status. Nursing is organized hierarchically so that, as staff progress, they move away from the basic bodywork of bedpans and sponge baths towards high-tech, skilled interventions; progressing from dirty work on bodies to clean work on machines." In a lower-resource setting such as Tanzania, nurses may still see the move away from basic body work as a move up the professional hierarchy. This occurs as nursing seeks to further professionalize and technologize to increase its value in fragmented health care settings that include more and more ancillary staff members (Sandelowski 2002). However, as nurses move away from "dirty work on bodies" there may not be "clean work on machines" to take its place. This leaves the patient in the unenviable position about which many of Mawingu's older nurses complained—lacking the close care and attention to their immediate needs due to younger nurses' desire to not engage directly with others' bodies that might be dirty in the physical (Strong 2018) or metaphorical sense (Sandelowski 2002), as through polluting taboos related to blood, feces, or other bodily fluids.

One of the other nurses, Furaha, told me that many years ago, earlier in her career, nurses took the time to cut patients' fingernails or help them wash their hair. In contrast, a passing nurse, of the younger generation, immediately scolded me the one time I was on the labor ward and tried to help wipe dried mud off the legs of a young pregnant mother who had walked through rain drenched roads for hours while in labor on her way to the hospital, arriving exhausted and on the brink of collapse. I related the story to Furaha during our conversation about the difference in nursing practices:

AS: You know, even me, one day last year, we received one mother, she had mud up to her knees, here. . . . She was completely exhausted. . . . I was washing her. One nurse came [imitating an angry voice], "Now what are you doing?! Tell her to get down [off the delivery bed], and go herself! Why do you want to help her?" She is really tired, why can't I help her? "Just leave her! What are you doing?!" I was shocked.

F: It's different now. Now, they are just there. . . . In the past, this thing wasn't there. We were braiding people's hair. You see here? And this wedding ring? You had it but if you enter into the [operating] theater there, you remove it. You see? But now, a nurse she can't enter the sluice room. Nor can she bathe a patient. Nor can she take lab tests. Another time they do this, they don't even take vital signs, isn't it so?

The tasks Furaha most frequently cites as those that nurses no longer do are those that put the nurses in the closest contact with the bodies of their patients. While some nurses may have objected to or avoided these tasks out of a distaste for these simple, humble acts of caring, others might genuinely have been afraid to be in close contact with patients due to the possible unknown infections their bodies might hold, against which the nurses had little protection (Strong 2018). I do not suggest that these infections were necessarily new but the younger nurses all came of age and trained in an era marked by HIV/AIDS and increased infection prevention control campaigns in health care. In contrast, one of the older nurses, Pili, remembered, "In the past, other sick-nesses were not there. For example, we didn't have HIV/AIDS." Other older nurses reminded me that they long felt it was their faith in God that had pro-tected them from occupational exposure to infectious diseases during the course of their careers when they often lacked personal protective equipment, another body distancing technology.

Rather subtler than her example of actual physical contact with patients' bodies, Furaha also brings up the example of a nurse's wedding ring and how she used to remove this item before scrubbing in in the operating theater. In the context of our conversation, I did not probe her further about this com-ment but I have now come to read it as an example of putting one's self after the patients and their care. This act of removing an item of important per-sonal value is a concrete example of the nurse subsuming her personal self into her professional, nurse-self, something that Furaha suggests, through this jux-taposition, the younger generation is less willing to do. This lack of willing-ness to fully become the Nurse in Florence Nightingale's image meant those in the field currently were moving further away from the ideals of the profes-sion as understood by their colleagues.

Some of this change in expectations and perceptions of appropriate nurs-ing duties might be attributed to the dramatic increase in the number of women arriving to give birth in the hospital. This increase is largely due to long years of public health campaigns encouraging skilled attendance at birth, almost exclusively meaning giving birth in hospitals and other biomedical facilities. As of 2019, the number of deliveries had drastically increased since I first visited the hospital in 2012, far outpacing the number of new nurses or doctors the hospital is able to hire or assign to the maternity ward, a trend common throughout Tanzania (Manzi et al. 2012). The demands of the work environment often preclude one-on-one care that includes the more menial tasks of hygiene, for instance. Women now must do this for themselves, or ask a relative to help them bathe during the brief visiting hours, if allowed. Furaha said,

> That is, let's say, that health care is coming to its end because [the younger nurses] treat it, health in general, like it is a job, like any other profession. They have removed that thing that was called *wito*, a calling. . . . Patients are there but other times [the nurses] are not engaged. The nursing of right now is different than that nursing of the past.

Here, Furaha seeks to highlight the important distinction between nurs-ing and other professions, in which people's lives may not hang in the balance to the same extent. When patients are treated in a routinized, impersonal way, without respect for their dignity as individuals, Furaha suggested that the overall quality of the care provided declines and so, too, do the hallmarks of nursing, and the profession as a whole. According to Furaha, patients are no longer at the center of this newer kind of nursing, much as Rosemary observed. These older nurses' observations about the state of nursing in Tanzania are similar to those Martin (2009) noted in Uganda, where older nurses and nursing educators lamented the declining quality of nursing students and students' choice of nursing as a last resort: "They generally saw the increasing professionalization—which discredited practical experience in favor of an accumulation of 'papers'—as devastating to the vocation of nursing and as one indicator . . . of a general move away from the 'true' altruistic nursing of the past towards a damaging commercialization" (Martin 2009, 79).

The ideal nursing care to which Rosemary and Furaha were referring includes selflessness, putting the patient first, engaging in intimate emotional and physical relationship with the patient (Kristoffersen and Friberg 2017), and ensuring the nurse provides care that is compassionate, as well as technically proficient and ethically delivered without neglecting or abusing patients. These ideals generally underpin nursing as it is taught and learned in locations throughout the world and across time (Fealy 2004; Malchau 2007; Liaschenko and Peter 2004; Sandelowski 2002).

Paths to Nursing
The Older Generation

The idea of a professional calling, *wito*, figured prominently in the older nurses' discussion of the differences between the generations. Nurse Neema, another of the older nurses still working on the maternity ward, explained the reason she decided to study nursing: "There was a time when you went to the hospital and if you see the nurses, how they are dressed, you like it. You ask them how do you become like them and so I said, 'And I, I will be a nurse.'" I asked Neema how she knew just from the uniform nurses wore that she wanted to be a nurse. She said,

> First there is a thing that if you see it, you like it. Then you start to dig into its interior so that you start to recognize that really it's like this and this . . . even while seeing that your heart is drawn that way. There can be another person who is drawn to the same thing but just for the appearance, she doesn't really have the heart for the work, but for others you're drawn to it.

While many of the older nurses thought this sort of story of their attraction to the nursing profession was unique to their generation, many of the younger nurses also related stories of being drawn to nursing because they had seen nurses working in their local health facilities while growing up. It was true that a few of the younger nurses had not initially wanted to enter the profession and, overall, students in Tanzania have not always perceived nursing as a first-choice career option (Achilles 2010). One male nurse, Samwel, who had been working on the maternity ward for about a year when I interviewed him, told me that initially, upon finding out that his secondary school exam results meant he could apply for positions in the police, nursing, or teaching, his father had wanted him to go into the police force. However, he was not accepted after he interviewed and was forced to consider other options. Samwel's mother then found a position for him at a nursing school and upon starting to study he found that he liked nursing. Another nurse whom I met in 2018 in Kigoma, Alika, was a cheerful hard worker who seemed to genuinely like her nursing job. I asked her why she had decided to be a nurse and she told me, as she laughed, "You know, us, you only do this thing if your other dream failed." I asked her what her original dream had been and why it had not been possible. She answered, "I wanted to be a doctor but it wasn't possible, because of my Form IV exam results, so I had to find a place to put myself. Really, I didn't want to be a nurse but that is what I went to study." I inquired if she had now come to like her job and she said yes, that she did. These types of trajectories confirmed Rosemary's suspicion that some nurses went into the profession only because they "lacked someplace else to put themselves" and that they had only come to nursing after failing to accomplish other goals. It is also possible that public perceptions of nursing as lacking professional autonomy and prestige, as well as being a feminine occupation, deter some school-leavers (Achilles 2010; Liaschenko and Peter 2004; Meiring and van Wyk 2013). Additionally, nursing work, in this era of increased patient loads, has become increasingly demanding but support for nurses has not increased at the same pace (Mselle et al. 2013; Tarimo et al. 2018). I asked another older nurse, Pili, about the idea of *wito* for the nursing profession:

AS: OK. I have also been told by other people that they think maybe those people who have been hired right now, they don't maybe have that calling [*wito*] like those people from before.

P: Eh, and I also can say the truth. Others, right now, to get work it is sometimes very difficult. She didn't want to be a nurse. . . . She has missed out there [somewhere else] so she says, "Wait, let me just enter in even here so that I get work." But if she comes and she encounters the work itself, of nursing, you should be going to care for the patient—but they don't have any mercy/empathy, they go to answer patients badly. For us, it was a taboo because your patient—well, again for me it was good luck that I studied with white nuns. They were teaching us a really high level of love . . . we were caring for [our patients] soul and body. We were really loving our patients. Yeah. But right now, I see that the love for patients has been lost. A person makes it like a patient isn't even a person. Even if you stand there and you watch them, you see what [the nurse] is doing. Even if it's your own patient that has been admitted, they *really* do badly until the point where you are feeling bad. Really honestly, *wito*—others, they will be only a few that have a calling, but not all. Many, they don't.

AS: For example, you, while you were studying and with others, in the past, were you able to choose any thing that you were wanting to study? These days I know if you have bad marks here they can refuse and tell you where you have to go. . . . Therefore, it means maybe a person these days feels like he wants to be a different kind of person but it is refused?

P: It is refused! After it is refused, he says, "Wait, just let me go here."

AS: But you, when you were studying how was it?

P: Us, when we were studying—but also it depends on what God has planned for you. You find that it just comes but then your heart likes it. Yeah. For example, me, when I was told that I would be taken for nursing, I was feeling very happy to go. Then I was liking nurses and if they wear [their uniforms] well, I was wanting that. Therefore, when I went, I saw that even me, I can succeed really, I am able. . . . When I saw that the Sisters loved me, those nuns, therefore I was just happy to keep studying because I saw that people loved me and whatnot. You continue to have a heart for loving the work.

For Pili, it is clear that her training with foreign nuns made a deep impression on her and her sense of caring as a nurse. She spoke about more holistic care that encompassed caring for a person's soul, in addition to their body, which she laments has been lost in this day and age when patients are barely even treated as human. She gave the example of bringing "your own patient" (a family member or friend) and watching how other nurses treat them because, usually, the nursing staff works hard to provide high-quality care and extra attention to the relatives of fellow staff members. Pili's saying that even when you are standing there, nurses can treat your patient badly, to the point that it hurts you as their relative who brought them, demonstrates how far she feels the standards of the profession have fallen from the time when she was undergoing her training. As in many health care settings in which I have worked in Tanzania, Andersen (2004, 2008) observes that in Ghana, as one informant said, "If a doctor or a nurse brings a patient, this patient is considered as a relative of the nurse or the doctor. Therefore [the treating providers] would want to treat that person nicely." This preferential treatment of one's relatives is, in fact, one of the biggest benefits of being a health care worker in these settings. This social capital leading to better and more expeditious treatment of one's family members and friends is a major subsidiary benefit that helps to make up for the low salaries many providers receive. With its erosion, or lack of respect for fellow providers' family members as patients, Pili is concerned the status of the nurse, or perhaps the older nurse, is beginning to slip.

The Younger Generation

For the younger nurses, those primarily in their twenties and thirties, their paths to the nursing profession tended to follow a slightly different route than those recited by the nurses nearing retirement. While some of these younger nurses' narratives confirmed the fears or suspicions of the older nurses about people "lacking a place to put themselves," others of the younger nurses had interacted with the health care system and been drawn to nursing as their first choice of a career, not a backup. On the whole, even those who had not chosen nursing as their first-choice profession had come to find it fulfilling. Samwel's (age 23, from above) explanation is representative of this evolution. I asked him why had he wanted to study nursing and he replied:

> My father wanted me to go into the police. I did the interview and I didn't make it. Now, this nursing college, it was just started and my mom found a spot for me there. So, I went except I was afraid. But the way we were being taught that nursing, I found that I have liked it. So, I said alright, wait, this indeed will be my work . . . so I am [now] living with the [fact] that I will do work as a nurse midwife.

In Samwel's case, his options for a future career were limited by his Form IV secondary school exam results. Those who score in the second lowest division (lowest being failing) are qualified to go into certificate programs in teaching and nursing, or into the police force. Alika also mentioned (above) that her poor Form IV exam results disqualified her from going directly to university to study as a medical doctor, leading her, instead, to nursing as a substitute.

Much like Samwel, Peninah, thirty years old, did not initially feel a strong calling to nursing but found herself studying it after she received advice from others upon completing secondary school:

> Mmm . . . nursing, you know, that age when we are finishing school, you finish Form IV, you didn't really have that strong feeling I will study this work or this work . . . sometimes you are advised. Those jobs that are easily available are nursing, teaching, and policing. Therefore, I decided to choose one among those, I entered into the side of nursing. . . . When that year came when we were divided, some to psychiatry, some to midwifery, I was interested in those things to do with caring for mothers and babies.

Rashida, age twenty-nine, had a different route to nursing because she had already been working at a health center. When I asked her about her motivations for pursuing nursing she told me:

> I liked something about nursing when I was there at the health center when I was doing the work of records keeper. The way in which the

patients, the way they were coming there and we were receiving them, the patients were comforted and the care they were getting really attracted me. . . . Me, I liked to help women.

In all of the above instances, the younger nurses found they liked nursing but, for the nurses nearing retirement, perhaps liking the profession and the work it entailed was not fundamentally equivalent to having a calling or *wito* for the professional. It may be that a nurse who *likes* her work does not go to the same lengths in order to help patients and is more likely to pursue his or her own interests than a nurse for whom the profession is a *calling* born of great commitment to the ideals of nursing and the broader goals of health care, more generally. Among those goals are a recognition of the dignity of all patients, close contact with patients, and a belief in the importance of health for all the country's citizens as foundational for a prosperous nation.

POINTS OF CONFLICT: TECHNOLOGY AND TRAINING

One of the biggest differences between the older and younger generations, not just a point of contention in Tanzania but also in a high-resource setting like the United States, for example, was how the nurses used technology and, particularly, their cell phones. Many of the younger nurses (and certainly several of the older ones) had smartphones and spent a good deal of time sending and responding to text messages via WhatsApp and SMS. They were on Facebook and email and online forums. They used Instagram and other apps. There were times when I would walk into the labor room and see many of the nurses on their cell phones with women in labor in close proximity. A former nurse in charge of the maternity ward, Nurse Kinaya, explained why she saw smartphones as a problem, linking them to globalization. She said,

> Another thing that I can say maybe is that it's these globalization things. When we say globalization . . . generally [it] is these things from TV, therefore you find a person that is seeing all these things on TV, she takes them and brings them to the side of her work. You find, for example, these phones. Especially these phones . . . there is a patient there making noise, the nurse, she sits, she is listening to the phone, she is chatting on the phone. That's a thing that's really painful for those who . . . have a love of nursing. Therefore, if you explain to a person, "Please don't listen to the phone, listen first to the patient," already that other nurse thinks you are bad. I was doing that and that's why they think I'm mean. There's a patient calling, "Nurse, help me, help me!" and there the nurse is just chatting on the phone.

Here, Kinaya also explains how the older nurses' different perceptions of things like cell phones could create conflict between them and the younger nurses if they tried to tell their younger colleagues to pay attention to patients present on the ward instead of being so engaged with their phones.

Reprimands led to resentment on the part of the younger nurses and increased the tension between the older and younger nurses.

Another difference between older nurses and their counterparts who had more recently begun working was a shift in the organization of nurse training programs nationwide. In Tanzania there are enrolled nurses, ENs, and registered nurses, RNs. The ENs historically underwent training for four years, including time spent in the classroom on complicated deliveries, in the case of midwifery students. One of the older ENs, Rukia, also explained that, in her time, before being sent out to run small facilities in remote rural areas, such as village dispensaries, the new nursing graduates first spent time in larger hospitals, gaining additional experience and skills. Samwel, the twenty-three-year-old, is also an EN but had spent just two years earning his certificate in nurse-midwifery. Starting in 2008, the EN certificate programs went from four years to two (S. Marwa, personal communication, September 26, 2018). Part of the reduction in training time was to keep pace with increased demand for health care workers as the country built more and more health care facilities to accomplish then-president Jakaya Kikwete's promise of a dispensary in every village.

While Samwel was posted at the regional hospital, others of his school-mates had been posted to rural dispensaries where they were the highest-ranking medical professional. When I asked Rukia what she thought could improve the health of the country, what she would want me to tell the Ministry of Health, she implored, "I mean, [Adrienne], I am sending you! If you go to the Ministry of Health, if you have only one request let it be to tell them just to return the nursing colleges to these four years! We will save the country. Deaths will decrease. But by this system that they have put in place, deaths will not be reduced, they are so many." Rukia was speaking generally about deaths here, but having inexperienced or incompletely trained nurses on the maternity ward presented a particular danger to pregnant women who might be at risk of developing complications. I spoke with the hospital's highest-ranking nurse, the Patron, about challenges facing the hospital. After telling me that the hospital was still lacking a large number of needed assistant nursing officers (RNs), I observed that these more highly skilled nurses were important and he elaborated on staffing decisions:

AS: And I see that these people are very important, especially for maternity. Okay, so we have received these ENs, they help us, but they have not studied complicated deliveries or there are other things they don't know or they are unable to do and others are brand new and they don't want to say [if they don't know].

Patron: And that is exactly the reason why I have more than twenty assistant nursing officers at the maternity ward. I knew there was a great need but if we had enough [assistant nursing officers], I was expecting that ENs there on maternity should be few, that is, their numbers there should decrease.

Their lack of a more comprehensive, four-year training program like that of the older ENs caused some of the older nurses, such as Rukia, to be suspicious of the newer nurses' competence. Worst of all, in the eyes of some of these nurses, the younger nurses fresh out of school sometimes did not ask for explanations if they were unsure how to do something. Instead, they simply proceeded as best they knew, which sometimes resulted in poor care, lack of monitoring, or even dangerous improvisation of standard procedures. For example, one of the new ENs on the maternity ward, Sofia, had consistently been leaving her work unfinished when it was the end of her shift. She would simply abandon what she was doing if any barrier appeared in her path, as in when she was near the end of her shift and, unable to find a working stethoscope (despite the one visibly hanging out of a nearby student's pocket), she changed her clothes and started to leave for the day without taking her patient's vital signs. The morning following that incident, one of the older, very experienced nurses, Gire, decided to give Sofia some dedicated attention by observing Sofia as she conducted a delivery. Gire repeatedly reprimanded Sofia or asked her to explain why she was doing what she was doing, as she was doing it, to the point that Sofia began to cry. Gire's point was that many of the young, new graduates lack supervision once they are hired and are then able to acclimate to bad habits or lax technique that they will carry with them throughout the rest of their career.

HISTORICAL MOMENTS AND NURSING

In the context of Tanzania, it is also important to consider the different historical moments in which the nurses were trained. Many of the older nurses started their schooling in the socialist period under then-president Julius Nyerere. Their memories of the Nyerere period were perhaps idealistic and were certainly nostalgic but also prompted me to further investigate why there might be such a shift in the way older nurses view their younger counterparts. One document from the National Archives, a memo from Minister of Health Bryceson on May 18, 1964, three years after independence, explains to health workers their roles in supporting Nyerere's five-year development plan. While none of the health care personnel with whom I spoke had begun their studies or practice in the 1960s, their accounts of their time studying or working under Nyerere reflect Bryceson's rhetoric in the memo. The health care sector was an important cog in the machine of Ujamaa socialism. Bryceson ends his memo to health workers by saying:

> We are responsible for the health of the nation. The attainment of the broad aim of an increase in life expectancy is dependent upon our efforts. The very target of an improved standard of living is dependent to a large extent on the success of our teaching. I know that our medical workers, of all grades both in the Ministry and in the Voluntary Agencies are already

hard worked. Nevertheless, I am asking for more time, more effort. (TNA No. HE 1172/67)

In light of my conversations with providers regarding their memories of working in health care during the Nyerere era, I am led to believe that this rhetoric, which invokes providers as key actors in nation-building, imbued them with a sense of purpose and responsibility that those currently working do not feel as strongly. The more diffuse twenty-first-century rhetoric of development and human rights simply does not resonate as strongly on the local level and therefore is not the same motivator for working hard under difficult conditions.

Another nurse who had started her career under Nyerere said, of the difference in attitudes, "Work accountability, people were really working very hard. People had respect and they had love. That is different than what you see [these days]." During this time period, health care providers were more focused on providing care instead of trying to make money. Enriching oneself for personal, rather than national or community, profit was antithetical to the mission of Nyerere's Ujamaa.

FROM NATION-BUILDERS TO ENEMIES OF THE PEOPLE

In contrast to the value Minister of Health Bryceson placed on health care providers in the important work of nation-building in the immediate post-Independence era, the present moment more often sees health care workers in the news or with radio DJs discussing them because of poor interactions with patients. Frequently prompted by a lack of supplies or brief interactions with brusque, overburdened health care workers, pregnant women's relatives often misinterpreted their interactions with providers as the result of the personal or professional failures of mean or corrupt hospital staff members (see also Martin 2009, 49). Nurses, particularly on the maternity ward, which had the highest patient load at the Mawingu Regional Hospital, bore the brunt of these poor interactions and sometimes had very bad reputations in the community. This lack of status in their communities might also be indicative of the shifts in national constructions of, or discourses about, the role of nurses.

One particular example of how the public's perception of the nursing profession has changed can be seen in the prevalence of satirical cartoons about the health sector generally and nurses in particular. One such image was circulating widely on social media in 2015 when I was in the field. The image depicts a nurse talking on her cell phone as a patient stands against the wall with his pants down, exposing his naked buttocks, with a syringe of medicine still sticking out of his exposed backside. The nurse looks unconcerned as she chats on the phone and the man has an expression of nervous pain and horror on his face as he turns to look at the nurse. The nurse's uniform is identical to the ones that nurses in Tanzania wear, though this does not necessarily mean the image originated there. It is entirely possible the image spread to Tanzania from another country in Africa, but its very presence, and quick circulation across media in Tanzania is a testimony to its relevance in the country.

In local newspapers, a quick search of their online sites produces dozens of stories from the last five years in which reporters and opinion writers discuss abuses occurring in health facilities, often perpetrated against pregnant women. One article from 2016 reports health care workers in a district of the Rukwa region neglected a pregnant woman, causing her baby to subsequently die after her husband was forced to help her give birth (Mwangoka 2016). A similar story was reported from another region in the same year, that time resulting in the death of newborn twins (Kofu 2016), and yet another from 2018 (Musa 2018). Another article published online in 2017 opens with: "Florence Nightingale would turn in her grave if she heard some of the stories circulating in Tanzania about how nurses treat their pregnant patients" and continues to list abuses (Makoye 2017).

CONCLUSION

In the current era in Tanzania, nursing is unmistakably shaped by an increase in demand for services. More and more pregnant women come to the hospital seeking high-quality maternity care but, because of various government policies, this care continues to lack sufficient financial support and it is difficult for the hospital to maintain supply levels or to pay nurses extra duty or overtime pay. These factors, plus a lack of recognition or positive reinforcement from the hospital administration, often meant nurses of all ages told me they felt frustrated and unable to live up to the ideals of their profession. It is not hard to imagine, then, how this frustration could combine with the enticements and escape of the world of social media or continuing education that took young nurses out of their wards, even temporarily, and offered them distance from the patients to whom they could often offer so little. These younger nurses, unlike the older generation, did not have memories of a time in which they had been more highly valued by their national government or the institution employing them, perhaps leading to more apathy and burnout without a deeper connection to a broader purpose.

Additionally, restructuring of the economy and workforce in Tanzania after the end of socialism shifted how nurses found their way into this work. Increased demand for nurses at the lower levels led to reduced training time, as well as relatively low qualifications needed for nursing study. These factors, combined with the excellent job security of most government employment, has led some younger people to nursing work less out of a vocational calling and more due to a need for job security and a desire for formal employment. The result has been, in the eyes of older nurses, the erosion of some of nursing's fundamental, nontechnical attributes, the loss of which has decreased the prestige of nursing and the close relationship between nurses and their patients.

CHAPTER 9

"We Work with What We Have, Not with What We Would Like to Have"

HOSPITAL CARE IN MEXICO

Vania Smith-Oka and Kayla J. Hurd

IN 1964, THOUSANDS of physicians across Mexico went on strike in response to changing health laws that affected their medical lives in hospitals. The strike lasted ten months, during which time they marched in protest in several cities, "painting it white" with their white coats and banners (Archundia-García 2011, S29). They demanded better labor conditions, better pay, and the agency to determine hospital training. They fought to wrestle control of medicine from the bureaucracies and state-level institutions and apply their own vision to their training and medical care (Soto Laveaga 2013). However, their efforts were ultimately unsuccessful. After months of negotiations with the country's president, their protests were violently shut down, the ringleaders imprisoned or fired, and the rest given the choice of being fired or returning quietly to work.

Fifty years later, in 2014, another medical protest erupted, this time in response to accusations of medical malpractice. Igniting a nationwide protest, physicians spoke out against the charges, blaming the abusive environments they labored in. Smaller, but equally vocal, protests in later years continued to address how doctors found themselves in the crosshairs of public concerns of health, human rights, and dignity. Participants in our ethnography in two hospitals in the city of Puebla, Mexico, repeatedly spoke about the difficulties of practicing medicine under such conditions, and how their ability to be physicians was greatly impacted by broader structures, financial allocation, and the violence from drug cartels.

Hospital ethnographies address important questions not only about hospital culture itself but also exploring topics specific to each locale, such as the unexpected presence of empathy and caring in medical training in resource-poor contexts (Wendland 2010), biomedicine as an incomplete solution for clinicians' decision-making within a growing cancer epidemic (Livingston 2012), or how clinicians and psychiatric patients struggle to maintain lives of dignity within dismal infrastructural conditions (Reyes-Foster 2018). They also discuss how a hospital emerges as a crucial, but hidden, mediator in the somatic relatedness and imaginings of national communities of blood donations (Street 2009, 194). Others show how surgical bodies—the bodies of surgery residents—come into being and how they learn to embody the expectations of biomedicine within American hospitals (Prentice 2013). The majority of these ethnographies examine the ways that things, practices, and people become knowable within biomedical interactions.

Hospitals have variously been defined by scholars as islands (separate from mainstream values, concepts, and practices), as part of the mainland (reflecting and reproducing society's values), or as ambiguous spaces (Long, Hunter, and van der Geest 2008). If hospitals are institutional spaces that replicate and reproduce a society's key cultural norms (Van der Geest and Finkler 2004), then these half-century medical protests we reference above provide a glimpse into how people belonging to a seemingly powerful profession can feel so abused and abandoned by the state. This paradox can perhaps best be explained by some scholars' suggestion that hospitals are ambiguous spaces that are simultaneously permeable and bounded, where the powerful can also be disenfranchised, and that are sites of social control as well as contestations (Brown 2012; Street and Coleman 2012). And yet, hospitals are both totalizing institutions as well as places where new and transgressive social orders are formed, a paradox that Street (2014, 12) argues in her ethnography of medicine in New Guinea makes hospitals crucial spaces to explore interactions between science, society, and power.

A country riddled with massive state-level problems, such as corruption, violence, and inequities, Mexico has struggled historically to provide appropriate health care to its population. Its public hospitals are a particularly illustrative example of these broader issues, which have faced increasing budget cuts and structural reorganization over the past few years. Mexican hospitals are teetering on the brink of a new relationship with clinicians, patients, and the state. Our aim is to trace how these broader structures are historically reproduced in health care institutions, which create abusive environments for hospital staff, ultimately enacted in abusive practices on the bodies of patients. Our analysis draws on scholarship that examines the creation of medical spaces and identities in hospitals and how these reflect and extend (social) hierarchies (Brown 2012); these reveal the day-to-day realities of hospital work (Finkler, Hunter, and Iedema 2008; Prentice 2013), as well as those that focus on the multiple ways by which hospitals and those who work in them mutually constitute one another (Street and Coleman 2012). We argue that while hospitals are spaces that reflect a country's concerns with nation-building (Street 2009; Soto Laveaga 2013), clinicians within these spaces are caught in a liminal state between being agents who can change the health of the nation and powerless pawns abused by the broader system. Their narratives interweave their paradoxical lives—love for the care work they engage in, powerful within hospital spaces, powerless outside the walls, and a deep anger at the broader system that routinely disenfranchises them.

DOING HOSPITAL ETHNOGRAPHY IN MEXICAN WARDS

To collect the data for this chapter, Smith-Oka (the first author) carried out in-depth ethnography between 2014 and 2016 at two hospitals in the city of Puebla, Mexico. Puebla has almost two million people living within the larger metropolitan area (INEGI 2017) and has over ten public hospitals, five large private hospitals, and dozens of smaller private clinics that provide a range of services and quality of care. Some of the large private hospitals are extremely luxurious, while some of the public hospitals are markedly understaffed and with decrepit facilities (stained medical gowns, third-hand equipment, poor plumbing, etc.).

The field sites for this research were two hospitals. Hospital Salud was a public hospital with 130 beds, 52 interns, and 104 residents in 2016. Hospitals belonging to these state systems provide medical care to government workers and were set up to safeguard a healthy labor force for the capitalist market sector (Finkler 2008); they were also part of nation-building efforts (Soto Laveaga 2015). As with many public hospitals across the country (see Reyes-Foster 2018), this hospital suffered from a lack of resources, such as the availability of laboratory tests or appointments for MRIs for cancer patients. As Lucero, one of our participants, said, "there are no [MRI] appointments for eight months, and these are people who need to get tests done right away."

Our second research location was Hospital Piedad, a small private hospital, with forty beds, in the city center, which primarily served people with private insurance. Our participants all emphasized that care at private and public hospitals was very different. Aarón, an intern at Hospital Piedad, said,

> From what I've seen of private [hospitals] they do seem to make a bigger effort . . . in interacting with the patient and with the family. [Doctors] take their time and even have the possibility of talking about stuff that is not so related to medicine. In the public ones they don't have that possibility of interacting with the patient. Instead it's like, "uh-huh, you come to treat this thing." They give the [patient] the prescription and the [patient] leaves. . . . They don't have time for anything else.

Some participants also made a distinction between the type of patients at each hospital, stating that patients at private hospitals tended to be more agentive, assertive, and asked more questions, while those in public hospitals were less agentive and "just let people do what they want to them."

We interviewed over sixty participants, including medical interns, residents, and physicians. The methodology included negotiated interactive observations (Wind 2008), ethnography, and deep hanging out where we investigated participants' interactions with peers and mentors, their ways of learning new skills, and their lived experiences in the hospital. We also carried out a historical analysis of the medical system in Mexico, delving into national protests by medical personnel that have occurred within the past fifty years. We analyzed our textual data by following systematic approaches to identify themes and recurring patterns (Bernard et al. 2017).

Ethnography is a deeply personal, self-reflective method. For most anthropologists working in hospitals, it is probably second nature to carry one's scruffy notebooks and pens, to sit down on gurneys to chat with participants, and to enter into procedures and stand out of the way of the clinicians doing their care work. As other hospital ethnographers have stated, many of us doing hospital (or any) ethnography balance emic and etic identities during our research (Zaman 2008). These identities necessitate a daily ongoing negotiation in our quest to develop trust and rapport with our interlocutors (Aberese-Ako 2016). In our case, our identity was sometimes a help and sometimes a significant hindrance. As we mentioned above, Smith-Oka carried out the ethnography for this research. Her multifold, yet ambiguous, identity tended to be confusing to our interlocutors. An Anglo last name, light-skin, and faculty credentials from a U.S. university projected a foreign identity; but a native ability in colloquial Mexican Spanish suggested a different, contrasting identity. Interlocutors often refashioned these multiple identities during our interactions. Some could not get past the phenotype and last name, and often complimented Smith-Oka on her good command of the language. Others accepted the Latinx identity, but they could not understand why someone with a PhD would be doing research—after all, most of them thought that research was to *complete* a degree. The prevailing assumption, therefore, especially among the older physicians and directors, was that Smith-Oka was a student and was doing research to complete a thesis; this identity of "thesis student" was literally laminated into the official hospital identification badges provided. Regardless of what identity is read by our interlocutors, as Inhorn (2004) reminds us, within hospital spaces any form of ethnographic gaze may be perceived as unwelcome.

"Why Me?": Life in the Hospital

"I had a patient who died just as I started the internship," said Paola as we spoke about some of the difficulties she had experienced during the year-long internship expected of all medical students. She was an intern at Hospital Salud and was known for her upbeat personality, easy smile, and cheerful Winnie the Pooh and flowered scrubs. All her peers respected her and regularly sought her out for advice. Only sometimes would she allow her vulnerability to emerge.

She described how her first rotation was in Internal Medicine, where the practice was to provide interns with more responsibility for patient care, almost like junior residents. She described her duties: "I was in charge of about twelve patients, well, not just me but alongside the attending physician, but I would write the medical notes, I would manage the labs, and I would do what had to be done with the patients." She continued, "There was a patient who just got worse. I first saw her and she was not that bad. But as time passed, she kind of got worse. A week passed, and she got worse and worse, until she died." Paola smiled wanly as she described how she felt,

> So, I just can't overcome what happened with that patient, I don't know why. I even feel it was kind of slightly my fault. I felt guilty because I would think, "Maybe we didn't do what we should have; maybe I didn't tell the doctor about the labs that I was meant to." And it really hurt me. That is when, honestly, I became depressed.

She said she would often ask herself "Why me?" and that her peers would tell her, "It was obviously not you; the patient's [case] was serious. If not even the [doctor] saw something, how were you to see something, having so little experience?" This patient's death had a significant impact on Paola, especially as she was present (and alone) when the patient passed away. She said she cried for a week afterward and still feels the pain in her heart. Research shows that practitioners experience powerful emotions when a patient dies, even when they are not close to the patient, like in Paola's case (Sorensen and Iedema 2009).

Paola's experience was not uncommon for most of the medical trainees we met. They all had "war stories" (Wendland 2010) consisting of death, fear, exhaustion, or personal feelings of failure. They all, of course, also had many exhilarating experiences, where they were allowed entry into the world of medicine and permitted to care for patients, to bring babies into the world, and to enter surgeries. Their everyday lives in the hospital often consisted of the seemingly banal practices of hospital medicine: taking biosamples (blood, urine, etc.), managing medical records, doing a basic physical examination, writing prescriptions, staying up late every third night for *guardias* (overnight shifts), shadowing doctors, and avoiding the ever-present *regaños* (scolding) from doctors. Their practices and care work thus revolved around the mastery of hospital processes and procedures (e.g., writing the charts) or proficiency in technology (e.g., taking samples or using a stethoscope) (Brown 2012; Rice 2010).

While our research investigated a variety of different themes in the hospital itself—the rotations, the *guardias*, the grand rounds, people's interactions with peers during downtime, and participation in procedures—here we focus on how the broader (Mexican) structures affect the hospital modes of organization and hierarchy. As Finkler (2004) stated, biomedicine in Mexico has been culturally reinterpreted, incorporating many of the values, but also constrained by many of the structures. Medical practice reflects the broader political and economic realities of the country (Finkler 2008). One of the questions that every participant in our study answered was, "If you had the power to change anything about medicine in Mexico, what would it be?" Their responses ranged from changing people's habits, to addressing a severe shortage of supplies, to dealing with the abusive issues in the medical hierarchy, to scrapping the entire medical system and starting again. But at the core of their answers lay a deep dissatisfaction with the medical system in Mexico and the ways that it played out in their hospital lives.

"You Pretend That You Are Working, and We'll Pretend to Pay You": Structural Concerns

Doctor Luna was an obstetrician in his late forties, with a florid face and whose glasses rested on protruding ears, framed by his thinning hair. He worked at Hospital Piedad, the private hospital, where, in contrast to all his other hospital peers, he solely attended to charity-funded patients. His salary, therefore, came from the hospital's foundation instead of from private patients and insurance companies. He said that most doctors made ends meet by working two (or more) jobs. Like many of his colleagues, he held a second job at a large public hospital where he worked three nights a week and additionally had a small private practice. During one interview we discussed the practice of medicine in Mexico, including workload and financial stability. Dr. Luna thoughtfully said, "All across the world medicine is very badly paid. Even we as doctors, with graduate degrees need two jobs just to be financially stable. . . . Here [medicine] is very badly remunerated."

Our data show that there was a significant dynamic between the state and the medical system. Several of our participants agreed that the three primary structural factors affecting their ability to provide good medical care were financial (such as the country's health care budget), governmental (perceptions of the government's corruption and/or inefficiency), and infrastructural (lack of hospitals or personnel). They saw these products of insufficient resources as key factors shaping their practice of medicine within the hospital, such as the medical hierarchy, the need to develop medical skills, the high patient load, the differences between public and private hospitals, the lack of supplies, and the ensuing poor service. All of these factors reverberated on their "daily ethical practices" (Finkler 2008, 175).

Historically, Mexico has undergone numerous reformations of their health care system to reach the state of health care today. In 1943, two institutions were created to provide care to the population: the Ministry of Health and the Mexican Institute for Social Security (IMSS) (Frenk et al. 2003). Amidst the changing epidemiological profile of Mexico, cost of care dramatically increased in the late 1960s, and health care officials sought reform to address these issues. In the 1970s, there was an increased push to certify more physicians, which created a surplus of unemployed doctors (Finkler 2004).

The three-tier system of access has continued in place until the present day: (1) the IMSS and the ISSSTE (the Institute of Social Services and Security for Civil Servants), which provide social security for citizens and their families that are formally employed and governmentally sponsored, respectively; (2) the Ministry of Health, designed primarily to provide care to the uninsured population; and (3) the private sector, with primarily out-of-pocket costs to patients who can afford it. In 2004, the Ministry of Health sought to provide medical insurance to the uninsured population through a health program called Seguro Popular. This program was criticized for not fulfilling its goal of universal coverage and not reaching underserved populations. Additionally, Mexico's ratio of providers to patients remains low, at 2.2 physicians and 2.7 nurses per 1,000 inhabitants (Juan López, Valle, and Aguilera 2015). These multiple and parallel public and private arrangements of health care impede the efforts to improve quality of care for Mexico's citizens.

All of our participants considered finances and the government's lack of investment in health care to be major impediments to providing good care. Many of them spoke about the need to increase health budgets, to increase funding to education, and to make medical care more accessible to impoverished patients. Julieta, an intern at Piedad, put it bluntly when she said, "They should channel the money where it's needed, right? . . . Mexico should provide more to the health sector than to *futbol*." Diana, another intern, argued that medicine should be the same in both public and private hospitals: "It's not as though we have public appendicitis and private appendicitis."

In our interview with Dr. Luna, he lamented the financial situation of health care, comparing medical salaries and workload in Mexico to the United States. He said that the Mexican system consisted of the hospitals telling doctors, "You pretend that you are working, and we'll pretend to pay you." For him, financial concerns intertwined salaries with the ability to purchase medical equipment. "It's difficult to buy an ultrasound. It costs like 200–300 thousand pesos (approximately US$10,000 to $15,000). As much as a car! Only if you have no kids, and you don't have to feed a family [can you buy one]."

In her research on Mexican health care, Finkler (2004) concludes that medicine as a profession has not achieved the power and prestige present in other countries due to a variety of structural factors. First, physicians are subordinate to government bureaucracy and hence have little power. Second, physicians find themselves competing for meager funds, thus fragmenting what little unity the profession might have; this process results in physicians feeling less identified with the profession. Third, the higher unemployment due to a glut of medical graduates we mentioned earlier meant that those who *were* employed as physicians preferred not to protest work conditions for fear of losing what they had. Finally, Finkler argues, Mexican medicine depends on U.S.-based medicine for its legitimacy, which is evidenced by Dr. Luna's words above. Invariably for our participants, the corruption of the government or its budgetary decisions about health were blamed for the health care landscape. Amanda, an intern at Piedad, stated, "Because the government steals the money, and there's no budget and there's not enough to buy medicines," Diana added, "I think that this comes from our corrupt politicians; if the government really cared about providing an adequate infrastructure to health care in Mexico, I think there would be many things that could be improved." Aarón, another intern, concluded, "Both doctors and patients are unhappy. But it's neither of their faults. This could be solved with two things: a budget and good planning."

Dr. Navarro, one of the administrators of Hospital Piedad, intertwined these broader structural concerns with the practice of medicine at hospitals. Giving us a hypothetical example one day in his office surrounded by dusty hospital records, he elaborated on what he perceived to be the main facets of health care. He said, "For example, I could have pain. I get to the hospital, and it's the appendix. They take it out and it turns out that it was not the appendix but some inflammation caused by something I ate, right?" With a laugh, he added, "When do I realize that? When I get the pathology results that tell me 'normal appendix.'" He then continued, "So, the problem in Mexico is that, first, health care is not equal, and the attention is still not quality attention." He pulled out a paper and pen from a drawer and diagrammed his view on medicine: "Health care expenditure in Mexico is disproportional, because if I do an analysis and I ask 'why do people get sick?' well, we might say because of heredity, right? An x percentage. We might say another portion is caused by problems in the health system; another portion because of environmental problems." He concluded his description by drawing all over the page, stating, "But behavioral problems cause *all* this, do you know what I mean? And what does the health system invest in? In this, which is the hospital, right? *This* is where most money is spent. But it is not even used for medications or for technology, but for its administration." The discrepancy between where the money needs to go and where it actually ends up structurally resonates with the broader system of Mexico, indicating that this structural violence has meandered from governmental institutions to the medical hierarchy to the livelihoods of every patient that the hospital treats.

"IT'S NOT GOOD FOR PATIENTS FOR US TO BE SO TIRED": HOSPITAL-LEVEL ISSUES

Besides the broader concerns with how health care budgets were allotted, our participants focused on a midlevel concern: the hospital itself. Clinicians emphasized three main problems: the medical hierarchy (i.e., the differences between ranks), the large number of patients at public hospitals, and the lack of supplies. The medical hierarchy seemed to reflect the abusive broader structure that disenfranchised those at the very bottom, and which, in many ways is what prompted the 1964 protests we described at the start of the chapter. Several of the interns we met emphasized that the hospital hierarchy was extremely marked and that these differences in rank were factors shaping their experiences within clinical training.

We spent many hours with our participants: entering into procedures, resting in their hospital barracks, observing classes and grand rounds, and meeting for coffee and meals when we knew they needed a break from their mental and physical load. One of our key informants was Julieta, a determined, iron-willed intern at Hospital Piedad whose dream was to become an obstetrician so she could intertwine rigorous biomedical care with home and water births. During one of the many coffees we had with her she elaborated on her anxiety about abusive interactions between ranks. Part of her narrative was on the ways that the senior interns bullied her own cohort when they started the hospital internship. "They're like, 'go for the paper, and do this; and you can't sleep in this bed; and go for that thing.' So, it's like mistreating people solely because they are lower on the ladder, on a lower rung; . . . It's having them do unnecessary things just to bother them." She concluded that many of these interactions were simply part of the culture of medicine, where, she claimed, people at each level of the hierarchy mistreated those below because, "you are an intern I'm going to treat you badly." She added that this sort of behavior was transmitted down the hierarchy and across the generations: "The attending physician is going to treat the resident badly, and the resident treats the intern [badly], like that." Perhaps because the broader health system was abusive and stripped doctors of power (Finkler 2004), many of them enacted these same abuses on those below them who were more vulnerable.

Diana, an intern at Piedad, connected this kind of mistreatment to a broader structural issue within all hospitals. She stated that in public hospitals, "The doctor is more exploited: excessive work days, and seeing no end of patients in a short period. I feel that many doctors in public hospitals are not sufficiently motivated to attend to their patients because they *know* that they don't earn well, that they don't sleep well, that they fight with everyone, and that the work days are excessive." She added that there was a significant difference between hospital types in terms of "salary, the magnitude of patients, and exhaustion (*desgaste*)." Her choice to use *desgaste* is interesting, as it can mean exhaustion but also to be worn out or eroded. Thus, it can convey an exhaustion from the hard work and long hours, a disillusionment in the system, and the inability to stand up for something because one's values and beliefs have been eroded and worn away. Dr. Valentina, a resident in the obstetrics ward of Hospital Salud, said that the *guardias* (overnight shifts) were not only exhausting but also problematic, "because, quite honestly, as residents they really do screw us. We spend a lot of time in the hospital, and it is sometimes not that good for the patients for us to be so tired." The converse seemed to be true in private hospitals, where people claimed that the work environment was very different, and was much more cordial and comfortable because, "They have well-established hours, salaries, and the hospital environment is different." In these private hospital spaces, the level of *desgaste*, and feeling worn out by the larger structure, was expressed very differently in clinicians. While they all worked long hours, had little sleep, and high stress (especially interns and junior residents), they had a lower patient load, a slightly more cordial relationship with their senior colleagues, and better infrastructure (better food, beds to sleep on, hot showers, etc.). Thus, in the long term they were much less *desgastados* than their peers at public hospitals.

Many of the clinicians we interviewed focused on the high patient load in hospitals, such as Julieta, who stated, "Many times there are so many problems in the public sector because there are *so many* patients, there are only a few doctors, and there are only a few things one can provide the patient." She added that when there is poor service, patients believe it is the physicians' fault, "but what they don't know is that there are twenty people in line after them, waiting; there are twenty people also waiting to be treated."

A significant factor in the medical care that reflected the broader structure was the very evident lack of supplies in some public clinics and hospitals. In our interview with Amanda, she mentioned how she had participated in a rotation at a government-funded clinic a couple of years earlier where they were so strapped for supplies that clinicians would use the same scalpel all day, only cleaning it with hydrogen peroxide between patients. She added that this shocked her because in medical school they had been taught "that there are some things that you use for one patient only, like a scalpel, a needle, and those things that you can get really sick from another patient." She said they also lacked gloves and other basic supplies, which meant that the interns and other clinicians had to buy them in order to attend to patients. Scarcity of supplies was only one part; there was a scarcity of medications, physicians, and specialists. Sebastián stated, "There are hospitals but they don't have physicians nor supplies. [Hospitals] are just decorative. They have nothing. . . . They don't have gloves, there are no face masks, no catheters; that's the problem: a lack of supplies." Diana added, "So we have to depend on or resign ourselves to what we have, and many times you can make a good diagnostic with a good physical examination. . . . And you know there are many things that could be improved, but that you know would be very hard to do." Dr. Marco, a resident at Hospital Salud, concluded, "Here we work with what we have, not with what we would like to have."

Humanized Care: Both Structural and Individual Level

In addition to mentioning the problems with the medical system, some of our participants also listed solutions. Some focused on a need to entirely change the broader health system, while others focused on the need for more humanized care for patients. Some of them apportioned blame on the patients themselves rather than on the system. It was common for the Mexican "*cultura*" to be blamed for the ways that medicine was addressed in hospitals. *Cultura* in colloquial Mexican parlance has a different definition than how anthropologists use it. It usually tends to be dismissive, derogatory even, and implies a certain intractability and reticence of impoverished, rural, indigenous populations to change and become "modern." As Duncan (2018) shows in her work in the southern Mexican state of Oaxaca, *cultura* is about indigenousness or ignorance and an absence of modernity. Like studies have shown (Reyes-Foster 2018), *cultura* is a socially relative understanding of culture that is very raced, classed, and gendered. Doctors in our study often lamented this *cultura*, especially people's reticence in going to medical centers, and thus, when patients were seen in the hospital, their conditions would usually be more advanced and harder to treat. César, an intern at Piedad, stated that in order to improve the quality of health care provided, and to overcome this *cultura*, physicians needed to "increase responsibility in patients, making them understand that [medicine] is not cheap and making them fiscally responsible. . . . Making them understand what it costs, so they can appreciate it (*valoren*), right?" His last phrase is interesting, as he uses the verb *valorar*, which can mean to appreciate. But it also can mean "to value," to understand that things, practices, and objects have value to those who wield them and re-create them through their knowledge and actions. We argue that this process of re-valuing objects and practices is similar to others observed by anthropologists in other medical contexts, such as mortuary spaces where dead bodies are constructed in multiple ways (Horsley 2008) or in the varied ways—tactile, auditory, relational— by which a fetus is constructed through ultrasound (Howes-Mischel 2016). Reyes-Foster (2018) identifies similar concepts of value among her participants in Yucatán, who emphasized a need for patients to have a greater civic engagement in order to modernize the nation. Rhetoric like César's is interesting, and paradoxical, as it clearly blames the government and the broader structure for corruption, while also implying that the root cause of this situation is the lack of participation and lack of knowledge and *cultura* in the population.

And yet, many interlocutors acknowledged that the ways that medicine was practiced was problematic for the patients, and thus wanted more humanized and more equitable care across the system, rather than the current system of significant disparity between public and private care. One of the interns at

Piedad explained why "the attitudes of physicians and medical personnel is generally not the best," stating that "maybe it's because, well, one is fed up of working so much." He added that things should not really be that way, "you should be grateful because, first of all, you have a job, and second, well, you're supposedly doing something that you like. So, yeah, I would change that." In another interview, Dr. Navarro stated, "A large percentage of Mexican medical care is costly; it's called catastrophic because the sickness is a catastrophe because, in addition to wounding the patient, it wounds their finances. Therefore, health is not egalitarian." He then went on to describe what he thought quality medicine consisted of: "One: . . . that the attention needs to be safe. It's not fair for you to come to me to be healed and I make you sick or create more difficulties, right? . . . And the second element is dignified care, respectful care." Ultimately, for many of the participants, the larger issues continued to be centered on the system itself, even though some of them, like César and others, blamed the patients for their own suffering. They considered that the only way forward was to, as one participant phrased it, "re-establish the Mexican health system completely."

Twitter and Protests

In 2014, Mexico began the gradual unrolling of a proposed Universal Healthcare System that would begin by having cost and service sharing between the major health systems we described earlier (IMSS, ISSSTE, and Ministry of Health). While in many ways a laudable move, many physicians were concerned about this new system, stating that it would amplify the current health care issues Mexico faced because it would stretch resources to their breaking point.

That very year also began an ongoing wave of medical protests. These protests had both structural and immediate causes. Their foundation was the ongoing and problematic labor conditions of hospital staff across the country. The immediate causes of the protests, however, were sparked by an arrest order issued by a judge against sixteen physicians in an IMSS hospital in the state of Jalisco in 2014 for the death of a fifteen-year-old patient (who had died in 2010). Two sides emerged from this situation—the doctors and their advocates on one side and the patient's family on the other. The boy's family argued that his death had occurred because of medical negligence and incompetence. They stated that the boy had entered the hospital in late 2009 with what seemed to be an asthmatic crisis, possibly caused by the H1N1 flu virus. Over the next two weeks the patient underwent more than a half dozen interventions, losing approximately four liters of blood and never regaining consciousness. Fifty-five days after admittance to the hospital, the boy died. An autopsy by a forensic medical service revealed that he had died from intestinal tuberculosis. The doctors, on the other hand, argued that they had done all they could for him but that they were stretched thin (through overwork, long hours, and lack of supplies) and so were not to blame for the death. They saw this situation as an effort to criminalize medical practitioners and as a way for the patient's family to make money from the lawsuit. The executive committee for the IMSS workers syndicate defended the physicians, stating that the boy's family took too long to bring him to the hospital, by which time he was cyanotic and in respiratory and cardiac arrest, needing to be revived through CPR and then interned in the Intensive Care Unit.

In 2014, arrest warrants were issued for the doctors involved in the case. Soon after, a group of doctors posted the hashtag #YoSoy17 (I am 17) on Twitter to support their colleagues. The idea behind the name is that any doctor could be the seventeenth member of the accused group because they had all been in that situation: exhausted, with few resources, too many patients, and few rewards for their effort. What began as a simple call to support their colleagues went viral, growing into a nationwide protest about problematic hospital labor conditions.

People posting on social media claimed that they were not at fault for patient outcomes because it was a system built against them, with long *guardias*, limited resources, corrupt politicians siphoning off funds, and with a high patient load. Posts on social media included phrases such as, "We're Doctors, Not Gods, Nor Criminals," "We owe ourselves to our patients; we're physicians thanks to them and for them!!" "Let's dignify our profession without forgetting our commitments to our patients," "For a more humane form of healthcare for our patients," "Come on indignant and victimized doctors, say your piece," and "Errare humanum est (To err is human)."

These online protests eventually shifted to real protests, wherein doctors marched in protest on June 22, 2014, in dozens of cities across the nation. As their past colleagues did in 1964, these protesters wore their white coats and carried signs; but they added a black ribbon around their upper arm as a metaphor for the death of their profession and the violence they faced from patients, the system, and the drug cartels. One national newspaper headline referred to this as "The death of a young man that unleashed a national movement" (Excelsior 2014).

An added facet of these medical protests was the feeling of insecurity pervading the medical profession. As other scholars have pointed out (Zacher Dixon 2015), the narco-violence of the drug cartels have made its presence felt and is filtering into the practices of medicine, fueling fears of what it is like to be a doctor in twenty-first-century Mexico. One of the primary requirements of all medical students is that, once they have completed their hospital internship, they have to do a year of social service, usually in underserved regions of the country. The participants in our study who were about to embark on their social service expressed significant fear about their safety during this year. Some sources suggest that anywhere from ten to twenty clinicians have either been kidnapped, killed, or disappeared during each of the recent years (O'Connor and Booth 2010). Clinics in some regions of the country stand empty, as clinicians refuse to staff them until their safety is guaranteed (Padilla 2018).

The doctors' marches have been repeated since 2014 and have sometimes also occurred in pockets across the nation on October 23 (National Doctors' Day in Mexico). These protests brought to the surface the longstanding tussle between policymakers and health care practitioners, and have increasingly added concerns for safety and life. Research has shown that the funds provided to the health care and education sectors are insufficient to combat both longstanding diseases and emerging ones. While government funds for health care have been reduced yearly making it harder for practitioners to do their work, there has been a simultaneous concern from policymakers and ministries with the quality of care provided to patients. One of the leaders of the protest stated in a speech, "We ask [the Minister of Health] to actually see the shortage of supplies, the scarcity, the lack of upkeep and maintenance of the [medical] units; we ask them to recognize the work conditions that forced our colleagues . . . to fall into that situation" (Enciso 2014). The speaker added that there is a recurring punitive action against "the medical class" that forces them to work under threat and in silence about a problematic medical system.

In 2016, in response to the proposed Universal Healthcare System, the organizers of the marches presented their demands to the Minister of Health. These demands included an improvement in labor conditions, increases in the budget for basic supplies, upgrades to the infrastructure of public hospitals, improvement in the safety of medical personnel, and guaranteeing health as a human right (Ureste 2016). For many of the protesters, the Universal Healthcare Law was emblematic of the nation's issues—a contested space between policy and practice that revived revolutionary promises while simultaneously breaking them on the backs of doctors and patients. Like its 1964 predecessor, this protest has also ebbed and flowed. Many of the older physicians we interviewed came of age during this tumultuous time. But, unlike the early movement, the 2014 protesters (and the yearly protests since) did not go on strike. They continued working, only marching as a group on one day. The protest has had greater visibility and activity in its online form, with postings and news almost daily about the situation between practitioners, patients, and policymakers.

Conclusion

Hospitals are a contested space between policy and practice where ideals (such as universal health care and humanized care) are developed within policies, but their enactment exists within a framework of rapidly diminishing funds and a system fraying at the seams. The contestations in our study also arise between clinicians and patients, who create and construct the value of medicine in different, and often opposing ways, and where perceptions of *cultura* (or lack thereof) shape these interactions. Clinicians continually re-create their identities and forms of practice as they navigate the health system. More junior interns and residents learn to navigate hierarchies, bodily exhaustion, and fears of failure or narco-violence. Those who work in public institutions also fashion their identity as capable, practiced, and experienced but also worn out. The clinicians in our research, and in broader Mexico, are caught within this system that aims to revive revolutionary and nation-building promises. But the system fails them (and their patients), not only in how funds are allocated and hospitals are built and staffed but also in the structural and infrastructural gaps that allow clinicians to fear for their lives. These problematic larger structures are reflected and replicated in the hospital practices—in abusive hierarchies that disenfranchise trainees, in gendered practices that exclude groups from leadership, or in allocation of resources where gloves and sutures are rationed. And yet, despite all these concerns shared by the clinicians in our study, almost all of them expressed a deep devotion to medicine and their lives within the halls of hospitals.

PART THREE

 Hospitals and the Patient

The Navigation of Public Hospitals by West African Immigrants with Cancer in Paris, France

Carolyn Sargent

AMONG THE THOUSANDS of immigrant patients consulting at public hospitals in Paris, France, those with potentially life-threatening prognoses such as cancer face particular challenges. Immigrant patients and families confront the deep meaning of a cancer diagnosis as well as difficulties engaging with the intricacies of French hospital bureaucracy and biomedical interventions. Clinicians and other personnel within the hospital struggle to offer comprehensible explanations of disease etiology and prognosis to a population with widely divergent understandings of cancer and its management. Meanwhile, interpreters play a liminal role, representing both the hospital and the patient in attempts to reach collective strategies for treatment decision-making. Drawing on a four-year study of breast cancer among immigrant women from West Africa in treatment in the Paris public hospital system, this chapter focuses on how sufferers, families, interpreters, and clinicians from this region conceptualize cancer and navigate the oncology system.

State policy and public sentiment in France reflect the ideological stance that health care is a human right—public hospitals are obligated to provide emergency care and to accept all patients, and national health insurance should eliminate financial barriers to medical care. This idealistic model does not reflect the obstacles patients face in accessing care. Immigrants, in particular, often are unaware of their rights to health insurance and hence to coverage for clinical interventions (Larchanche 2012). Navigating the complexities of the health bureaucracy is challenging for the most informed and experienced patients, and especially so for those with language constraints or who lack experience with biomedical institutions. While accompanying patients to hospital consultations, discussing these consultations with the patient afterwards, and interviewing interpreters, we concluded that translation problems dramatically affect patient understandings and treatment strategies. Interpreters reported difficulties translating for oncologists, given the absence of relevant vocabulary in patients' local languages. The dissonance between patient expectations and clinical discourse, especially biomedical prioritizing of "truth-telling," leads to patients' interrupting or categorically stopping hospital interventions in favor of ritual specialists, who emerge as options preferable to the hospital (Sargent and Kotobi 2017; Sargent and Benson 2019).

Accordingly, in this chapter, I address these fundamental questions: how does the cancer patient's engagement with hospital personnel and cancer treatments play out in creating an identifiable "hospital experience"? This is particularly salient for patients whose societies of origin in West Africa often lack high-functioning hospitals, and for whom French hospitals represent both hope for a cure and fear of the unknown. In addition, I ask how prospective patients and their families determine that a hospital is the appropriate health care site for diagnosis and treatment, when many immigrants are unaware of their rights to access hospitals. This question is especially pertinent given the state ideological premise emphasizing egalitarian health care—how do patients come to realize their rights to health care by virtue of living in France and suffering from a life-threatening disease?

The broader research project on which this chapter draws addressed the following issues:

1. The implications of a constitutional right to health care and a national health system for immigrant health care access
2. The features of clinical communication regarding end-of-life care and the prioritizing of truth-telling in a diverse patient population
3. The meanings, discourse, and experience of suffering associated with a cancer diagnosis among West African immigrant women
4. The navigation of the public hospital system, from diagnosis through treatment (biopsy, chemotherapy, surgery, radiation, and follow-up consultations) by women from an immigrant population

This research project is situated in a burgeoning anthropological literature on cancer in transnational perspective (Livingston 2012; McMullin 2016; Mathews, Burke, and Kampriani 2015; McMullin and Weiner 2008). Our findings resonate with McMullin and Weiner's contention that "cancer has a past and a present steeped in metaphors that reveal inequality, stigmatization, and struggles to control the uncontrollable" (2008, 9). As McMullin (2016) observes, anthropological studies of cancer have evolved from a U.S.-centered focus to a global cancer discourse, including such concerns as stigma, the dominance of biomedicine, and the implications of cancer for social and material relations. In this study, I examine the construction of meanings surrounding cancer in a population with little historical precedent on which to build an understanding of a disease variously imagined by West African immigrant women in France as a product of European contact with Africa, colonization, contagion, poverty, social conflict, or sorcery. The structures of inequality that shape the life trajectories of these women and their families are amplified in the context of life-threatening sickness, in this instance, breast cancer, whose treatment is inextricably linked to perceptions of the French hospital system.

NAVIGATING PUBLIC HOSPITALS

The French public health system is organized by sectors, in which hospitals target particular geospatial regions. Accordingly, two hospitals where we conducted our study, Avicenne and Delafontaine, are located in the 93rd department, Seine-Saint-Denis, where their target populations reside. Avicenne is a university hospital, affiliated with the AP-HP (Assistance-Hopitaux de Paris). Delafontaine is a general public hospital (Centre Hospitalier), but it is not in the university system. However, it is in partnership with hospitals in the AP-HP such as Avicenne, and with private institutions such as the Institut Curie.

Despite the organizational feature in which hospitals have designated target populations, patients may choose the institution they prefer for consultation and are not restricted to the hospital closest to their residence (Observatoire Régional de Santé 2013). Some patients prefer to seek care at especially distinguished private institutions known for cancer treatment, such as the Institut Curie or prestigious university hospitals such as the Hopital Européen Georges Pompidou. However, success in obtaining care at a favored hospital may depend on insurance status, illness criteria, finding an oncologist who accepts the case, and other features of the patient's health and social circumstances. Patients may try to obtain care in more than one hospital before finding clinicians and social workers who enable them to "enter the system." There is variation by hospital and by personnel regarding admission criteria for cancer treatment, although theoretically, all public hospitals should be using the same determinants for access.

The region of Seine-Saint-Denis is notable for its relatively high cancer mortality compared to other regions and relative to national statistics. With regard to breast cancer mortality, Seine-Saint-Denis also exceeds the national average. Similarly, recent statistics indicate that patients accessing care for breast cancer in the Seine-Saint-Denis department are diagnosed at a stage where their condition is more advanced than the national average at time of diagnosis, with larger tumors, and more often present with metastases (Groupement Hospitalier de Territoire Saint-Denis et deGonesse 2018). Approximately 25 percent of the population of this administrative department is classified as low income, a significantly higher level than in France or in Ile-de-France (metropolitan Paris), with 13.5 percent and 14.2 percent, respectively.

Despite the national health system and the constitutional right to health care in France, health disparities exist along axes of social class, geospatial location, immigration status, and type of insurance (Sargent and Kotobi 2017, Saint-Martin 2004). The adoption of a new management model for hospital financing also has had negative implications for vulnerable populations. According to this budgetary policy, national, uniform reimbursement rates are set to reflect services delivered, putting pressure on professionals to provide more medical "acts" in less time. The tariff system does not facilitate coverage of linguistic and social costs associated with patient care, such as use of interpreters or assistance in addressing patients' legal, financial, and family crises (Kotobi, Larchanche, and Kessar 2013, 75). In this regard, the organization of budgeting by classifying charges as medical acts works to the disadvantage of vulnerable and marginalized patients, as our cases demonstrate.

Because of national restrictions on the collection of ethnic statistics, there is limited data available on the epidemiology of breast cancer among immigrants. However, two innovative studies (Rondet, Lapostolle, et al. 2014; Rondet, Soler, et al. 2013) demonstrate that breast cancer screening is much less likely among women of immigrant origin or whose parents were immigrants and living in the Paris metropolitan area. Social isolation, lack of formal education, and no insurance were also associated with a low probability of breast cancer screening.

To supplement this limited scholarship on immigration, ethnicity, and cancer, we focused on an immigrant population, from a West African region with a history of migration to France dating to World War I (Lorgeoux and Bockel 2013). We engaged in intensive ethnographic research with a vulnerable and marginalized immigrant population confronting cancer and seeking hospital care in Seine-Saint-Denis, where they also lived. We designed the study specifically to explore the experiences of breast cancer patients living in a geospatial zone known for its history of immigrant migration, economic vulnerability, comparatively high breast cancer mortality, lack of breast cancer screening, and late onset of hospital treatment.

Hospital as Sites and Case Studies

Attending oncology consultations at two public hospitals in the northern region of Paris, Seine-Saint-Denis, enabled us to represent the lived experience of suffering for a marginalized population of breast cancer patients attempting to negotiate the hospital system (Thornber 2018, 165–167). A team of four researchers (two anthropologists, one sociology graduate student, and one retired midwife–public health educator) conducted the broader study. Two team members, an anthropologist (CS) and the recently retired midwife (MB), interviewed thirty-six breast cancer patients to elicit their experiences undergoing breast cancer treatment.[1] We adapted the McGill Illness Narrative protocol to frame questions concerning how women with breast cancer living in the metropolitan Paris region progressively define, understand, and manage cancer. In addition to these patients, we interviewed caretakers, kin, clinicians, and interpreters. The sample consisted primarily of immigrants from the Senegal River Valley countries of Mali, Senegal, and Mauritania, as well as Guinée and Côte d'Ivoire. Using semi-structured interviews and participant observation, we assessed the experience of breast cancer as constructed in the French public hospital context and influenced by close kin and friends in Paris and in West Africa. We also conducted observations of patient consultations with six oncologists in the two hospitals over a two-year period.

Of our overall sample, ten patients were intensively followed over one-year periods, by means of regular home visits, at least monthly and often weekly. Although we had intended to engage in home visits from the inception of the project, we encountered unanticipated acceptance and encouragement by women in our sample. They actively sought our participation at their oncology consultations, before and after surgical interventions, during chemotherapy, and as part of diverse everyday activities associated with their illness. These included shopping for a wig, making appointments with assorted clinicians and therapists, attending women's association meetings, visiting during a meal to raise questions about breast cancer or to express illness anxieties, but also to discuss problems with spouses or family in France and "at home in Africa," financial and housing difficulties, and so forth. The remaining twenty-six women were interviewed, in sessions lasting one to two hours; most were interviewed on two occasions, including follow-up by telephone.

We found that women who had completed or were about to complete treatment were reluctant to continue speaking about their illness. The principal reason for reluctance to continue discussion was (a) intention to place the illness in the past by terminating illness discourse and (b) intention to avoid future misfortune that might result from persisting in thinking of or talking about cancer. Despite hospital publicity for support groups, we found that the concept of "cancer survivor" was of minimal interest to this sample. All women, with one exception, emphasized the importance of a return to their pre-illness identity, the widespread conviction that "cancer is a disease which cannot be cured" notwithstanding.

THE IMPLICATIONS OF POSITIONALITY

Given her thirty-year career in the public health system, her experience as a midwife in West Africa, her history as the organizer of three public family planning clinics in Paris, and as a clinician herself, MB occupied a space in the research project that we had not foreseen. Accordingly, I underscore the relevance of positionality for this project. At each of the four hospitals where we interviewed during the four-year study, MB (although retired) was perceived by clinicians as "of the hospital" as well as a "patient companion." In both Seine-Saint-Denis hospitals, she observed consultations during a two-year period, and clinicians frequently asked her to explain procedures, trajectories, and prognoses to patients. Nurses at one hospital invited her to sit in on group

meetings, while patients asked her for reassurance and clarification of pro-
nouncements they failed to understand and were afraid to question directly in
the presence of doctors or nurses. Because of her own professional history,
patients and clinicians constructed a complex identity for MB, which we had
not envisioned but with which all concerned seemed comfortable. The intensity of MB's interactions with women in our sample produced rich ethnography, and we hope these long-term relationships also provided support for
some patients in extremely precarious and vulnerable circumstances.

Madame D, whose case I describe below, was one of several patients who
sought to engage MB as fully as possible in her treatment. She also relied on
her to listen attentively and propose solutions to her numerous dilemmas of
everyday life. For example, when she arrived in France, Madame D initially
lived on the street and experienced continuing difficulties in finding long-
term housing. Her oncologist proposed various alternatives in the Seine-
Saint-Denis area, such as living in a residence for patients in circumstances
such as hers. Madame D did not reply, and the oncologist asked the researcher's opinion. MB suggested that they talk about the possibilities after the
appointment. As Madame D's treatment evolved, her relationship with MB
intensified. She asked her for help increasingly as she became more fatigued.
Similarly, the oncologist and nurses also asked MB to intervene on behalf of
Madame D. Subsequently, MB learned that Madame D did not have enough
money to pay a nurse who would give her an injection within forty-eight
hours. MB, in consultation with the oncologist, offered to give the injection
herself (as a trained clinician) while visiting Madame D at home.

It was striking that Madame D rarely asked questions of her doctor during
her first months of treatment. As she experienced more advanced treatment,
and underwent a mastectomy, she routinely questioned MB and occasionally
asked questions of her doctors. She systematically followed up by asking MB's
interpretation. Regarding treatment efficacy, when Madame D experienced
side effects that made her doubt the wisdom of continuing, MB reminded her
the doctor had told them both that after each session (chemotherapy, radiation) her tumor diminished in size. Madame D's oncologists encouraged and
indeed depended on MB to convey instructions and provide some oversight
of Madame D's capacity to follow the treatment schedule, arrange transportation, and so forth. The case of Madame D is particularly sensitive in that she
was briefly homeless and periodically at risk of losing the temporary lodging
she found. She was in an ambiguous relationship with the man who helped
her find housing but to whom she felt obligated and even coerced. During a
conversation with CS, she described how desperate, lonely, and frightened
she had felt until she met MB—who made her laugh and made sense of the
incomprehensible.

On one occasion, Madame D expressed her frustration with the trials of
clinical communication at the hospital. She said that doctors do not explain

anything and if one asks nurses, they tell you to ask the doctor. In contrast, she lauded MB, who explained things in language that is clear. In principle, patients can ask questions and express their concerns to the nurses whose specialized task is to meet with the patient one week after the cancer diagnosis (*infirmières d'annonce*). However, in Madame D's experience, one has two appointments with the *infirmières d'annonce* but their primary responsibility seemed to be to schedule appointments for chemotherapy, surgery, radiation, and for complications that may arise. On the other hand, the nurses who manage day chemotherapy are technicians and not responsive to overtures from patients who seek information or reassurance. It can be difficult not to feel lost in the system, with no routinized nurturing or support within the hospital. It is not surprising that women in our sample highly valued MB for her willingness to offer support in many ways. A larger issue that underlies the value of MB is to identify the structural constraints, which left so many of the women we interviewed bewildered, afraid, and uninformed about their condition, its management, and the dilemmas of everyday life. In addition, we see the implications of their unexpected reliance on the random presence of a research team committed to offering support when approached for assistance.

Cancer Discourse in Immigrant Associations

In addition to breast cancer patients, their social networks, and clinicians, we met with leaders of fifty immigrant women's associations. The objective of these gatherings was to engage in focused discussions regarding cancer in general, and breast cancer in particular. We sought to determine the extent to which informants conceptualized "cancer" as a single disorder or rather as a set of related conditions (for instance, breast cancer, colon cancer, prostate cancer, and lung cancer) and the salience of the terms "metastasis" and "biomarker." We also attempted to elicit shared constructs of breast cancer etiology and the prevalence of breast cancer in women's countries of origin.

The combination of semi-structured interviews and extended participant observation allowed us to determine ease of access to oncology services and how patients entered treatment in the two Seine-Saint-Denis hospitals, Avicenne and Delafontaine. For the patients we interviewed at Avicenne Hospital, the initial point of entry into the hospital system usually began elsewhere at a maternity clinic or with a neighborhood general practitioner. A common scenario involved a woman finding a breast lump and seeking advice from a midwife or doctor with whom she was already familiar, who would refer her for a mammogram and/or biopsy. Following a positive biopsy, the patient would be referred to the oncology service at Avicenne. The medical oncology service at Avicenne offers day and inpatient chemotherapy, regular oversight of patients in treatment, and hospitalization as necessary. The medical oncologists at Avicenne treat approximately two hundred new cases of breast cancer annually; this represents thirty-five to forty patients in consultation per week per oncologist, of an estimated 1,500 cancer cases of all types per year. Patients are referred to other hospitals such as Jean-Verdier for mastectomy, breast reconstruction, lymphedema, and comorbidities. Radiation therapy is available at Avicenne.

Patients consulting at the second Seine-Saint-Denis institution, Delafontaine Hospital (Centre Hospitalier Delafontaine), benefit from an affiliation established in 2013 and reaffirmed in 2016 with the private cancer hospital, the Institut Curie. As at Avicenne, women usually begin their illness trajectory at a maternity clinic or in consultation with a general practitioner. Clinic personnel then refer patients to Delafontaine for mammography, biopsy, surgery, chemotherapy, and radiation therapy. Approximately eighty cancer patients undergo surgery at Delafontaine annually and continue with follow-up consultations at intervals determined by the severity of their condition. Oncologists at both hospitals have heavy patient schedules, with waiting periods as long as two hours per patient. Increasing budgetary constraints and the new management model add to administrative and organizational difficulties in accommodating the numbers of patients in treatment and under surveillance.

MADAME B: A THERAPEUTIC ITINERARY

The case of Madame B illustrates a possible circuit of hospital care for a diagnosis of breast cancer and the external influences on treatment decisions. She was first interviewed at Avicenne Hospital, on the day of her second chemotherapy session. She expressed considerable trepidation about chemotherapy but agreed to describe her illness experience nonetheless, while waiting. Her narrative began with finding a breast lump, which she thought was the result of anxiety. She perceived her stress to be caused by marital tensions and difficulties with her import-export initiative in West Africa. Eventually, she consulted a general practitioner near her home in Seine-Saint-Denis, who referred her to Jean-Verdier Hospital, where she was diagnosed with breast cancer and underwent a mastectomy. She subsequently began chemotherapy at Avicenne. As she recounted her illness narrative, she described her immigration and family history. She arrived in France from Bamako, Mali, in 1994, hoping to continue her education and study medicine. But she was not admitted to university and eventually became a nursing aide. She currently works at a residence for the elderly infirm. She has French nationality and hence full health insurance in the national health system. However, because of her illness and the rigors of chemotherapy, she was unable to continue working and faced increasing financial insecurity.

In the midst of our discussion concerning her recognition of a breast anomaly and consideration of what to do about it, she abruptly began to discuss her marriage, as an important link to the precipitating factor in her breast cancer episode. Upon her arrival in France, she focused especially on finding employment in the health sector. Then she met a man who seemed amiable and married him. They have one son. Her husband, she explained at length, is 100 percent religious and devoted to prayer. His sole charitable act is to give money to the imam at the local mosque. Responding to her own perception of charity, she began to collect medications for women living in precarity in Mali. In this initiative, she relied on her employer, who provided her with surplus medications for distribution to impoverished Malian women with serious health issues.

She was in the process of organizing her humanitarian initiative when her plans were interrupted by her cancer diagnosis, surgery, and chemotherapy. We followed her as she finished chemotherapy and was scheduled to commence radiation therapy. However, she decided to temporarily stop treatment to visit family in Mali. She still pondered the cause of breast cancer, asking, *what is this sickness?*—it had never been "known" in her family. We discussed terms for cancer in French, in Bambara, and in Soninke, languages of her society of origin. She noted that some (in Mali and in France) use the French word "cancer," others use a word such as "*bon*" (Bambara term for a curse), referencing sorcery or a sent illness. She added that she does believe that breast cancer may be a "sent" illness, but not in her case. Rather, she attributed her illness to stress associated with family relations and business problems (CS Interview AB, June 7, Avicenne).

In addition to her consultations at the two hospitals, Madame B also attends workshops and meets with a psychologist and a social worker at a local association, which provides support services for those with serious illnesses, such as cancer or diabetes. In this, she is typical of many patients who find that hospital social workers are unable to assist them with the array of services they need; such patients look to private or quasi-private humanitarian associations, which increasingly take on these responsibilities. At this association, she was able to obtain advice from a psychologist for ameliorating relationships with her husband and son, as well as clarification concerning which hospitals offer certain clinical services and how to make an appointment. Given her inability to continue working during her treatment, the association was able to intervene for her and demonstrate her eligibility for a daily indemnity from the state. In this regard, Madame B represents the many immigrants who rely on nonprofit associations to supplement or substitute for the direct health care services ostensibly offered in the public hospital network (Sargent and Kotobi 2017; Sargent and Benson 2019).

MADAME D: A STRUGGLING PATIENT

Madame D, age forty-three and an immigrant from Conakry, Guinée, participated in our study for two years. She met MB during her second chemotherapy session at Delafontaine and immediately expressed interest in discussing her illness and her immigration history. She arrived in France in 2015, hoping to obtain health care. She came on a short-term visa but had no health insurance or possible residence permit. Her only contact in Paris was "a man" who had known her sister when they lived in the same village in Guinée. Madame D grew up speaking Sosse, a language related to Bambara, the principal language of many of our informants. She attended secondary school but was forced to leave when her parents died. She then worked in the restaurant business until pain and swelling in one breast led her to France. Her quest for treatment began when she consulted Doctors of the World (Médecins du Monde, a humanitarian organization). They referred her to a gynecologist at Delafontaine the same day. There, she underwent a mammogram, then a biopsy, and an MRI. Subsequently, she met with a surgeon who informed her of her diagnosis, advanced breast cancer. He scheduled her immediately for an appointment with a medical oncologist for a prompt initiation of chemotherapy. She had no health insurance, but cancer is a condition included on a national list of serious, chronic illnesses that merit coverage for all.

On the occasion of the first home visit with MB, Madame D cried, describing her fears and uncertainties. She was terribly tired, and she was extremely afraid because "*c'est grave un cancer*" (cancer is serious). She described herself as a devout Muslim, who prayed regularly, hoping for divine intervention. She was plagued by existential questions: *why me, what is the cause of this sickness, will I survive?* She had heard of cancer in Conakry, but she thought it only affected elderly women. She was lonely, and her family lived in a rural area of Guinée; they expected her to send money home. She had only told her older sister about her cancer to avoid worrying other family members. Another blow: the woman who had housed her learned that she had cancer and told her she could no longer live at her home for fear of contagion. She would once again need to find lodging.

Madame D's understanding of breast cancer was similar to that of Madame B, as reported in the first case, and of most of the women we interviewed. Madame D commented on a conversation with her sister in Mali by phone. They agreed that breast cancer is a grave condition; it cannot be cured. Although reluctant to pose this question to the clinical staff at the hospital, Madame D asked MB if it is true that cancer is a disease with no cure. She frequently asked, "Where does this disease come from?" finding no reassurance in any answer. During numerous conversations during her treatment, she asked: *How does this treatment work? Does it make the tumor smaller? How do I know if the treatment is effective?* She asked, as did most of our informants, for the origin of this disease, and observed that she knew the names of many sicknesses (which she listed): malaria, hepatitis, diarrhea, AIDS, but not "this one."

NURSE SPECIALISTS: THE ANNOUNCEMENT

According to the oncology service organizational structure, a category of nurse specialists, knowledgeable about the trajectory of cancer care, meets as needed with patients to reformulate the diagnostic, treatment, and prognostic information presented to patients at their first consultation. It is this category of nurse whom Madame D dismissed as unavailable to answer questions or to address patient needs. In contrast, discussions with three nurse specialists at one of the hospital sites offered a different perspective on the idealized construct of the nurse specialist who "announces" the cancer diagnosis (Interviews June 19–20, 2018).

The oncology service at Avicenne has three such nurses who are expected to do consults for all forms of cancer. This is a demanding role, in that there are approximately 1,500 patients in treatment for some form of cancer each year at Avicenne. In theory, the same nurse should continue with a patient throughout treatment, but this is not always possible, given that each nurse has fifteen to twenty new patients each month.

In an open-ended conversation regarding their responsibilities, the nurse specialists pointed to inadequate staffing relative to a heavy patient load, which prevented them from engaging in intensive interactions with each cancer patient under treatment. Although according to their job description they present the cancer "announcement" to the patient, in reality, most patients are already aware of their diagnosis. They usually have had a mammogram and a biopsy at Jean-Verdier Hospital or elsewhere, in which case a surgeon gives them at least a minimal diagnosis. Alternatively, they may have met with their neighborhood generalist physician (if they have one), or they may already have met with an oncologist at the hospital. Thus, the orderly presentation of information as designated on a flow chart does not represent the much more chaotic transfer of detailed information to the patient. In one instance, for example, a nurse specialist met with a patient to determine what questions he had about his cancer treatment as he was waiting for his first chemotherapy session to begin.

The announcement or discussion of diagnosis, treatment, or prognosis are intended to be held after the RCP—a pluri-disciplinary committee composed of doctors, surgeons, and a secretary—have met to agree on the treatment trajectory. The committee decisions need not be unanimous, but rather depend on the staff hierarchy (for example, the chief of service has a more authoritative voice). The committee secretary is supposed to prepare a form, summarizing the diagnosis and treatment plan, and pass it on to the nurses, in preparation for their first meeting with the patient. However, given the shortage of staff and scheduling difficulties, some patients have already spoken to at least one doctor or surgeon and may have had a session of chemotherapy before meeting with a nurse specialist.

If arranged correctly, the meeting of the patient and nurse specialist should be adapted to the questions and needs of that patient, and a one- to two-hour period is reserved for this encounter. The concept of the "announcement" is that the initial communication with the doctor, typically following the biopsy, is usually brief. Doctors are aware that the nurse specialists will subsequently provide additional details. Because the cancer diagnosis is shocking to most patients, they are likely to retain only random information from the communication with the doctor, sometimes the color of the doctor's shirt or the view from the window, rather than the schedule of chemotherapy, surgery, and radiation. The nurse specialists' objective is to ascertain whether the diagnosis was understood, and whether the patient is in denial. They reiterated that one needs considerable experience in oncology to determine what constitutes "denial" and whether the doctor needs to start anew with the details of the diagnosis. During the first meeting with the patient, the nurses pose questions about issues that may require support, such as marital relations, finances, nutritional status, housing, child care, or whatever concern the patient may express.

An important consideration for these nurses is determining the most effective language and vocabulary to use in exchanges with patients. They evaluate whether the patient understands terms used by the doctor, and if not, try to correct misperceptions and teach new vocabulary. One patient, for instance, referred to his condition by saying "I have pimples" rather than I have cancer. Whether this has significance, and whether it is necessary to modify the patient's terminology, is an ongoing topic of debate.

One nurse uses whatever term the patient uses, adapting the technical to everyday language. Many find chemotherapy a frightening word, so over time, she has decided on the term "treatment" as a substitute, which is less loaded. The three nurses noted that breast cancer often has a long evolution, during which time many patients begin to read the Internet or ask literate family members to do so. In this way, they become more comfortable with certain terms, for example, "markers" or "biomarkers." Learning the cancer lexicon is an indicator of chronicity and of disease evolution.

One nurse who has worked at the hospital for thirty-four years noted that even now, many immigrant patients do not speak enough French to communicate about a complex issue such as chemotherapy or radiation therapy. The nurses deal with this by checking for family members who do speak French well, then searching for hospital staff who are bilingual (this is especially successful when seeking an Arabic-speaking staff member), and finally, calling an interpreter service for a telephone translation. Interpreter organizations such as Inter-Services Migrants will send interpreters to the hospital, but the cost is usually prohibitive and arrangements complicated (Kotobi, Larchanche and Kessar 2013).

Collaboration between the nurse specialists and social workers is presumed but not necessarily enacted. As in other domains of hospital services, budget cuts have reduced personnel. The nurse specialists, in addition to their designated task of explaining "the announcement" to cancer patients, find themselves taking on the responsibilities of social workers. The impact of staff shortages inevitably leads to diminished time available for each patient. In one case, the nurse specialists met when possible with a patient undergoing chemotherapy and eventually learned that he had lost his job because of the time commitment to treatment, and then lost his apartment because he could no longer pay his share of the rent. Normally, a social worker would have been assigned to the patient and dealt expeditiously with this "social" problem. Finding themselves faced with a patient problem that was both medical and social, the nurses created a solution by placing the patient in post-acute care and rehabilitation, until he died.

Given the insufficient personnel and limited budget to attend to dilemmas of everyday life that confront immigrant women, the nurse specialists now give patients their cell phone numbers. In this way, they can intervene with problems that would not normally be in their realm of responsibility, such as making appointments with specialists, advising patients on where to go for imaging or lab work, and referring patients for family conflicts and diverse issues ostensibly dealt with by other categories of personnel. Women with breast cancer with whom they establish rapport, later in the evolution of their illness, may introduce the "problem of sex" (Interview CS, June 20, 2018). For women who have undergone mastectomies, the nurses argued that reappropriation of a woman's body after this surgery is imperative. Women report that they do not want to touch or even look at themselves. And they complain that men are afraid to touch them, but at the same time they minimize the importance of the mastectomy. The nurses agreed that there is the potential for considerable bonding among women around "the body," if there were time, space, and leadership from the administration.

Women in our sample who underwent mastectomies echoed these sentiments. Madame D, for example, expressed her distress following surgery, and described her sense of mutilation when she first removed the bandage covering her incision. "It's horrible," she said. "You realize that nothing is there. It is not death that is the issue, we all die," she shrugged. "It is *this* sickness" (unknown to us, with no history, no language or shared experience). Many women whom we interviewed lived in fear of abandonment by their husbands or partners if they did not become pregnant. For women like Madame D, who had no living children, pregnancy loomed as her highest aspiration. Despite her excellent French, she was unable to grasp why taking the medication tamoxifen would be incompatible with pregnancy. This proved to be an enduring topic of conversation with MB, who tried repeatedly to explain why Madame D's age, forty-three, and her fragile health made pregnancy an unwise decision.

Like Madame B, Madame D involved herself in the social support association in Seine-Saint-Denis for those with cancer or other serious, chronic diseases. At last contact, Madame D had enrolled in yoga, in an attempt to comply with her oncologist's encouragement to lose weight, and attended cooking workshops and chat groups, all sponsored by the association. She had also made a new friend, a Malian woman with breast cancer, in similar circumstances. The association had succeeded in helping her obtain AME, health insurance for undocumented immigrants having resided in France for at least three months.

ONCOLOGISTS IN CONSULTATION

Cancer patients at both hospitals interact with diverse clinicians and staff—secretaries, laboratory technicians, administrative assistants, social workers, nurses, surgeons, and most regularly, with medical oncologists. MB and CS observed consultations with women in our sample, but they also sat in on other consults to assess the organization of appointments, the style of communication, and the mode of imparting complex information to a minimally educated patient population. At each hospital, oncologists hold consultations two days a week. Six oncologists, three at each hospital, invited us to observe their consultations at our convenience. In addition to accompanying women in our sample to their appointments, MB attended surgical consultations for one year, weekly, at Delafontaine, and accompanied nurses at the same hospital. She also attended consultations at Avicenne one day per week for comparative purposes. CS observed consultations at Avicenne two or three days weekly over a five-month period, alternating among appointments scheduled with three oncologists.

A typical day might follow this sequence: each morning, the secretary gives the day's files to the doctors. Appointment hours are approximately 10 A.M. to 3:30 P.M.; on this day, the oncologist sees seventeen patients in that time period. The doctor goes to the waiting room and calls the name of the patient, accompanying her to his office. Often, he knows all the women, some since 2009. He seats the patient and companion, if there is one, directly across from him. Although he has a desktop computer to his right, he does not enter data during the appointment. He has the patient file open in front of him, and the patient often has duplicate copies of lab reports or scans. He generally writes a few comments in the file and uses a Dictaphone after the appointment to record significant details. When asked about the computer, he says that he decided long ago if he had to choose between looking directly at the patient and looking at the computer screen he would look at his patient's face. In our collective observations (CS, MB), we noted that he is attentive to each patient, always asks if she has any questions, but as he is usually at least two hours behind on his schedule, he may close the file and pick up the next patient's file. There is often a "*temps blanc*," an empty space with no words, until the doctor says, "Madame, you may leave now . . ."

Despite the exigencies of the daily schedule, each oncologist has both a personal political agenda and idiosyncrasies. For example, one oncologist, at the end of an over-scheduled day of consultations, began to laugh as the last patient departed. He laughed, it seemed, from the frustration of smiling and responding with reassurance to a dozen patients who suffered too much: they were too unhappy, too alone, too poor, too sick, too hopeless (MB field notes, July 2018). It had been a day of excess and of meetings with disagreeable patients for whom he tried to generate empathy.

An oncologist at the other hospital was known for his disparaging behavior with immigrant patients, including two women from our sample. He criticized the irrationality of a West African patient who stopped chemotherapy after one session, because she thought her tumor had decreased in size. In another instance, he disagreed with an oncologist colleague about the appropriate treatment for a woman we were accompanying and argued vehemently in front of the patient, who was outraged and felt ignored and marginalized (MB field notes). Similarly, he debated the intervention of choice for a Malian woman with advanced breast cancer, speaking to a colleague and looking over the patient, directing his gaze at the other oncologist. They discussed the patient as if she were not present or not capable of comprehension. In fact, she was quite aware of her lack of agency and objectification during this encounter, as she later recounted.

Most oncologists, however, were respectful and attentive to all their patients, despite over-scheduling and inadequate resources. Indeed, the physicians who work in the public hospital system seem particularly committed to providing health care for low-income patients. They acknowledge the communication constraints they confront with immigrants, especially those with chronic, life-threatening conditions, and regret the lack of interpreters. As one oncologist said, "how could one work with a population like this [West African, North African] without wondering about their lives, their histories?"

At the same time, budgetary constraints over the past decade have increasingly decreased the capacity of hospitals to hire on-site interpreters to enhance communication with immigrants and refugees. In four years of hospital-based research, we observed only two consultations where interpreters accompanied a patient—one, a Punjabi speaker, and the other, a Bambara speaker. In other instances, difficulties in communication are dealt with using family members or hospital staff, or by contacting interpreter services by telephone. Observations during oncology consultations suggest that most West African patients understand sufficient French to convey agreement with treatment suggestions but not enough to discuss the complicated personal, existential, and social issues surrounding their illness. These patients rarely ask questions of doctors and have few opportunities to question nurses, but women in our sample relied heavily on our researchers to explain and reassure. This reflects in part the new management model of hospital financing, which emphasizes "medical acts," each of which has a fixed charge, and diminishes the coverage of "social" expenses. Such costs might include taxi or ambulance transportation from home to hospital for low-income patients too fatigued to travel by other means, or making available on-site interpreters. Hiring freezes, which reduce the number of nurse specialists or social workers, also have direct effects on patient access to assistance with comprehension of diagnosis and treatment, and with social issues such as inability to work, pay rent, or arrange child care. Thus, the structures of hospital management and budgetary organization eventually play out in the lack of access to supportive services for vulnerable patient populations.

In the course of treatment, most oncologists found themselves in the position of explaining to patients that a change of medication would be necessary, that their laboratory results were problematic, or that their condition was not responsive to treatment. Discussions of palliative care, although not pertinent in the two cases presented here, arose with other women in our study, three of whom died. In these instances, one woman stopped treatment temporarily and two expressed outrage at doctors who conveyed negative prognoses. The first patient concluded that if her doctor spoke to her of death, there would be no point continuing chemotherapy. The two others asked of doctors who raised the subject of imminent death or lack of hope for a cure, "who do they think they are? God?" In contrast, the oncologists participating in this project perceived themselves as appropriate communicators, performing responsibilities for patients at the end of life who might need to "make plans" for those left behind.

CONCLUSION

West African patients with breast cancer uniformly feared their disease. Madame B and Madame D both commented that even the word "cancer" causes fear and is conflated with "death." Hence, the widespread understanding is that cancer is a disease without a cure. The case of Madame D illustrates fear of contagion, when her proprietor evicts her because of her cancer diagnosis. In our broader sample of patients, kin, and association leaders, the consensus was that those diagnosed with cancer should not inform anyone other than immediate family because of ensuing gossip, stigma, and the possibility that sorcery was implicated in the manifestation of the disease.

For many West African immigrant patients, especially those who are undocumented, breast cancer is not only life threatening but also a challenge to household economies. If chemotherapy or radiation therapy render the patient unable to work, unemployment may make it impossible to afford rent, food, transportation, or child care. For some, the choice is to stop treatment in order to continue working, or to remain in treatment, with ensuing financial risk. Those with no health insurance are particularly imperiled. Accordingly, serious chronic illness intrinsically intersects with economic vulnerability. The growing reliance on social support associations by cancer patients reflects the need for institutional recognition of unmet needs. These range from initiatives to assure that patients are aware of rights to health care coverage and access to public hospitals, to financial assistance for those unable to work, and to social services in the midst of health crises. Public hospitals, overburdened and understaffed, are now less likely to take on such responsibilities, formerly central to their mission of serving a vulnerable and marginalized target population.

ACKNOWLEDGMENTS

This research would not have been possible without the support of Laurent Zelek, MD, head of medical oncology, Avicenne Hospital; Vincent Levy, MD, head of oncology research, Avicenne Hospital; Anne Festa, director, ACsante 93; Joseph Gligorov, MD, professor of medical oncology, Tenon Hospital; and Pierre Chauvin, MD, PhD, social epidemiologist, University of Paris 6. We also gratefully acknowledge the support of the National Science Foundation (Grant 1354336).

NOTE

1. In addition to Sargent, the research team included Stephanie Larchanche (anthropologist, director of research, Centre Minkowska); Martine Beauplet (midwife, cadre supérieur, retired); Thomas Huet (doctoral candidate EHESS); Samba Yatera, associate director, GRDR, Research Group on Rural Development; Bintou Baradji, mediator; and Oumou Traore, interpreter; as well as the interpreters of Inter Service Migrants).

CHAPTER 11

Each Child Is Unique

THE RESPONSIBLE U.S. PARENT'S TAKE ON
HOSPITAL CARE GONE WRONG

Elisa J. Sobo

HOSPITALS ARE CORE sites for mass biomedical care provision.
People from the Global North tend to see hospitals through a development
lens, as an exportable Western invention, amenable to replication elsewhere
given proper funding and training. This mainstream vantage begs questions
regarding the hegemonic intentions and unilinear progressivist ideals embedded in the global dissemination of Western- or biomedicine's material assem-
blages, aims, and practices. It offers, simultaneously, an easy explanation for
why hospitalized patients and their families might supplement care in various
ways, from self-supplying food and linens in systems where funds for those are
lacking to providing their own bandages and drugs—including adjunctive or
even alternative treatments. Regarding the latter, the development purview
also provides an opening for inferring that local ignorance or a knowledge
deficit and related belief in so-called folk medicine (culture) distorts the fidelity of hospital instantiation.

Yet, patients and families in well-resourced settings also augment hospital
care in various ways that give expression to aspects of culture running counter
to the scientific ideal. As well, biomedicine itself—including its priorities and
practices as well as its undeniable benefits—has cultural dimensions.

These two facts pull at the seams of conventional understandings of hospital medicine as a self-contained, stable, fully authoritative, flatly objective,
exportable entity. Notwithstanding, they do not dislocate it, for reasons I
shall explore with reference to U.S. cultural models regarding the parent's
role in pediatric medication management in hospital settings and, by extension, at home for chronic care. These cultural models affect parents' experiences of their children's medication regimens, their own culpability as
caregivers, and the culpability of biomedical providers in charge when their
children experience adverse events. Moreover, they do so in ways that take as

foundational and in turn shore up the aforementioned figment: the bounded, objective, authoritative biomedical ideal of and for curative efficiency—"The Hospital."

My inquiry into how this circle of cultural self-reinforcement works entails a retrospective discussion of three projects in which Southern Californian families supplemented hospital care, superficially disrupting but ultimately upholding biomedicine's hegemony. Two involved parents of patients at Children's Hospital of San Diego (CHSD), in the United States, where I was employed from 1999 (see Sobo 2009), first as a research scientist, and eventually as associate director for research, in the Center for Child Health Outcomes. "Medical errors" had just emerged as a crucial concern (Kohn, Corrigan, and Donaldson 2000). The projects highlighted here—two of many—focused on parents' experience of medication administration before and during inpatient pediatric cancer care (Sobo et al. 2002) and parents' perceptions of children's risks for medical errors in day surgery (Sobo 2005). The third study to which I will refer is a more recent community-based project undertaken with parents whose children have what biomedical doctors term "intractable" (i.e., pharmaceutically uncontrollable) epilepsy, and thus spend a lot of time hospitalized or in specialist clinics. These parents were pioneering cannabis as a cure (Sobo 2017, 2021). In all three projects, parents confronted the culturally contextualized specter of something that is not supposed to happen: biomedical failure.

Findings invite us to attend to how parental nonconformity to biomedicine's expectations or directives can serve a structurally supportive function, particularly for those in highly dependent positions. That is, they show how, even when parents do not follow doctors' orders, their refusals can signal not rejection as such but a desire to hold the system accountable for and support it in providing the kind of high-quality, science-based care that one is supposed, ideally, to receive in hospital. As I hope to demonstrate, parental nonconformity (e.g., use of alternative medicine or nonadherence to a prescribed pharmaceutical regimen) often is meant by parents to bolster biomedicine's assumed and ostensibly culture-free curative prowess or to help hospital care be at its anticipated best. Nonconformity now can also be intended to support conformity later, or overall. That is, although parents may take aspects of care into their own hands when things go wrong or to ward off errors, ultimately, most would prefer to leave things with the experts: their faith in The Hospital abides (see also Sobo 2004, 2017).

RESPONSIBLE COMPLIANCE

This assertion may sound counterintuitive in the context of the contemporary emphasis on active, informed health care consumerism, in which patients—or their parents—should eagerly self-educate in preparation for making wise health care choices (e.g., Henderson and Petersen 2001, 2–3; E. Lee,

Macvarish, and Bristow 2010). Such self-responsibility tracks back in part to the structural conditions of postindustrial life, which both privatized child-drearing in ways that make parents accountable for child health (see Reich 2014) and created vulnerability and stimulated doubt in expert systems (see Beck 1992; Giddens 1991). Distrust of massified (mass produced, mass marketed, routinized) goods and services followed for many who came to understand that corporations prioritized profits over public health and safety in ways that extended longstanding patterns of worker exploitation into the consumer marketplace.

Although the expression of consumer agency was at first perceived as a threat by health care, it was seized upon after a pivotal report from the Institutes of Medicine came out in support of "shared knowledge and the free flow of information" and "the patient as the source of control" (Institute of Medicine Committee on Quality of Health Care in America 2001, 8). The shift was justified through the rhetoric of rights as well as improved health outcomes and cost-savings data (e.g., Bottles 2012; Greene and Hibbard 2012).

In the mid-1990s, influenced by Foucauldian thought and Latourian language (Barry, Osborne, and Rose 1996, 12), critical theorists began referring to how internalized self-responsibility could be leveraged to serve corporate (including state) agendas as "responsibilization." Mothers are the main target for responsibilization in discourses on child health. Indeed, they are held "uniquely accountable" by definition (i.e., in light of gender ideology); "good" mothers are duty bound to invest in their children's well-being and protect them from potential harms (Reich 2014, 699). In tension with this, however, is the fact that responsibilization should, from the view of corporate entities promoting it, lead us toward the decisions that clinicians themselves would prefer; in this equation, the "responsible" health care consumer/"good" parent should also be "compliant."

Intersecting this angle on biomedical hegemony and increasing the tension between compliance and our celebration of active, informed, engaged health care consumerism, there is the fact that some consumers (or, in pediatrics, their parents) do not *want* to take an "'activated" role. As laypeople, they would prefer to be able to rely on biomedical experts. They may further hope that whatever ails them is commonplace and that its treatment is routine and so perfectly amenable to the efficiencies of The Hospital.

There have been some intimations of a preference for submission in the literature. For instance, Lupton mentions having been involved in a survey of three hundred individuals (Lupton, Donaldson, and Lloyd 1991, as cited) that found high levels of "unwillingness to approach the medical encounter from a position where they distrusted the doctor" (Lupton 1997, 375). Intrigued, she interviewed sixty more people regarding their experiences with health care providers. Older participants who had been with their doctors for decades were most likely to express a preference for deference, but participants of all ages still displayed respect for doctors and faith in medical science and provided examples of times when an authoritative clinician would be preferred. While knowledge asymmetry ("I'm not the expert") does explain in part people's active resistance to health care's invitation for patient engagement, because the doctor knows more, a preference for an authoritative clinician additionally relates to the emotional and physically dependent aspect of the relationship. Wynne also has commented on dependence as the root of expressions of trust in scientific authority (Wynne 1996).

Brunson has found some people prefer a docile stance even for preventive care. Although dependence here could be seen as indirect (because one's decision today might impact future service), it is of note that many parents in Brunson's research had *not* internalized the activated, engaged patient–consumer role in which planning for the future might figure in: they simply accepted "doctor's orders" (Brunson 2013). I saw the same in regard to pediatric vaccination acceptance (Sobo 2016) and, looking back, it also was present in my earlier hospital research. Exploring deviations from this form of "compliance" will shed more light on cultural aspects of biomedicine, including not just the partiality of a self-responsible consumer model of and for health care but how health care consumer behavior that appears to counter biomedicine (e.g., use of alternative medicine) can, in fact, aim to serve a structurally supportive function. As I hope to demonstrate, the agency shown in parents' small and large acts of refusal was in each study meant to help biomedicine live up to its culturally constructed promise to make their children better.

STUDY 1: MEDICATING CANCER

The first project addressed the fact that cancer patients are extremely vulnerable to medication errors because of their frequent hospital and clinic visits, complex and evolving medication protocols, toxicity of medications, and use of multiple care providers at multiple sites. My project team[1] worked closely with clinical and social work staff as well as the parent liaison (herself a parent whose child had had cancer) to find out from parents which part of the medication process worried them, how well the discharge medication education they received served them, and what they would have liked CHSD to have done or do differently. We also asked whether they used any complementary or alternative medicines (CAM) to supplement hospital care, and if so which and why; and for this as for almost all my studies at CHSD parents were encouraged to bring up issues that the questions overlooked (Quinn 2005).

Given patient numbers and our practical goals, our recruitment target was twenty parents. Most San Diegans speak English or Spanish, so we recruited from both these groups. Parents were not always approachable because of the ongoing clinical needs of their children or because they were at work or caring for others. When parents agreed to participate in the project, we invited them to sit and talk in the hospital's gardens or elsewhere, away from their child. This option would enable a parent to speak freely, without concerns about being overheard by the child or a care team member. But none was willing to leave the child's bedside.

Data analysis began with the first interview and was ongoing, using a simplified adapted version of Grounded Theory (Glaser and Strauss 1967; Strauss and Corbin 1998). My extensive day-to-day experience of the lived ethnographic context of care in this hospital was central to the analysis (Sobo 2009).

The inpatient medication process included administering chemotherapy to destroy cancer and other medications to support this. Parents did worry a bit about side effects due to the potency of chemotherapy medication. Seven, or one in three, reported some CAM use—most commonly vitamins, massage therapy, and brewed mint or chamomile tea—to combat this. The buildup in the child's body of toxic chemicals also was at the root of much of the CAM use. One parent intended to use milk thistle for protecting (cleansing) her child's liver: "The kidneys are flushed out with water but the liver cannot be cleansed that way." Another told us that she sometimes did not administer the doctor-prescribed medication because the child's little body "could not take it." In ways such as these, parent-led CAM administrations helped them tailor the hospital's pharmaceutical offerings to better suit their individual children.

Only after mentioning their worries about side effects did parents mention concerns about medication delivery problems, most related to hitches in efficient care systems. Some had personal reasons to worry: in one case a nurse had in fact given wrong instructions, telling a parent to administer a medicine when the child was symptomatic when, in fact, the drug should have been administered on a regular basis during the stay. When the doctor realized the error, he told the family not to listen to the nurse, although the nurse might have made the mistake due to poor documentation.

Parents knew, as one said, "They don't intentionally want to harm my daughter." The hospital had their allegiance, ultimately. Still, vigilance was needed. One father reported a nurse prerecording in his child's chart that the next dose of medicine had been given, without telling the next nurse that she had done so. The next dose thereby could have been missed had this responsible parent not flagged it. In another case, a child needed surgery and the surgeon was ready to do it. However, a new doctor wanted to do more tests, likely to ensure that the preoperative medication regimen had been effective, and this delayed the surgery. The primary doctor was not informed of this until the mother called and told him.

Indeed, most parent stories focused on the assistance they gave in assuring provider–provider communication went well. Hospitals offer efficiencies, sure; but their very complexity also creates opportunities for in-system information slippage. Provider–parent communications, too, could be problematic. For instance, although most parents found the formal medication review process done on discharge helpful, the nurses' approaches to these reviews seemed inconsistent. Some parents received types of help or information that others may not have. The reasons for this were unclear but potentially linked to variations in time made available to nurses to do the review as well as cultural biases regarding how much people from certain backgrounds were able to understand (Sobo 2004).

The practical ramifications of this and other information collected notwithstanding (process improvement being the project's aim), some interesting theoretical ground regarding expertise and culpability as well as parents' roles as adjunct healers and system supporters was opened in the discourse. Threads that pop up again in the next study I describe will be pulled at then, and revisited as the third project brings these and related major issues further into focus.

STUDY 2: RISKING ANESTHESIA

The second study took place in day surgery's discharge ward, where recovering patients were reunited with their parents or guardians and given time to "wake up." The public had just learned that every year, hospital errors result in more deaths than car accidents, breast cancer, or AIDS (Kohn, Corrigan, and Donaldson 2000). I was curious about how this and related reports had affected the parent experience in day surgery.

In tandem with a patient satisfaction initiative, parents' perceptions of their child's chances for experiencing a medical error during day surgery were queried using rapid open-ended interviews in the discharge room. This method (adapted from the "five-minute speech sample" approach developed by Gottschalk and Gleser 1969; and see Sobo 2009) allowed us to collect data as near to the event in question as possible. Respondents would thus be able to directly reference situational knowledge, and their discourse would reflect immediately salient issues without the bias introduced by memory decay. The focused question we used was: "Please tell me: What worried you about your child's operation?" All English- and Spanish-speaking parents whose children came through surgery and the initial recovery phase without complications were eligible to participate.

Parents received their children in a ward longer than wide, with an alcove to one side, furnished mainly with movable visitor chairs and the patients' rolling beds; this emphasized throughput. The low hum of nursing activity and murmuring parents alert to their groggy, recovering children's needs comprised the soundscape. To ensure ample time for reunion, potential interviewees were approached about one-half hour after their children had been wheeled out. When we reached data saturation, twenty English- and fifteen Spanish-speaking parents had been interviewed.[2]

The analysis relied on methods similar to those described for Study 1. By this time, however, my involvement in the hospital had been augmented with personal experience of having a young child in day surgery myself.

Most children underwent high-volume procedures that most parents saw as low risk. One parent explained, "Tonsillectomy is typically a routine procedure, so I really wasn't concerned." Another said, "My nephew and niece both had it done, and two friends, their daughters just went through with it. So [there was nothing to be worried about]."

Many parents did worry, however, about their children's emotional well-being and whether they would cooperate, partly because of the children's hunger (children generally fast prior to surgery) but also because of the unfamiliar setting. As one parent said, "Our biggest worry is that . . . he gets to calm down so he doesn't get scared. . . . He is terrified of masks and when the doctors have masks on, that stuff scares him." One noted, "If you don't explain well to them what is next, what are the steps then they don't understand and start to cry and they don't want to go in."

But also: nobody wanted to be judged an insufficient parent whose child therefore caused disturbance. Reputational worry dovetailed with the disempowerment or lack of control many parents reported feeling, for instance regarding speaking to clinicians. As one parent told us, "It is traumatic or actually you feel powerless, you feel useless." Parental feelings of inadequacy stemmed partly from their lack of fluency in the language of biomedicine and in simple status differentials between laity and experts, but they were intensified by the fact that their maternal or paternal power to fix their child's ills had been ceded to or usurped by hospital workers, who were now in loco parentis. Their children were now as if wards of the institution.

The primary hazard parents feared was posed by anesthesia, without which surgery could not take place. As one mom said, "You hear of other kids, you know suffering or having problems with it so it is always in the back of your head. . . . Some kids can die under anesthesia, they get too much, they have brain damage. Those kind of things."

Parents referred to stories heard on the news and through the grapevine to justify the fear of an anesthesia administration error, generally because of too much being given (it was never from too little). But they also referred to information they learned during the intake process itself and when signing the anesthesia consent form: "If you read the risk sheet even up to even death, so that is why it was really scary for me," one parent said. Another remarked, "When you go to sign the document that says there are so many things that can go wrong you just worry that those things will happen to your child, that is what scared me the most." For example, "On the paper it says that there could be people that won't wake up from the anesthesia, that is my main worry." In this way, standard consent forms operate as technologies that create and sustain doubt (a la Giddens 1991 and Beck 1992; see Carey and Pederson 2017).

How did parents justify taking these risks or enduring such worry? One way was to consider the benefits to be gained. "She needed this done; she couldn't breathe," said one parent. "I was more worried about the problem that she had," said another.

But the notion of risk also could be refuted, for instance when they praised CHSD and its staff, referring to the hospital's or their doctor's reputation, whether mythic or real, for providing safe, high-quality care, or to the opinion of a respected individual. For example, one father said, "I know that the doctor is a good doctor. The wife really like him." He also said, "If anything atypical happened here, this was the staff to deal with it." Another parent said, "We heard some good things about Dr. [Smith] from some other parents"; another sweepingly confirmed "they are well-recommended doctors." Parents also referred to the routine nature of the surgery, clinicians' professionalism and training, and previous examples where surgeries had good outcomes. In offering such declarations, they affirmed their existence as "good" parents— careful parents who would do all they could to minimize their children's exposure to potential harm—and good consumers—informed consumers able to make and exercise wise choices regarding care.

A related method of risk refutation entailed selectively offering evidence that CHSD was not a risk-ridden place. For instance, some referenced information that CHSD began providing, in response to an earlier day surgery study I'd done, affirming there had been no deaths at CHSD due to anesthesia. Parents also could refer to "seeing them [clinicians] checking and checking and checking" patient identification and instructions. Parents deployed such testimony to justify the decision to bring the child in.

In addition, faith sometimes entered the picture directly. "You trust in God I guess to make sure everyone is—make sure that the doctor is doing his job," one parent offered. Along the same lines, parents appealed to a cultural belief that children are inherently vulnerable beings. Most saw potential mishaps as stemming from the children's as-yet uncharted natures rather than failures on biomedicine's part: children are not typical adult patients with established health histories; their bodies are still in flux (see also Castaneda 2002), so anesthetizing them is inherently risky. "Since it is the first time that she gets any, I didn't know how she would be," said one parent.

Unknown allergies were often blamed: "Being at his age you never know if he is actually allergic to anything yet, he might not have had that drug that he is allergic to, so you always worry. . . . When he is four years old he hasn't had a life yet to know if he is allergic to anything, so and we would never know." The allergy theory was complemented by ideas relating to other idiosyncrasies. For instance, one parent feared "just [that] there is something that goes wrong that is not typical." With all its efficiencies, hospital care does not work well when problems presented are unique. A somewhat related fear was that "the surgery would be more complicated than they thought and they wouldn't be able to fix the problem."

The construction of children as naturally vulnerable, with unanticipatable frailties has been critiqued as involving the "mistaken concretization of essentializing concepts" (Frankenberg, Robinson, and Delahooke 2000, 586) when, in practice, vulnerability is situationally and relationally determined. As Frankenberg and colleagues argue, it is contagious rather than an essential property of individual (children's) bodies: When children are present, certain types of vulnerability can be produced in adults as well. For example, day care providers are vulnerable to accusations of negligence or abuse. Likewise, the parent of a child in day surgery may feel vulnerable to being judged (e.g., by day surgery staff or providers) for how well—or not—they meet parental role expectations.

Regardless, and although U.S. popular culture offers countervailing images of children's physical resilience, plasticity, and compensatory ability (Castaneda 2002), parents focused on concealed, unanticipatable weaknesses. This figuration, in which the body is its own worst enemy, deflects attention away from social and political-economic causes of ill health. Further, it deflects responsibility for what may be provider-driven error onto the child's own (immature and defenseless) body. It rationalizes marketplace massification. It also takes hospitals off the hook, helping to preserve official organizational accounts regarding what happens on the operating table or elsewhere backstage in hospital settings by not shining light on it. Parent vigilance and use of CAM in Study 1 did the same, keeping near misses from turning into bad outcomes that might become public knowledge.

In Study 2, the focus on children's potential, hidden vulnerabilities seemed to have the benefit of increasing comfort levels regarding what might otherwise be cast as system-driven procedural risk. It also could feed the sense of powerlessness reported by some parents—for example, in relation to handing the parent role as the child's protector over to the surgical team or hospital when the child is taken away, particularly if a team or hospital was chosen by an insurance plan or the state. Still, the ideals of "wise" health care consumption and "good" parenting nevertheless held sway and, at least when we spoke with them, their children's surgical outcomes seemed to confirm this.

Study 3: Cannamoms

The third project concerned parents for whom in loco parentis arrangements and mass care technologies did not suffice: in contrast to the first two populations, hospital care had not supported good outcomes for this group's children, all of whom suffered from epileptic seizures. Indeed, biomedicine had classified their children's conditions as "intractable": pharmaceuticals could not control their seizures. They faced the threat of early death and/or profound disability as a result (Wirrell 2013). So, the parents elected to explore options that might not have appeal otherwise: cannabis-based preparations which, at the time of the project, were highly illegal, even in California.

The plant's criminalization in the early twentieth century put the kibosh on its medical use and on scientific research into its potentials, but small-scale clinical studies overseas (e.g., Israel, Brazil) and amassing case, laboratory, and animal studies set the stage for the public's rediscovery of cannabis's antiepileptic potential in the 1990s (Friedman and Sirven 2017; Russo 2017). Public access to research findings expanded with the Internet, and adults with epilepsy began to experiment (Chapkis and Webb 2008; M. Lee 2012, 300–303).

A small pediatric groundswell followed, stemming mostly from research on one cannabis chemical, cannabidiol (CBD), which could be offered in a liquid tincture containing little to no THC (tetrahydrocannabinol), the cannabis chemical directly associated with getting "high." CBD, which entails no high, seems crucial to limiting seizures (Devinsky et al. 2017). The growing understanding of this reflects the efforts of parents who took cannabis treatment research and development into their own hands (e.g., Warner 2014; Vogelstein 2015; Maa and Figi 2014).

In 2016, a heavily engaged parent—a "cannamom," as many participants would say—invited me to work within this community. Use of cannabis was only legal then in California for verified and approved medical reasons. It was relatively easy by 2016 for an adult with funds to get a verification letter, but getting one for a child was exceedingly difficult due in part to ideas about child vulnerability referenced above but also to normative links between cannabis and family dysfunction as well as criminality. Although perhaps difficult to remember given today's leniency, procuring medical-grade cannabis let alone CBD was harder still. Given this cultural climate, I wondered: *how radicalized were these parents?*

My study (Sobo 2017, 2021) targeted English-speaking, Southern Californian parents using, interested in using, or who had used cannabis for a minor child's intractable epilepsy or seizures. I implemented a snowball (word of mouth) sampling protocol starting with a post on a grassroots pediatric cannabis website focused on epilepsy (pediatriccannabissupport.com, created and maintained by Allison Ray Benavides, MSW). Data became redundant by the time twenty-five parents had enrolled.[3]

The protocol included a brief demographic survey as well as a set of eight interview questions based on the existing citizen-science literature and then-current knowledge regarding pediatric CAM use. The average interview lasted sixty-six minutes. Analytic methods were similar to those previously described. My ethnographic immersion did differ, however. I attended relevant community events (e.g., the annual family education conference of the local epilepsy foundation) and visited social media and product information websites. I also conversed informally, in person and by email, with local cannabis referral doctors, care providers who supported use of the drug, growers, product makers and distributors, laboratory personnel, and dispensary workers ("budtenders") as well as the scientific communication officer and the medical affairs director at GW Pharmaceuticals, a company with vested interests in the medicinal cannabis market. I attended, by invitation, two pediatriccannabisupport.com meetings and participated in various industry events (e.g., a cannabis "'workshop" sponsored by a local entrepreneur).

Parents in the study had sought to control their children's seizures for an average of eight (median = 6) years each. Notably, only three children had epilepsy alone. Eight also had autism; five also had cerebral palsy. Many had developmental delays, and some were profoundly disabled. Spontaneous testimony revealed that at least six children had feeding tubes. A number had rare ailments, disclosure of which would compromise privacy. Although household incomes ranged, average earnings were below what is necessary to afford a median-priced home locally (Horne 2014).

Prior to cannabis, the sixteen child users had taken an average of seven pharmaceuticals. Now, they took an average of one, with eight of the sixteen on none. I cannot confirm clinical research suggesting that cannabis works best for certain forms of epilepsy (see Devinsky et al. 2017), although three of four children in the sample with Dravet syndrome were said to benefit. For Lennox-Gastaut syndrome, it was three of six.

Most parents learned about cannabis (then still highly illicit in the dominant culture) via word-of-mouth, on television (e.g., CNN), and through social media. Many did not pursue it immediately—because, as one father said, "As a parent, you're just hoping any of these FDA-approved drugs are gonna help. You don't wanna go that [non-approved] route." Like this dad, many parents were keen to show in their discovery narratives that they were not prone to "noncompliance."' Broad anti-biomedical or anti-science views were notably absent. In the words of one mother, "If any of these [pharmaceuticals] had worked for my son, I wouldn't be in any way think that it was a bad thing or that I was a bad mom or that I need to get him more organic or some crap." Like many, she hoped cannabis would be "pursued as an actual medication that someday will be in a pharmacy and prescribed as an epilepsy drug. . . . All we want is safe medication for our kids."

Many parents also avoided cannabis initially due to stigmatized associations between "pot" and pleasure (getting "high"), criminality, and laziness. Referring to an infamous "dopey stoner" comedy duo, one mother said, "We all got the Cheech and Chong image in our head." Parents also feared what one termed the "gray area of the legality" and the potential for harassment from Child Protective Services (CPS), such as the whole family having to undergo drug testing or, worse, having one's child taken.

Beyond the common refrain "nothing else was working," certain antecedents emerged as key to parents' interest in cannabis, such as prior biomedical letdowns. These included adverse events from seizure treatments ("pharmaceuticals almost killed her more than once"); seizures' iatrogenic onset; the failure of expensive, hard-to-get biomedical treatments that required relocation or otherwise stressed a family; and being given pharmaceuticals to use in non-FDA-approved ways. The latter practice, called "off-label prescribing," is not that uncommon, particularly for children (American Academy of Pediatrics Committee on Drugs 2014). Nonetheless, parents felt that doctors who prescribed off-label but justified refusal to talk about cannabis with the axiom, "It's not FDA approved," were holding them to a double standard.

Unsuccessful pharmaceutical experimentation, in which doctors "keep trying and trying and trying," often "writing prescriptions without solid clinical trials data or FDA approvals," diminished expectations parents held for cannabis, supporting only cautious optimism. "I thought it wouldn't work," said one mother; "I thought, 'How is this going to be different from the other thirty medicines?'" Pessimism was mitigated by the idea that, eventually, with perseverance (if money held out), they would identify an individualized medication regimen that worked for their child. The unique bodies theme seen in Study 2 also was present here, but in reverse: their children's bodies *had* failed them, annulling their candidacy for the routine, massification treatment regimens of The Hospital. Accordingly, some critiqued depictions of cannabis as a one-size-fits-all cure ("everybody's chemical levels are different, everybody's reactions to either pharmaceuticals, cannabis, diet, all that stuff is all different for every single person").

Participants felt that if one cannabis preparation did not work, another might. Like their flummoxed doctors, they practiced trial-and-error—only without limiting their experiments to pharmaceuticals. Also like doctors, to find a regimen, parents considered like cases. For instance, Cari consulted "parents that had the same diagnosis as my son . . . males specifically, but [also . . .] on the same medications." In this way, parents landed upon formulations (brand, ratio of CBD to THC, carrier oil type) that they thought might work.

Then, parents verified ingredients, both to safeguard their children and provide experimental control. Regarding an initial purchase, one dad said, "We got it tested for strain to make sure what he was selling us was legitimate in terms of strength and ratio [of CBD to THC]. Also, we had it tested for pesticides or any chemicals like that." Parents with means often tested repeatedly to verify a supplier; parents tested when they changed brands, too. Parents also asked other parents about reputable sources and gaged legitimacy through packaging quality, customer relations techniques, and whether quality controls are imposed at source.

After verification, parents decided how much to give and when, generally following the axiom "start low and go slow" and using a weight-based formula. Most reported asking other parents where to start and/or using dose calculation information found online. But products come in different forms and dilutions, droppers vary, and dose suggestions often seemed arbitrary compared to pharmacy's scientific precision. For instance, one mother was told, "start out with a grain of rice. What the heck is a grain of rice? We needed exact milligrams to weight." As another noted, "All of the bottles say on it 28:1 and 25:1 [CBD:THC] but that's not saying how many actual milligrams per milliliter that you're giving . . . and how much is a drop or ten drops? How many milliliters is that?" Like the other parents, she said, you "just try."

Primed by extensive prior experience managing their children's health, parents experimented with cannabis as any new medication and in keeping with versus in ways contrary to the ideals they'd learned from biomedical clinicians. That is, they did it carefully, methodically, and patiently. They procured baseline blood tests and determined baselines for seizure activity, sleep, and other variables of interest. And they tracked. This was nothing new for parents: data collection in notebooks, on a computer, or in a phone app often began with the initial diagnosis anyhow; "it's like a job" said one mom. The reason for tracking was self-evident: "If you don't, how are you gonna know if it's positive or negative?" Control was favored similarly (e.g., "We were very careful . . . about making changes, only one at a time").

Parents knew, from prior experience with pharmaceuticals, how to measure variables and they knew which variables to measure. Sounding not coincidentally like a scientist, one mother reported seeing "immediate decrease in the length, frequency, and duration of the seizures within the first month. The seizures were shorter, less severe, and less frequent." How did she know? "We timed [my daughter's] seizures [and] they were shorter. The frequency we chart and calendar them. So, we were able to see objectively that there were less of them. They were decreased by 50 percent and then 75 percent and then 80 percent."

Through discursive strategies such as avoiding street language, employing scientistic jargon, and referring not to "marijuana" but to chemical isolates (e.g., CBD), parents emphasized a self-identity as scientific thinkers and in keeping with mainstream hospital care consumers while distancing themselves rhetorically from recreational users. For instance, many referenced "titrating" to describe how they arrived at an effective quantity; one mother explained the term as "the same thing doctors are doing." In short, rather than rejecting the system because it had failed them, these parents saw it as foundational to their work.

Their dedication aside, most parents were overwhelmed ("It takes me twenty minutes to load my kid in the car on a good day"; "I'm always sleep deprived. . . . You're in survival mode"). Further, most saw pharmaceuticalization as preferable (in keeping with scientization) and inevitable: "It's just capitalism." In one mother's words, corporations "are gonna try to get in on it, are gonna synthetically modify what's a natural thing because they gotta put their brand on it because that's the only way they can get it FDA approved." She added: "if that's what it takes to be able to legally give that to my kid . . . then I'm thankful."

Most parents were pleased when Big Pharma recognized the market, and excited about the prospect of buying cannabis medicine at the pharmacy, thus reentering the patient–consumer mainstream (e.g., "being able to go to the drive-through at CVS [drugstore]"). A subset hoped that this would not mean limited, monolithic formulations (the government controls strains for studies), or medicine with "too much junk in it." However, even they did not object to having their groundwork co-opted ("anything that's going to make it more accessible and easier for parents . . . I'm all for that").

Having internalized a preference for hospital-authorized care, including its preferred drug fabrication and dosing processes, most dreamed of a pharmaceutical-grade supply. Self-governed so, they would, when this day came, make model health care consumers. They wanted The Hospital to work. Only the lag in antiepileptic science kept them waiting.

CONCLUSION

I opened my inquiry by observing how explanations for local differences between hospitals around the world generally focus on resource shortages and cultural factors that undermine the fidelity with which the idealized Western hospital can be replicated. But hospital medicine everywhere—even in the North—is subject to local modification. Moreover, the very idea that The Hospital exists as a flatly objective exportable unit or thing is itself a cultural invention. In other words, this explanation for variance stands on false premises. Yet, these premises are widely held to; and they play a generative role in shaping how those who adhere to them experience hospital care.

The idea that The Hospital, and that the biomedical care it efficiently delivers, stands apart from culture is leveraged in U.S. cultural models of and for pediatric expertise, health care consumerism, good parenting, and even pediatric vulnerability. Findings from the studies just described illustrate this in relation to parents' experiences of their children's medication regimens, their own culpability as caregivers, and the culpability of biomedical providers and their organizational employers when children experience adverse events. The findings illuminate how and why parental experiences reflect and reinforce, rather than dislocate their faith in and hopes for, The Hospital.

In each of the studies described, parents expressed their fitness as health care consumers and their status as "good" parents in their discourse regarding their children's medication-related regimens and risks. U.S. cultural expectations for "good" parents and "wise" health care consumers supported a high degree of vigilance over medication administration to ensure things did not go wrong as they were churned through the inpatient system, with its shift changes and medical note handoffs, or routed through the routine of day surgery. These expectations also supported a willingness to use complementary and even alternative medicines to augment the care offered—and to fend off near-misses in which children might come to harm due to system or individual worker failures. Their preventive action coincidentally supported the official safety narrative commonly cultivated by hospitals.

In addition, constructions of children's individual uniqueness, and childhood as an inherently vulnerable state, affected interpretations of certain forms of risk (e.g., during anesthesia administration). They also colored how parents viewed a portion of side effects (e.g., during cancer care) and routine pharmaceutical failure (e.g., in "intractability"), deflecting blame away from the system and its materia medica, reinforcing again the rosy official narrative in support of hospital efficiency.

Further, in all three studies, behavior that looked on the face of it subversive (e.g., skipping a medication dose or giving mint tea), if not revolutionary (offering cannabis to children), was shown instead as helping parents maintain their identities as activated, educated advocates for their children—as good parents willing and able to follow the doctor's orders and who endorsed The Hospital ideal. That is, parents made adjustments when needed in support of the larger care plan, shoring up biomedical authority through, for instance, ancillary quality assurance efforts, nonbiomedical practices adjunct to hospital medicine, redirective blaming, and scientized efforts to support expanding the pharmaceutical formulary. They did all this despite deep desires that biomedicine would work as advertised—without such assists.

Affirming that one's biomedical care providers are highly reputable experts or come well-recommended offered another way to shore up a preference for hospital medicine, making the "choice" for care an index of one's status as a savvy health care consumer and responsible parent. Although some parents did self-authorize more than others, for instance deciding to skip a pill or, more than that, by bringing in cannabis, biomedicine still held as their standard.

Crucially, and again even among the "cannamoms," a full and overt rejection of what The Hospital offered was not an option. Radicalization was foreclosed by the fact that most families were already highly vested in and dependent on The Hospital, whether for cancer care, surgery, or in the last case for comorbidities, partial seizure control, and certain social services. An anti-biomedical position would too greatly damage a parent's (and child's) rights to these services. Further, casting errors as commonplace would implicate parents as having failed at their jobs as savvy health care consumers and as responsible parents because a good parent would never have placed their child in such danger (Wynne 1996 also discusses such accountability gaming). Finally, in contrast to ailments like HIV/AIDS, none of the conditions that children whose parents participated had are implicated overtly in identity politics: none indexed directly a disenfranchised status that might predispose someone toward radicalization.

Instead of turning on the system or desiring to redraw it, then, parents—even those whose children biomedicine failed—felt an imperative to support The Hospital and to help optimize its potential. As a touchstone, The Hospital was both incorporated into and leveraged in relation to models for good parenting and wise health care consumption. An expressed commitment to The Hospital was central to how parents actualized themselves and safeguarded their children, any critique parents might have offered notwithstanding, The Hospital was the entity from which even the most nonconforming parents wanted their children to receive care. Culture affects not only the ways people augment hospital care but also their allegiance to it.

NOTES

1. My team included research assistants Lilian Lim, J. Wilken Murdock, Elvia Romero, and the medical safety officer Glenn Billman, MD.
2. Leticia Gelhard collected the data.
3. Research associates were MarkJason Cabudol, Tiyana Dorsey, and Gabriella Kueber.

CHAPTER 12

Making Ethnographic Sense of Cesarean Rates in Greek Public Hospitals

Eugenia Georges

AT OVER 60 PERCENT, the cesarean rate in Greece is one of the highest in the world. Survey data from public hospitals indicate, however, that the rate for immigrants is half that for ethnic Greek women. In this chapter, I explore this seemingly paradoxical difference through the lens of my long-term research in and of public sector hospitals in Athens, Greece. I argue that these marked disparities in cesarean rates represent a local manifestation of the widespread phenomenon of stratified reproduction, which refers to how reproduction and reproductive practices are hierarchically and mostly invidiously "structured across social and cultural boundaries, particularly at local/global intersections" (Ginsburg and Rapp 1995; Colen 1986). The Greek example suggests that in certain contexts, however, stratified reproduction can also confer a degree of protection to vulnerable Others. Thus, the majority of ethnic Greek women experience cesarean births at levels criticized both within Greece and by global health organizations (e.g., UN Convention on the Elimination of Discrimination Against Women [CEDAW] 2013 as excessively and unnecessarily high, while poor and immigrant women give birth vaginally at rates closer to those recommended by the World Health Organization (WHO 2015).

The chapter is based on ethnographic research conducted in a public maternity hospital in Athens between 2012 and 2014, and in 2018–2019. Fieldwork comprised daily observations across several sites in the hospital, in-depth interviews with thirty ethnic Greek women who had given birth in the previous two or three days, and formal interviews as well many informal conversations with seven obstetricians and eleven midwives. Descriptions of maternity care for immigrant and refugee women are based on my observations, interviews, and informal conversations with the midwives who provided their care and conducted their births. I also observed prenatal visits at the weekly clinic midwives had recently established in the hospital to provide culturally appropriate prenatal care to immigrants and refugees.

APPROACHES TO ETHNOGRAPHIC RESEARCH IN/OF HOSPITALS

Over the last two decades, studies in and of hospitals have cumulatively advanced and refined medical anthropological understanding of hospital ethnography both in terms of theory and method. Conceptions of hospitals as bounded sites of homogeneous or monolithic biomedical authority have been challenged and refined as ethnographers have described the various ways in which hospitals are permeable to, and reflective of, social, cultural and political-economic forces at once local, national, and global (Van der Geest and Finkler 2004; Long, Hunter, and Van der Geest 2008). Research focusing specifically on childbirth (Davis-Floyd and Cheyney 2019; de Vries et al. 2001; Jordan 1993), moreover, has demonstrated how medical specialties also reflect and reinforce these forces, with obstetrics and maternity care showing the greatest range of cross-national variability—not surprisingly, given their intimate association with a society's understandings of gender, sexuality, family, and kinship (de Vries et al. 2001).

More recently, medical anthropologists have also called attention to the ways in which hospitals may comprise multiple, stratified, and internally differentiated spaces across which medical knowledge, authority, and modalities of expertise and technologies of care may be unevenly distributed. Street and Coleman (2012 6), for example, argue that conceptualizing hospitals as heterotopic spaces—that is, as comprised of diverse and contingent sites that coexist in dynamic relationship to each another—helps attune the ethnographer to how hospitals can at the same time be "sites of control and spaces where alternative and transgressive social orders emerge and are contested" (5). This coexistence of layered and uneven hospital spaces can also generate "gaps" in the medical gaze (Gibson 2004). That is, the technologies of medical surveillance that produce and sustain medical knowledge, power, and authority in the hospital may operate inconsistently across contexts in which access to care is hierarchically stratified. As Gibson shows for South African hospitals, the result is that "there are people in different wards in different hospitals who supposedly fall under the scope of the gaze, but who remain invisible" (2004, 2014). Often, in this example as in other resource-poor contexts (Sullivan 2012; Street 2014; Brown 2012; Mulemi 2008), gaps in medical surveillance lead to neglect that puts the most vulnerable patients at risk. The Greek context I describe in this chapter offers an example of how the invisibility that ensues from such gaps may, in certain intensively medicalized contexts, offer a degree of protection to vulnerable Others. As I hope to show, a focus on the forces that differentially allocate space, professional authority, and modalities of birth care within the hospital ultimately enhances our understanding of the generative and unpredictable "frictions" (Tsing 2005) that can occur when universals such as biomedicine, global and national health policies, and the like, encounter the uneven political, social, and cultural terrain of particular local contexts.

THE LANDSCAPE OF MATERNITY CARE IN GREECE

The fundamental features of maternity care in Greece diverge in a number of ways from those found in much of the rest of Europe. Many of these distinctive features can be traced to the influence of American foreign policy on Greek society in the postwar period. In the aftermath of World War II and the long civil war that followed, Greece began the process of rebuilding its devastated institutions. Greek national recovery took off in the context of the Cold War, a time when the United States was determined to contain the influence of the Soviet Union, and to prevent the "dominos" of southeastern Europe from falling under communist influence. Under the emergent policy of American soft power inaugurated by the Truman Doctrine, Greece was identified as a frontline of Soviet containment. Massive amounts of nonmilitary aid poured in to help rebuild the nation, and at least partly as a result, by the early 1960s, the Greek economy had one of the highest growth rates in the world (Kalyvas 2015, 105).

In the "American Era" that ensued, the United States exerted a strong cultural influence on the institutions being rebuilt as Greece recovered from war (Carpenter 2003). Medicine was no exception. Before the war, Greeks had looked mainly to Germany and France for models of the most advanced and modern medical practice and training. After the war, the authority and prestige of European models were eclipsed by U.S.-style biomedicine. Under the Truman Doctrine, doctors, nurses, and other health care professionals were given stipends to study in the United States with the proviso that they return to practice in Greece. By the 1960s and 1970s, many young doctors, such as the former director of the Maternity Department in which I conducted my fieldwork, preferred to do their specialized training in the United States rather than Europe. The imprint of U.S. influence on the development of Greek obstetrics was decisive and remains so. In contrast to much of the rest of Europe, childbirth in Greece reflects the technocratic model of American birth as classically described by Davis-Floyd (1992). As in the United States, "normal births" are not distinguished from those that are "high risk." All births are generally understood to be pathological or potentially pathological events that should properly take place under the surveillance of physicians and be equally subjected to an intensive array of technological interventions.

Health care in Greece today comprises a mix of the public sector and a growing private sector. In 1983, Greece's social democratic government resisted prevailing neoliberal trends to establish a National Health Service (ESY) to provide universal and free access to health care to Greek citizens. In 2016, refugees and asylees also formally gained the right to free care in the ESY system. Greece as a whole enjoys low rates of maternal (3.3) and infant mortality (3.6) and birth outcomes are considered to be roughly the same across public and private sectors. However, because ESY hospitals are chronically underfunded, facilities can be basic and hospital visits may involve long waiting times and other inconveniences. For these and other reasons, women who can afford to do so may opt to give birth in the comparatively more luxurious private clinics and hospitals where about half of all births now take place. Still, some ESY hospitals, including the one I studied, enjoy strong reputations for good doctors and modern technology that attract a broad range of women, many of whom could afford private care.

Across Greece, all but a handful of births take place in hospitals and clinics, and women's range of choice in childbirth is essentially limited to deciding on whether to go to a public or private facility. Immigrants, refugees, Roma, and poor ethnic Greek women overwhelmingly give birth in the public hospitals. Built into the design of Athens's public hospitals is a hierarchical arrangement of space, in which rooms are divided into three tiers, called "Alpha," "Beta," and "Gamma." Ethnic Greek women typically pay an extra fee out of pocket to stay in an Alpha private suite or a Beta semiprivate room. Immigrant and other poor women are concentrated in the more basic Gamma rooms that may contain up to eight beds, though due to Greece's very low fertility rate, only about half are occupied on any given day (Kaitelidou et al. 2013, 28). Reflecting older medical beliefs in the therapeutic effects of light, air, and sun, Gamma rooms are relatively spacious, with high ceilings and tall windows, architectural design features that along with the lack of crowding help make them relatively pleasant spaces.

Across public and private sectors, childbirth in Greece is dominated by obstetricians and their technologically intensive regimes of maternity care. In the decades following World War II, professional midwives attended births in rural areas throughout the country, often in fulfillment of the compulsory rural service that was part of their training and certification. By the 1970s, several trends combined to effectively end their brief stint of independent practice. Postwar migration to the nation's largest cities, particularly of young people, helped depopulate the countryside, diminishing the need and opportunities for rural service. At the same time, the supply of obstetricians began to expand rapidly as Greece experienced unprecedented economic growth and social mobility. During this period, many new universities, including new faculties of medicine, were founded throughout the nation. Doctors have long enjoyed high status and prestige in Greek society, and the new medical faculties attracted (and continue to attract) large numbers of students. Since 1990, for example, the number of medical school graduates has more than doubled. Obstetrics and gynecology was a particularly attractive specialty, in part due to the extra income that could be made from performing (technically illegal) abortions for which there was strong demand (Hionidou 2020). In response to such incentives, the number of ob-gyns grew by one-third, the greatest rate of increase of any specialization (Mossialos et al. 2005). As the birth rate plummeted to historic lows during this same period, the supply of obstetricians inevitably outstripped demand. By 2000, Greece's ratio of obstetricians to inhabitants was roughly double that found in the other countries of the European Union, and Athens alone had four times the number of obstetricians per capita as London (Kaitelidou et al. 2012). Inevitably, given the significant oversupply, competition between midwives and obstetricians and among obstetricians themselves, intensified. Given the substantial political influence exerted by the organized medical profession in Greece (Nikolentzos and Mays 2008, the intense competition for pregnant clients has resulted in the almost complete elimination of midwives as independent practitioners.

Midwives do play a role in maternity care, but almost always as auxiliaries to a particular doctor—a dependent status clearly indexed by the fact that pregnant women and their families may refer to them as "the doctor's midwife." Midwives who work in hospitals are essentially restricted to teaching childbirth classes, providing doula-like support during labor and delivery (doulas are rare in Greece), and promoting breastfeeding among new mothers. Their exclusion from the birth process itself belies the fact that Greek midwives are all highly educated professionals who undergo a rigorous four-year program of university coursework and clinical training. Upon completion, they become certified as direct-entry midwives with the right to practice autonomously. Almost all, however, find work in hospitals or as part of an obstetrician's private practice. For example, in Athens, a city of over three million people, only three or four midwives practice autonomously, mainly serving a select clientele of well-educated ethnic Greek women who espouse an alternative lifestyle, Greeks returned from the diaspora and a few celebrities who seek out a low-tech, holistic birth experience. Not surprisingly, many midwives felt that the kind of work they typically performed did not make use of the extensive training and professional skills they acquired in midwifery school.

The erosion and de-skilling of practical midwifery practice may be at least in part accounted for by the historical absence of organized oppositional or alternative movements that seriously challenge the hegemony of obstetricians and the rigid and technologically intensive protocols of hospital-based birth. Elsewhere, pressure from feminist activists has helped protect, promote, or revive midwifery and push back on rising cesarean rates (Georges and Dallenbach 2019). The Greek feminist movement, which peaked in the late 1980s, was instrumental in effecting profound cultural, social, and legal changes (Papagaroufali 1990). However, much of the movement's energies coalesced around the urgent task of revoking Greece's repressively patriarchal family law (the now defunct "Family Code") that had effectively defined adult women as minors and enshrined their subordination to men in the judicial process. Issues in women's reproductive health, while also of concern, were not at the top of the feminist agenda.

Due at least in part to the historical absence of organized opposition, the provision of maternity care throughout Greece is remarkably uniform. Whether Greek women give birth in a posh private clinic or a no-frills public hospital, they experience very similar protocols and procedures, including almost identically high rates of cesareans. When I began my research over twenty years ago, pregnancy and birth were already thoroughly medicalized (Georges 2008). Since then, the use of technological interventions has steadily intensified, even as media reports of evidence-based critiques of conventional obstetrical practices have proliferated. Greece's cesarean rate, for example, which stood at 25 percent in 1990, reached 60–65 percent by 2017, prompting the UN Convention on the Elimination of Discrimination Against Women to declare it "the highest in the world" (CEDAW 2013).

There is widespread acknowledgment from women and their families, the media, midwives, and doctors themselves that the cesarean rate is excessively high. Explanations vary markedly across audiences, however. Popular opinion in general points to physician's economic self-interest (cesareans are more expensive) and the convenience and expediency of the operation (cesareans take minutes instead of all day and can be arranged to fit the doctor's schedule; Mossialos et al. 2005). The argument for convenience has gained traction through stories in the media that periodically report on findings that cesareans are more likely to be performed on Saturdays in the ESY hospitals, as doctors clear their schedules in preparation for their Sundays off. Doctors, on the other hand, typically attributed high rates to demand on the part of women, prompted in particular by their intense fear of childbirth. As one doctor put it, "Greek women suffer from tokophobia," using a technical term derived from the Greek for "fear of birth" that began to circulate in the global medical literature in the 1990s, "and so they ask for or even demand, the operation" in order to avoid the pain and trauma of vaginal birth.

Unfortunately, both quantitative and qualitative research on cesareans in Greece remains scant. Systematic national statistics are not available as until recently reporting of hospital outcomes to the Ministry of Health was done on an essentially voluntary basis and access to such information remains uneven. As a result, researchers must rely on the occasional survey, making it difficult to track changes in the national rate and distribution of cesarean sections (and other health outcomes) over time. However, the surveys available confirm my observations that rates have risen steadily over the last few decades. More intriguing, however, are the studies that suggest that regardless of whether they give birth in a public or private hospital, cesarean rates for ethnic Greek women are roughly identical (Mossialos et al. 2005). I discuss this finding, unusual in cross-cultural perspective, in greater detail in the next section.

In both ESY and private hospitals, vaginal births are routinely subjected to a similarly intensive array of technomedical procedures. Although women refer them as "natural births," (*fisiologikos toketos*) they are in fact more accurately described as "operational deliveries." Episiotomies, surgical incisions into the perineum, are nearly universal, and the women I interviewed were well aware that they would "cut either above or below" (as in Brazil, Diniz and Chacham 2004). Women give birth almost exclusively lying flat on their backs in the lithotomy position (another legacy of postwar U.S. influence). The use of electronic fetal monitors and IV Pitocin drips is routine and universal, effectively immobilizing women during labor. Most have their contractions induced and augmented by stripping the membranes (amniotomy) and administering labor-enhancing drugs and/or prostaglandins by the thirty-ninth week before their calculated due date. Few reach forty or forty-one weeks. Until recently, epidural analgesia was generally unavailable, and few anesthesiologists had acquired the training to administer them. Today, private clinics offer epidurals, but at the time of my fieldwork, they were only sporadically available in public hospitals due to cost and a chronic shortage of anesthesiologists. Most doctors enter one of just seven specializations; historically anesthesia has not been a popular choice (Kaitelidou et al. 2012, 726).

Although nearly all of these interventions intensify the pain of labor and birth, sometimes considerably, women who gave birth in the public hospitals could only rely on getting substantial pain relief by undergoing a cesarean section, which is typically performed under general anesthesia.

One ostensible difference between the public and private sectors is the ability to choose one's physician. By law, most ESY doctors are prohibited from seeing private patients. Pregnant women, however, regard choosing their obstetrician as the most critically important decision they can make to ensure a good outcome. To finesse the restrictions on ESY doctors, patients and their families resort to the widespread practice of informal payments. As I discuss in the next section, the shadow economy of health care in which ethnic Greek women and their doctors are enmeshed effectively blurs the boundaries between private and public care. Ultimately, the blurring of the lines between the two sectors has resulted in the effective semiprivatization of public health care and, with the exception of availability of epidurals, near uniformity in regimes of care.

CESAREANS AND THE SHADOW ECONOMY OF HEALTH CARE: BLURRING THE BOUNDARIES OF PUBLIC AND PRIVATE

In Greece, the provision of health services in the public sector is subtly and sometimes profoundly affected by the existence of a pervasive shadow economy of care. Across the public health sector, patients often resort to making informal payments of various kinds to bypass the formal structures intended to prevent ESY doctors from seeing patients privately. By giving cash and gifts to their health care providers, women and their families strive to realize the kind of care they value and actively desire: continuous attention from the doctor of their choice, shorter waiting times for appointments, and personalized support from the midwife during and after the birth.

In practice, the term "informal payments" encompasses a range of practices, each embedded in distinctive logics, meanings, and contexts. At one end is the *fakelaki*, or "little envelope," an extra fee that doctors may demand in advance to expedite a procedure, usually a surgery (Colombotos and Fakiolas 1993, 140). At the other are culturally appropriate gifts embedded in a moral economy of reciprocity, such as flower arrangements, boxes of pastries, chocolates, and the like, made to doctors and staff to express gratitude and appreciation for the care they received. By far the most significant informal payment in maternity care, however, is the lump sum of cash that most women and their families give their doctors around the time of the birth. Although such informal and extralegal practices are notoriously difficult to document, in a recent survey of Greek maternity hospitals three-quarters of patients admitted to making such cash payments (Kaitelidou et al. 2013).

Typically, when women learn they are pregnant, they consult their family, friends, and the Internet for the name of a good doctor and may shop around across private and public sectors until finding one they feel they can trust and "bond with." Francesca, who had just given birth to her first child, explained that she had found her doctor after careful deliberation, ultimately picking him because of his responsiveness and his willingness to "help her" in terms similar to those expressed by many other women:

> My doctor helped me a lot. I could ask him about anything. He gave me support. That's why women say, "You've got to be bonded, *dhemeni*, with your doctor." Me, I go to my doctor with my eyes closed (*me ta matia klista*), with complete confidence. He's very good—he helped me a lot.

Francesca's confidence in her doctor did not, however, reflect blind and unreflective trust in doctors in general. Women and their partners often criticized the medical profession as a whole, and many readily pointed to the greed and self-interest of other obstetricians as reasons for the high cesarean rate. Like many women, Francesca, who gave birth by cesarean, believed that some doctors performed the operation largely for their own convenience: "That's why you see that most of the babies in the public hospital are "Saturday-born" (*savatogenimena*)," she explained, echoing the popular view that ESY doctors resort to cesareans to protect their Sundays off. But also like most women, she did not impute these sentiments to her *own* doctor, with whom she and her husband had cultivated a relationship of trust.

For their part, doctors strive to foster trust and closeness as a way to gain and retain patients in a highly competitive environment, even if they might also complain about the inconvenience and overwork that results from the extra time and effort such closeness entails. One highly respected ESY obstetrician who had practiced in both the United States and Greece compared his experiences in the two countries:

> My patients want an exclusive relationship with me [and thus, as he went on to explain, would not accept a group practice as his U.S. patients did]. They are very tied to me, very dependent, even compulsive [*psichanangastikes*]: they can call me thirty times, at my office or on my cell phone, at any hour, midnight even. . . . That's the kind of relationship a Greek woman has with her doctor. It's very tiring, unbelievably tiring. I'm tied down, whereas in the U.S. I had more free time. But if a doctor doesn't do these things for them, they don't stay, they will go elsewhere.

Left unspoken in this doctor's narrative is why—however overworked and tired he may be—he is willing to go to these lengths: the implicit cultural expectation of receiving an informal payment from his patient. Although it is difficult to estimate how much money doctors derive from informal payments whenever the practice occurs (Cohen 2012), the effect on the total income of ESY doctors appears to be substantial. Recent studies, for example, calculate that cash gifts amounted to approximately two and a half times their annual salaries. Women interviewed in a public hospital reported giving their obstetrician an average of 921 euros for a cesarean (US$1270) and 755 euros (US$1040) for a vaginal birth (Kaitelidou et al. 2013, 26).

The widespread practice of making informal payments to ESY doctors has often been denounced as another example of the corruption and clientelism endemic to Greek bureaucracies. From the patients' perspective, however, it has also been interpreted as a culturally appropriate tactic of resistance to the "externally imposed depersonalization to relations" represented by huge public bureaucracies like the ESY (Tsoukalas 1991, 14). By cultivating relationships of reciprocity with their doctors through informal payments, women and their families are able to personalize ostensibly rigid public bureaucratic structures to achieve the kind of care they want. Nonetheless, even if sometimes celebrated as an index of citizen agency and resistance to an unresponsive state, such payments are not without their negative consequences. As critics point out, informal payments in health care represent an individual response to a social problem and their effects tend to be regressive (Cohen 2012; Salmi 2003; Souliotis et al. 2016; Economou et al. 2017). After the economic crisis hit Greece in 2009, for example, the size of informal payments actually increased as ESY doctors strove to compensate for austerity measures that cut salaries across the nation's public sector (Souliotis et al. 2016). An additional, though less obvious, issue is the potential impact that the close and trusting patient–doctor relationships cultivated through informal payments may have on the cesarean rate when there are unspoken incentives for doctors to perform the operation.

ETHNIC GREEK WOMEN'S PERCEPTIONS OF CESAREANS

In this section, I focus on ethnic Greek women's narratives as a lens through which to explore the dynamic complexity of their attitudes and perceptions toward modes of giving birth. Although the majority of the women I spoke with expressed a preference for vaginal birth, most (60%) ended up with a cesarean anyway once they entered the hospital. Important to understanding women's perceptions of cesareans is a socio-historical context receptive to the notion that technologies of all sorts are essential to the management of the array of manufactured risks associated with modern life. Reproductive technologies such as genetic testing, prenatal diagnosis, fetal ultrasound imaging, cord blood banking, and in Greece, cesareans as well, are understood as means by which doctors can assist women to reduce such risks and take responsibility for the medical futures of their children (Rose 2007, 9). As I have described in detail elsewhere (Georges 2008), for Greek women, acquiring knowledge about risks and using technologies to reduce them also serve as vehicles for enacting and crafting desirable identities as modern pregnant subjects. Alongside the political-economic context of health care described above, this historic dynamic has also helped promote the adoption and intensification of medicalized maternity care in Greece (Chatjouli 2015).

Women held a range of perceptions about cesareans, but two themes were particularly salient across their narratives, whether they had given birth vaginally or not. First and foremost was the widely held perception that cesareans reduced risk of harm to the infant, and thus were a safer and more prudent way to ensure the health of what, after all, might be the only child a couple will have (or at most, one of two). Cesareans were also regarded by doctors and women alike as the safest option for older women. Since the average age of the women I spoke with was thirty-five (tracking the national trend toward delaying marriage and starting families), many told me that the operation had been justified because of their age. This perceived safety in turn allowed women to regard it as a viable option when considering issues relevant to their self-care: avoiding the pain of childbirth and safeguarding their own health and bodily integrity.

Although when asked, women most often expressed a preference for vaginal birth, their narratives typically revealed a mix of positive, negative, and ambivalent perceptions of both vaginal and cesarean options. The most commonly mentioned undesirable aspects of the cesarean that women wished to avoid included postoperative pain, longer recoveries, and a fear of anesthesia—notably, all fears for themselves and their own well-being. These concerns, however, were often outweighed by the aura of reduced risk for the baby that perceptually accrued to the cesarean. Doctors, along with women and their families, often used the word *taleporia*, which means hardship or suffering, to describe the process of labor for women and their babies. It was commonly felt that the risk of injury or other harm to the fetus's health only increased as labor dragged on and the infant was squeezed and stressed (*zorizete to moro*). Thus, Magdaleni, thirty-four, told me that she initially wanted a vaginal birth but that when her doctor recommended a cesarean because the fetus was too big for her small pelvis, "I accepted gladly." She had been present at her sister's vaginal birth "from beginning to end," and, as she explained, witnessing her sister's fear and insecurity had left her "with a very bad feeling. It was a diffi-cult birth and I saw the fear in her face. She didn't express it, of course, but I saw that she didn't feel fully safe. I didn't want that." The perception that cesareans were generally safer was also surprisingly common among those closest to the birthing woman. Many women referred to the stories of difficult vaginal births they heard from their mothers, sisters, and others close to them as reinforcing a positive inclination toward the operation. Husbands were occasionally present during interviews and sometimes offered their perspec-tive as well. Niko, whose wife Georgia, had given birth by cesarean the day before, had this to say about the operation:

> I believe that women who prefer vaginal birth haven't realized that the cesarean is an advancement of medicine that we have now [*mia ekseliksi tis ghiatrikis pou ekhoume tora*]. They believe that it's better to give birth vagi-nally; they don't accept the medical developments that are now part of our lives.

Georgia, who expressed satisfaction that her cesarean had been necessary to ensure a good outcome, agreed with her husband's views, but, significantly, went on to cite additional advantages of the operation:

> There are some women who don't want to give birth vaginally because of the pain. . . . I believe that the way of birth is a woman's choice. If she believes that she can't stand the pain, and she doesn't want it, she says to the doctor, "I don't want to." It's her choice, because she's the one who will give birth.

As this exchange between Georgia and Niko hints, women and their families have come to attribute positive dimensions to cesareans on multiple, often overlapping fronts. Reflecting at least in part the intersection of a modern liberal discourse of "choice" with the longstanding ethics of maternal moral responsibility for their children's health, the cesarean can be interpreted as another modern reproductive technology that prudent women must consider to ensure an optimal outcome (Paxson 2004; Rose 2007). Thus, when their doctor recommends a cesarean, women like Magdaleni are disposed to agree, and even, on occasion, to "agree gladly."

Georgia's excerpt also reflects a concern with self-care that was the second major theme that emerged from my interviews. Although vaginal birth in Greece is popularly referred to as "natural birth," given the intensity of medical interventions involved, it is in fact more properly described as an "operative delivery." Thus, when women considered the options of cesareans versus "natural" birth, they were essentially comparing two sets of technomedical procedures and interventions—in effect, two modes of operative delivery. When compared to the invasive and often painful procedures that inevitably accompanied a vaginal birth, a cesarean was seen as protective of valued aspects of a woman's bodily health and function. In this calculus, stories of other women's adverse experiences with episiotomies appear to have been particularly influential in shaping perceptions about mode of birth. Women told me of family and friends who had not being able to sit, go to the bathroom, or have sex for weeks or months after the procedure without discomfort or pain. One woman had not been able to forget the doctor sewing up the wound (typically done without anesthesia) even years later. Thus, many women recognized the protection a cesarean offered from the risk of iatrogenic damage (both corporeal and psychological) that could result from the episiotomy. Ultimately, the women I interviewed knew that they would be surgically cut, either "above" or "below." They were also well aware that they would experience pain, as they put it, either "during" or "after" the birth. They considered the tradeoffs to each medicalized way of giving birth, which they pragmatically evaluated in light of their own experiences and the embodied experiences of others in their networks of female kin and friends. With the cesarean, the pain was expected to be temporary, lasting a few days or so after the operation. The side effects of the episiotomy, in contrast, might be longer term and negatively affect their marriages, as well as the healthy routine functioning of their bodies. In sum, the cesarean had acquired a *relative* value within the intensely technocratic regime of Greek maternity care. Thus, to the medical reasons their doctors gave them when recommending the operation to ensure the safety of the baby, women added their own considerations centered on the care and protection of their own embodied well-being.

EMERGENT POSSIBILITIES: IMMIGRANTS AND MIDWIVES IN THE GREEK PUBLIC HOSPITALS

Over the past three decades, transnational migration has transformed Greece from a relatively homogeneous society into one that is ethnically diverse and multicultural. After the collapse of the Soviet Union in 1991, a first wave of immigration was launched as unprecedented numbers of people crossed Greek borders from neighboring post-socialist countries of the Balkans and Eastern Europe, and increasingly from Africa and Asia as well. By 2011, over 1.2 million immigrants were living in Greece. Today, immigrants comprise over 10 percent of the total population of eleven million—one of the highest proportions in the European Union. In a second, more recent wave, large numbers of refugees and asylum-seekers have arrived on Greece's shores fleeing war and dislocation in Syria, Afghanistan, and elsewhere. Given their large numbers, relative youth, and higher birth rates, immigrants and refugees have played an important role keeping Greece's very low birth rate from falling lower still (Cheliotis 2016). In the aftermath of the economic crisis of 2009 and the austerity measures that ensued, the decline in the birth rate intensified once again as many Greeks began to emigrate in numbers not seen since the 1960s and couples put aside their plans to start a family or have another child. That the national population has not experienced a net decrease is due largely to the presence of substantial numbers of immigrants and refugees.

In the margins of the public hospitals, the social and demographic changes that have recently transformed Greece have also had an impact on the provision of maternity care. Most influentially, as described in this section, they have generated new spaces and opportunities for midwifery practice within the hospital. Immigrants, refugees, Roma, and poor ethnic Greek women who can seldom afford the cost of private clinics, overwhelmingly tend to give birth in the public hospital. The Gamma rooms in which they are concentrated have now become largely the province of midwives and the midwifery students they supervise and train. With the exception of the occasional medical resident, patients in these rooms are rarely visited by obstetricians. As one midwife bluntly explained, "the immigrants are poor, so they are left to the midwives." In other words, because immigrants do not have the economic means—and perhaps also the insiders' intimate cultural knowledge (Herzfeld 1997)—to participate in the shadow economy of care, they provide no incentive and hold no attraction for the obstetricians, who focus almost exclusively on their ethnic Greek clientele whom they treat as their quasi-private patients. As a result, midwives have been left to fill in as the primary birth attendants for immigrants and other subaltern women. Given that midwifery care generally tends to be associated with higher rates of vaginal birth (Mander 2004, 79), one striking consequence of this division of labor is that these women undergo far fewer cesareans than ethnic Greek women: about 25 percent versus 65 percent, respectively (Mossialos et al. 2005).

While the shadow economy is critical to understanding the stratified division of professional labor, space, and care in the hospital, the popular perception that immigrants have different, and by implication, inferior, needs compared to Greek citizens may also play a role (Lawrence 2007). In the popular imagination, immigrants may be stigmatized as backward and culturally lagging "behind" Greeks by a couple of generations (Psimmenos and Kasimati 2003). By this logic, immigrants are typically perceived as able to endure conditions that Greek citizens can no longer withstand and hence not to require the same level of modern consumer goods and services (132). By the same reasoning, it is possible that doctors implicitly deem cesareans, positively associated with risk reduction, pain relief, and technological modernity, as more suitable for Greek citizens. Conversely, midwifery, with its low-tech, "less-than-modern" connotations, may be viewed as more appropriate care for immigrants, refugees, and poor others. Whatever the combination of reasons, the outcome is that birth for Gamma patients is typically vaginal. As one exasperated midwife declared, with some overstatement, "in Greece, you have to be an immigrant, a gypsy, or have no money to have a vaginal birth." Ironically, subaltern women, who are subject to multiple forms of discrimination, stigmatization, and even violence outside the hospital (Cheliotis 2016), tend to be less susceptible to what birth activists and other critics have identified as the "obstetrical violence" of unnecessary cesareans. Maternity care in Greece thus offers an example of how stratified reproduction can in particular contexts confer a degree of protection to vulnerable others.

In addition to acting as obstetricians' assistants during birth, midwives in the public hospital are also responsible for supervising the hands-on experience of midwifery students. Typically, students are present only as observers during the births of ethnic Greek women as doctors strive to maintain an exclusive relationship with their patients; as a consequence, opportunities to acquire hands-on experience are significantly restricted. However, in order to obtain their certification, midwifery students must participate in a total of forty births under the supervision of an experienced midwife-instructor. In the past, they easily met this requirement over the course of their obligatory service in rural areas. Today, this number of births would be difficult to achieve without the Gamma patients. By leaving them in the hands of the midwives, doctors have inadvertently opened up a pedagogical space for the training of the next generation. Thus, another unanticipated consequence of stratified reproduction in the public hospitals is that midwifery students are able to obtain the practical experience needed to fulfill to the letter their degree requirements. Not all students actively desire this kind of experience, I was told by one midwifery professor, and many are content to graduate with less training and make a comfortable living working as a "doctor's midwife." Those students who do, on the other hand, actively seek out the hospitals known to serve the largest numbers of immigrant women.

CONCLUSION

In sum, in filling the gaps in medical surveillance presented by the Gamma patients, midwives have been able to expand the practice of their midwifery skills and transmit these to the next generation. Outside the scope of the obstetricians' gaze, the Gamma patients have opened up a space at the margins of the public hospital that shelters the devalued and stigmatized knowledge and bodies deemed out of place in the central and dominant spaces and practices of the hospital. Because obstetricians have tacitly "left" the care of these patients to the midwives, they in turn have been able to take the opportunity to teach and supervise their students the hands-on skills to conduct vaginal birth. Of course, this degree of freedom from the purview of obstetrical power is precarious, contingent and largely restricted to the heterotopic spaces of maternity care reserved for poor and immigrant Others. Still, there are some indications that the experiences and confidence midwives have garnered in these spaces may have begun to translate into organized efforts to increase their professional autonomy.

One example of such efforts is their successful initiative to set up a weekly prenatal clinic within the hospital exclusively for immigrants and refugees. Through the nonprofit they established in 2017 called "ORAMMA" (an acronym that means "vision" in Greek), a group of activist midwives secured funding from the European Union to design and implement a project to offer maternity care that was "woman-centered, culturally appropriate and evidence-based" (https://oramma.eu/the-project/). A highly innovative component of the project was the recruitment and training of immigrant and refugee women to work as cultural and well as linguistic mediators between patients and providers. While setting up the ORAMMA clinic represents an unprecedented achievement, it remains the case that midwives have not substantially increased their professional autonomy or their ability to practice midwifery across *all* settings within the hospital. At the same time that the presence of large numbers of subaltern women has enabled midwives to apply their expert knowledge and skills, it has also reproduced the broader conditions of subordination to doctors, and thus may offer little or no sustainable possibility of overcoming or even blunting the subordination of the midwifery profession in the longer term. At least for the present, however, the heterotopic spaces within the hospital remain open and productive of alternatives to the prevailing model birth dominated by cesareans.

CHAPTER 13

The Nightside of Medicine

OBSTETRIC SUFFERING AND ETHNOGRAPHIC
WITNESSING IN A PAKISTANI HOSPITAL

Emma Varley

NIGHTSIDE ('NAIT,SAID)—NOUN

1. Astronomy: the dark side (of a planet); the side of a planet, the moon,
   etc. facing away from the sun
2. The dark or evil side (of a person's character or of a thing's nature)

During four years of fieldwork in a northern Pakistani hospital, I bore witness
to the cumulative impact of medical neglect, misadventure, and predation for
childbirth and its outcomes; these haunt me. Provoked by this haunting, my
chapter dwells on medicine's darker side and details how it can operate *otherwise*, or against its own standards, and take nightside form. Here, I qualify
nightside medicine as that which deviates from, and even defies, the medical-
bureaucratic norms expected to undergird and hold fast hospital services; the
standards that regulate personnel's dispensation of care, and, by defining medicine's allowable outer limits, work to protect patients and ultimately also
their treating providers from birth's calculable risks, and the dangers posed by
medicine gone awry, off-the-books, and off-protocol.

Through a bedside focus on the everyday violence of labor and delivery
care, I revisit frontline providers' misuse and mishandling of protocols and
confront the suffering, maiming, and death it produces. In trying to understand how clinical iatrogenesis, or "the injury done to patients by ineffective,
toxic, and unsafe treatments" (Illich 1976), comes into being, I invoke the
ways that conditions of want and wrongdoing become encoiled, and attend to
the watchful vigilance and defensiveness necessitated by precarity in medical
settings and services. Habituated by experience to expect diverse kinds of
medical harm, maternity patients and their advocates were alert to the imperilments posed by the hospital and its dysfunctions and providers' missteps or
misdeeds—ever-ready to intervene to prevent or mitigate risk and bad outcomes through acts of resistance, disruption, and refusal.

In coming to grips with nightside medicine, my chapter takes us to Gilgit, the capital of Gilgit-Baltistan in northern Pakistan. Since 2004, I have explored the wide-ranging determinants that either drive improvements or underpin lags in women's maternal health. My research has been tied to critical moments in Gilgit's recent history: the 2005 and 2012 "tension times," which consisted of the worst Shia-Sunni sectarian strife in living memory, and the 2010 floods, when Gilgit's civil infrastructures, and government hospital services, were devastated by torrential summer rains. While the tension times signaled the enactment of disadvantage across sectarian lines of affiliation, and against maternity patients by treating providers (Varley 2016), the damages incurred by the 2010 floods exacerbated preexisting clinical insufficiencies and brought into stark relief the state's failure to protect patients, providers, and health systems overall from either (Varley 2019). In answering why the dangers faced by women in Gilgit were not only poorly remediated by but could also result from medical services, my ethnography speaks to the content, texture, and limits of public health infrastructures and maternal and newborn interventions, and the global paradox of the Safe Motherhood Initiative (SMI) in particular.

Since 1987, the Safe Motherhood Initiative has tasked signatories with the responsibility to reduce treatment delays, identify high-risk pregnancies, implement faster clinical referral mechanisms, and charge hospitals with final responsibility to avert obstetric crises (Benagiano and Thomas 2003)—feats typically, if only also marginally, accomplished through varied reforms, such as deepened investments in primary and preventive health care services, and the reorganization and redistribution of technical expertise (see Dawson et al. 2014). Yet, thirty years of Safe Motherhood Initiative interventions in Pakistan (Jafarey et al. 2008) have yielded only modest and slow reductions in the rates of maternal injury, illness, and death (Nisar et al. 2017). The story of the District Headquarter Hospital (DHQ) in Gilgit may help answer why.

With the vast majority of deliveries in Gilgit being hospital based (Government of Gilgit-Baltistan and UNICEF 2017, 13), and roughly half of these taking place at the DHQ, its services are not incidental to the story of maternal morbidity and mortality in Gilgit-Baltistan. Rather, the austerity, dysfunction, and precarity bound up with obstetric care at the DHQ's Labour Room affords compelling insights into the reasons why maternal illness, injury, and death rates across Gilgit-Baltistan remain high. Notwithstanding steady increases in the accessibility and use of regional maternal health services since the late 1970s, and a near-total transition away from community-based midwifery, the regional maternal mortality ratio is upwards of 450 per 100,000 live births (Government of Gilgit-Baltistan and UNICEF 2017), far higher than the national average of 276 (Jafarey and Rabbani 2014). With Gilgit having among the highest rates of clinical uptake in the region, if not all of northern Pakistan, why did it also have one of Pakistan's highest reported morbidity and mortality ratios? With pregnancy and delivery occurring against the global backdrop of widespread development and the medicalization of childbirth, how had one set of progressions failed to lead to another?

Gilgit-Baltistan's Maternal, Newborn, and Child Health (MNCH) and Safe Motherhood Initiative proponents characterized persistently high maternal morbidity and mortality as the outgrowth of patient-side treatment delays. However, even with clinical services for pregnancy and childbirth having reduced the number of deaths caused by a number of preventable complications, such as placental abruption, eclampsia, or obstructed labor, it was impossible to ignore how women's use of resource-poor, under-staffed and inadequately supervised clinical settings placed them at high risk of nosocomial infection and childbirth injury. Providers' sometimes-necessary improvisations on medical protocols emerged as the source of a host of risks and harms. More than this, hospital insufficiency was not the only reason for protocol revisions. Interlaced with providers' reworking of medical protocols were other kinds of intentions and pursuits. Maternity patients and, to a notable degree, their treating providers routinely emphasized the contribution of negligence, malpractice, and even corruption for poor outcomes.

In tracing nightside medicine's features and consequent effects at the DHQ, this chapter seeks to answer a series of interrelated questions. How can anthropologies of clinical services provide insights into the efficacy, unevenness, or even outright failure of global maternal health interventions? How can hospital ethnography provide insights otherwise eclipsed by economic and political evaluations, institutional audits, or public health policy, and which explain the persistence of high morbidity and mortality rates irrespective of hospital services? As importantly, how can critical exploration of hospitals as sites of dangerous clinical dysfunction generate the evidence needed to enhance anthropological as well as global public health advocacy and activism?

"Nightside" Precedents and Methods

In unpacking the complex ways that nightside medicine comes into being, unfolds, and leads to harm, this chapter deprioritizes analysis that reconfirms medicine's ability to resolve obstetric crises in favor of attention to its contributions to and worsening of the same. There is no doubt that poorly resourced, under-regulated, and unevenly administered hospitals generate risk; iatrogenesis' likelihood is exponentially increased by system-side deficits, oversights, and neglects. The global literature confirms how often medical deficiency and even wrongdoing can be linked back to many hospitals' fraught circumstances (see Prata 2009; Livingston 2012; Rivkin-Fish 2005; Strong 2016).

Women delivering at the DHQ faced a daunting array of intervention-linked risks, including overdosing, cross-contamination, nosocomial infection, and surgical error and injury. As their accounts and my case observations confirmed, iatrogenic acts and outcomes ranged significantly by degree and form, from that which was so normalized as to become largely invisible, to that which was so spectacular or exceptional that it was impossible to ignore, and even criminalized. At the DHQ, and innumerable hospitals across the globe, such incidents are underreported (if they are reported at all; see George 2007, 91, and Grünebaum et al. 2015), statistically under-enumerated (Wendland 2016; see also S. Davis 2017), and qualitatively underexplored.

In pursuing this tack, my ethnography draws on a rich precedent of work focused on reproductive injustice, in the form of neglectful, disrespectful, and abusive maternity care (Castro and Savage 2019; Chadwick 2017; D'Oliveira, Diniz, and Schraiber 2002; Jewkes, Abrahams, and Mvo 1998; Smith-Oka 2013; Van Hollen 1998); uneven care and medical mismanagement (Fikree, Mir, and Haq 2006; Jaffré and Suh 2016; Knight, Self, and Kennedy 2013), and "unnecessary" medical violence (Shapiro 2018; see Diniz and Chacham 2004). Growing attention is also paid to the nonmedical—or, gendered, socioeconomic, political, and racial—factors contributing to clinical iatrogenesis (Illich 1976) in hospitals (Dastur 2016; Jaffré and Prual 1994) and obstetric medicine in particular (D.-A. Davis 2019; Dixon 2015; Jaffré 2012; Jeffery and Jeffery 2010; Smith-Oka 2013; Towghi 2018; Varley and Varma 2019).

Even with the literature confirming how hospital services reflect and repeat structural violence, the iatrogenesis borne not only of idiosyncratic neglects, omissions, or accidents but acts that are demonstrably deliberate, is largely under-investigated, or is obliquely cast as "invisible" violence (Diaz-Tello 2016; see Bourgois 2010). Too often, ethnographers' expositions prioritize exculpatory explanations at the expense of attention to the inculpatory empirics by which providers and systems alike can be more fully evaluated and held accountable, evidence that remains poorly captured by national and global maternal death surveillance systems (Gutschow 2016; World Health Organization [WHO] 2016).

Because ethnographies of medical harm run counter to the stories that health systems and hospitals tell about themselves, claims of neglect, incompetency, and malpractice require robust corroboration. My efforts to not only document medicine gone awry and its iatrogenic aftermaths but also confirm the degree to which clinical interventions are undergirded and even impelled by a dense constellation of nonmedical forces, entailed close, comparative analysis of the narratives, hospital case reporting, and Labour Room observations specific to individual cases. My fieldwork included interviews with women and their families, health service providers, and hospital administrators, and observation of prenatal, labor and delivery, and postpartum care. My findings were triangulated with the hospital's records, including ten years' worth of Labour Room registers, clinical pro formas, doctors' "Call Books," and patients' own medical records. The rigor of my efforts was in many ways tactical, intended to preempt and destabilize public health critiques of ethnographic evidence as anecdotal and inactionable, rather than empirical and actionable.

What the Ethnographer Saw

The DHQ's Family Wing—which includes the Labour Room, Operating Theatre, Intensive Care and Female Medical Wards, and Outpatient Department—sits on the crest of a small hill, backed by the steep slopes of the mountains encircling Gilgit. In 2013, when I last undertook extended field-work at the hospital, its gynecological and obstetrical services were provided by an all-female staff, led by ob-gyns, who provided specialist treatment, and Lady Medical Officers (LMOs, the equivalent of general practitioners), who, along with several nurses, managed the outpatient, inpatient, and intensive care medical wards. With nearly four hundred patients daily attending the Wing's Outpatient Clinic, and high-risk and postoperative patients to manage in the ITC, physicians only rarely attended Labour Room deliveries, for which Lady Health Visitors (LHVs), the equivalent of nurse assistants, were primarily responsible.

During my fieldwork, the Labour Room handled the highest annual number of hospital-based births in Gilgit-Baltistan; during a 2017 field visit, upwards of thirty-five women delivered there each day. The Labour Room's social and structural contributions to maternal risk were first and foremost a product of the institutional organization of clinic personnel. Holding two-year diplomas in the safe management of uncomplicated pregnancy and child-birth, LHVs' are, in essence, skilled birth attendants whose duties, elsewhere in Pakistan, are confined to community- and clinic-based antenatal care and delivery support. Because of the dearth of physicians and nurses, Gilgit-Baltistan's Secretary of Health provided special dispensation for LHVs to manage the Labour Room. Though physicians were supposed to supervise and intervene as needed, the reality has been that LHVs handle the vast major-ity of delivery cases without specialist support, no matter the degree of com-plication. Many women arrived already disadvantaged by the health effects wrought by structural violence: malnutrition, iron-deficiency anemia, tuber-culosis, and hepatitis were commonplace. Daily, patients included women undergoing early- or late-term miscarriages, stillbirths, and fetal abnormali-ties, or who were suffering from potentially life-threatening post-abortion complications like sepsis.

The chronicling of iatrogenesis that follows is intended neither to be unduly bleak, nor engage in ethnographic catastrophizing. Rather, the evi-dence on which I rely is mundane and commonplace, typical of the treatment provided for deliveries. In tracking the mechanics generative of maternal injury and even death, the content and contours of nightside medicine emerge.

To begin, expediency and convenience rather than expectant manage-ment or clinical indication defined LHVs' practice of obstetric medicine.

Patients newly admitted and reporting contractions were brought into the Labour Room and checked for cervical dilation. In this first exam, irrespective of the stage of labor, strength of contractions, and even also before confirming the due date, LHVs often injected oxytocin or inserted tablets of Misoprostol, each a synthetic hormone stimulating contractions. If misused during childbirth, especially when they are used simultaneously, oxytocin and Misoprostol are strongly associated with uterine rupture. Once dosed, contractions increased dramatically in strength and duration. If pain made patients "unmanageable"—noisy, uncooperative, demanding—LHVs administered intramuscular injections of Buscopan, a muscle relaxant they said would soften the cervix, speed dilation, and hasten delivery. Until they were ready to deliver, women labored in adjacent rooms, where they received neither active management nor support from on-duty staff, nor pain relief. Weight and blood pressure were not assessed. Blood chemistry and urine were checked only when women hemorrhaged and crossmatching for transfusions was necessary, or when they suffered hypertensive seizures. Fetal well-being was assessed only intermittently, for seconds at a time, by use of a fetoscope. Fetal distress's signs—diminished heart rate, movement, and meconium-stained amniotic fluid—were often missed during rushed initial exams.

When birth was imminent, women returned to the Labour Room where, to reduce the time and effort spent managing them, LHVs inserted cannulas, a shortcut in case transfusions were needed. To these were connected IVs, into which more oxytocin was injected. Oxytocin overuse risked precipitous labor, and all the cascading complications that come with it: neonatal asphyxia and hypoxia, cervical tear, uterine rupture, and hemorrhage (see Berglund 2012; Brhlikova et al. 2009; Jeffery and Brhlikova 2009). Over-dosages were commonplace: the IV-solution given to women frequently already contained high levels of the drug—sometimes upwards of five times the standard dose of 10 units oxytocin per 1 liter of normal saline. The oxytocin-infused IV solution for one patient was almost always reused with subsequent patients, for whom the dosage was repeated, leading to overdosing. For delayed or obstructed deliveries, the LHVs pushed heavily on the top of the uterus to help force the baby out, risking rupture, tears, and fistulas. Upon delivery, more oxytocin was given to prevent the hemorrhage made more likely by the drug's overuse during labor. LHVs used controlled cord traction to remove the placenta, tightly coiling the umbilical cord around and around a set of clamps. LHVs' heavy-handed use of the technique risked uterine rupture, inversion, or even prolapse, which then required surgical repair, and exposed women to additional iatrogenic risk in the Operating Theatre.

There was also the danger of cross-contamination. The Labour Room's gas-powered sterilizer was regularly inoperational and its boiler sterilizers irregularly used. Instead, instruments were washed with or briefly soaked in Biodine, a disinfectant. One IV bag and line and set of surgical gloves were used for multiple patients, even when fresh resources were available. LHVs routinely shook the blood from used IV lines before reattaching them, and the unfinished IVs to which they were connected, to the cannula in the next patient's hand. The hospital's critics, including former administrators, physicians, and nurses as well as patients and their allies, described the Labour Room as a key regional vector for blood-borne diseases:

> At the DHQ, they will use the same equipment on woman after woman, without doing more than washing it with soap and water, or boiling it quickly, which is not adequate protection. . . . . Hepatitis B infections are at their limit. Mothers pass them to their infants, during pregnancy and after birth, and the Hep B in these children becomes malignant at some point in their late teens. (Dr. "Zahir" [pseudonym] July 2005)

Even though LHVs lamented physicians' absences when obstetric crises had evolved past the point of easy or effective management, they were often also resentful of physicians' intervention. Doctors' authorities undermined the expansive powers LHVs ordinarily held over the Labour Room and its patients, while their very presence prevented some LHVs from engaging in illegal acts of economic predation. Save for those patients with whom they enjoyed close affinities or to whom they were previously obliged, many LHVs solicited informal payments from women and their families, usually under the guise of the *mubaraki* (congratulatory) monies traditionally and voluntarily offered to providers in exchange for successfully handled deliveries. These were secured through extortive threats of treatment delays, denials, and withdrawals, as one former patient described:

> When women have babies at the DHQ, it happens that [the LHVs] won't let the family into the Labour Room to take the baby until the family has given them money. When this happened to us, we said we would report them to the police, so then they gave the baby to us. If we were to give them PKR 300 or 400, they aren't accepting it. They're asking for PKR 500 or 1,000. If it's a boy, they're asking for even more. If they see the patient is rich, they're taking care; if a poor woman comes in, then they're not look after her. . . . [b]ecause the rich women can pay them more. ("Shamim" [pseudonym] July 2012)

Added to this, the more urgent the delivery and the greater its risks, the higher the gratuities claimed. Herein lay among the most important reasons for expediency: speed ensured LHVs' during-shift capture of the monies extorted from patients and their families during labor and delivery, sometimes before any care was provided at all. Many LHVs were divorced or widowed, or they were the primary earner for their families. LHVs' economic, social, and professional vulnerabilities not only facilitated the pivot toward informal, exploitive economic practices but also ensured they were the least able to protest their working conditions, or agitate against the health care system to effect necessary change. In turn, physicians more often than not consented to their exclusion by LHVs. Distance from the Labour Room's poorest outcomes afforded them an important measure of protection and less culpability and liability. It therefore worked to hospital administrators' and physicians' advantage that highest-risk care was provided by the lowest-skilled providers; paraphrasing Jaffré, "every department organises its work according to its own constraints" (2012, 8).

NIGHTSIDE OUTCOMES

The stories of deliveries gone spectacularly, though not unusually, wrongly illustrate nightside medicine's direst effects and help explain patients' and their attendants' hyper-attentiveness to medical neglect, abuse and fault, and readiness to intervene and disrupt care—sometimes violently so—if the situation demanded. In spring 2009, a long-term interlocutor, "Anila," delivered her firstborn, a stillborn daughter. The circumstances of the delivery haunted her mother, "Haleema," who twenty years prior had lost her youngest son to stillbirth because, she believed, she had been given a "wrong injection" by Labour Room staff.

> Last year, do you know what happened to my daughter and her stillborn girl? They cut her in two different places [for an episiotomy] and took the girl out that had died inside her. They didn't let me inside the room. She was screaming. I could hear her from outside and was going crazy. . . . Afterwards, they . . . told us her uterus had come outside with the baby.
>
> After they cleaned her up, they [LHVs] . . . stitched her up. After labor, we took her home and were looking after her, giving her medications and cleaning her stitches. We thought she would get better, but she wasn't feeling better. . . . She was saying, "There is a smell coming from inside" and she asked me to look at her urine because she had a strange discharge.
>
> For fifteen to sixteen days afterwards, she didn't get any better and I brought her to my home to care for her. She was here another twenty days and wasn't getting better at all. I told my daughter, "There may be something in your uterus, otherwise why would you get this smell?" . . . We took her to the DHQ again and again, and the LHVs said, "Why are you disturbing us, coming over and over? There's no problem." But my daughter was very sick and saying, "'Something like a big ball is rolling around in my pelvis." Twice we took her to the hospital, but they didn't check her [internally].
>
> She said there was still a foul smell and then began fainting . . . so we took her to Dr "N"'s clinic. Dr N checked inside and found a huge ball of cotton gauze packed against her uterus, sewn up inside, and it was rotten. There was lots of infection and smell, so she gave Anila medication for infection and pain and a few injections for germs. This was after forty days. (July 2010)

It was for these reasons, Haleema "never left the Labour Room" when her daughters and daughters-in-law were delivering, and she paid such vigilantly close attention to every clinical intervention. Haleema's cousin "Sairah" soon after shared her own story of loss at the DHQ the year before.

> My maternal uncle's daughter, she died [because] of doctors' negligence. She was having labor pains but there was a failure [to] progress, [so] the doctors decided to operate her but, in the end, they didn't do that. Finally, they [LHVs] delivered the baby forcefully vaginally. They delivered the baby girl, but she died soon after birth. I don't know exactly what happened, but probably the uterus got ruptured. She was bleeding heavily, and then became heavily swollen, and then died. (August 2010)

Two years later, another interlocutor's account of maternal death almost exactly repeated Sairah's:

> In our neighborhood, a woman died because her uterus was broken [ruptured]. . . . At the end of her delivery, they gave her an injection for her contractions; they gave her Syntocinon [synthetic oxytocin]. When they put the injection in, then she had the pains and delivered almost right away. For contractions, the injection is bad because of its effects on the uterus; it's better if the baby comes naturally, right? (July 2012)

In 2010, "Zunaira," a close relative of Haleema, died of complications following a series of medical errors. After LHVs' forceps delivery of her seventh child, who died in the process, Zunaira's uterus was perforated following a too-fast placental removal. She began to hemorrhage; even after recognizing they'd failed to control the bleeding, LHVs delayed calling the on-call ob-gyn to come to the DHQ to perform an emergency hysterectomy. Though the surgery eventually took place later the same day, the surgeon left swabs and scissors inside Zunaira's pelvic cavity. Even though these were soon removed, sepsis set in. Concerned that providers at other hospitals would confirm the extent of her iatrogenic injuries, her treating physician initially delayed her referral to a better-equipped hospital, where aggressive antibiotic therapy and follow-up surgeries to remove necrotic tissue kept her alive for another month. Before dying, Zunaira told her story to all who would listen, arguing that LHVs' "cruelty" and refusal to promptly summon specialist help, then the medical specialist's errors and deferred referral were *the* causes of her impending death. Later, not a trace of her story could be found in the hospital's Labour Room register. With providers' professional security contingent on the clinical outcomes they achieved, case details were managed defensively: the labor observed was rarely if ever the labor that was recorded.

Even with the starkest outcomes irregularly captured or excluded by LHVs' recordkeeping, the data that remains paints a grim portrait. In January 2011, 9.7 percent of 391 deliveries were fresh stillbirths, suggesting demise during active labor, while women were under medical supervision: 9.7 percent versus an average of 0.5 percent in the United Kingdom. The same month, only 5.6 percent of deliveries were cesarian sections, rather than the optimal 10–15 percent recommended by WHO. When considered against highly reported incidences of eclampsia, intrauterine death, birth asphyxia, face and hand presentation, uterine prolapse and rupture, the infrequency of LHVs' C-section referrals spoke to the habitual mismanagement of complications. Hospital records also showed how physicians were called only when obstetric crises, especially those that were undeniably iatrogenic, had escalated to the point that women could be irreparably injured or die, and disciplinary sanctions and criminal charges become more likely for on-duty personnel.

The Labour Room therefore served as the jaggedly unreliable interface between women and the health systems purported to serve them. It was no wonder that for patients, medicine appeared Janus-faced: its nightside demanding vigilance by women and their families who were well-enculturated to the difference between medicine as it ought to be, and as it actually is. Paraphrasing Brenda Walter, for patients the hospital was transgressive and duplicitous; its services a failed promise, even a lie (2014: 57). And, yet return again and again for delivery women did. In answering why they continued to rely on the DHQ, even in the aftermath of traumatic deliveries or loss, women patients and their families offered three broad explanations.

First, as a no-fee public sector facility, patients avoided the high out-of-pocket expenses associated with private and nongovernmental sector labor and delivery services. Such services are especially exorbitant for complicated deliveries and C-sections. Second, after several generations' worth of experiences of labor and delivery care at the hospital, women and their allies described themselves as "well prepared" to recognize and act to mitigate—though not always prevent—missteps and misdeeds both in the execution of medicine and the care expected from treating providers. Third, others described how over time they had developed longstanding social connections with Labour Room staff; these, they hoped, would hold LHVs to act in their favor and achieve better medical results. In turn, through the mechanism of informal payments, LHVs made themselves more available to be influenced by their patients. Even if the quality of medical services was no safer, patients perceived "better" care as being gentle and compassionate. (Conversely, LHVs were more likely to be described as "'corrupt" when treatment was predicated on excessive informal payments or accompanied by physical or verbal abuse.) By relation, LHVs' efforts were less likely to be characterized as "wrong" or "dangerous" (khattarnak) if patients felt that their services were altruistic or even heroically provided. For instance, LHVs' surreptitious use of hospital facilities and resources for "criminal" abortions—no matter the illness or injury that ensued—were often viewed positively by women facing unwanted or "illegal" (premarital or extramarital) pregnancies, which risked their families' honour (izzat) and, by turn, their lives.

EXPLAINING NIGHTSIDE MEDICINE

When asked to discuss the factors contributing to maternal and neonatal illness, injury, and death, the DHQ's health care providers first laid blame on distal and anonymous structural forces. They sourced poor outcomes back, not to clinical decisions and acts, but, rather, to infrastructures and systems at-large—what Hamdy (2008) refers to as political etiologies. They pointed to the hospital's acute resource and personnel constraints, and argued that, under these fraught circumstances, they were unable to fully adhere to clinical protocols. Here was a partial truth. More often than not, even when the resources supportive of protocol adherence were present, LHVs instead followed the informal, unwritten indigenous protocols that had evolved over several professional generations. These were the outgrowth of deep institutional memories concerning the practices that worked best under the hospital's difficult circumstances and helped offset the specific risks posed by the DHQ for patients and providers alike. When considering LHVs' approaches to case management, I never lost sight of the ways that nightside medicine was, first, a response to structural deficits, clinical gaps, and absent specialist support. The DHQ's insufficiencies produced unmet need and precarity, which necessitated creative contouring of high-resource protocols to fit low-resource medicine. Yet, in the process of amending protocols' procedural elements and sequences, opportunism and enrichment became enmeshed with LHVs' evolving preferred practices. Inasmuch as their strategies grew out of conditions of want and peril, they were oftentimes-risky distortions, undergirded by impulses that could be nonmedical in the extreme.

Conscious of their medical liabilities, LHVs defensively encircled themselves with like-minded others and those obliged to protect them especially. LHVs knew many of their superiors' secrets—having observed firsthand the misconduct and malpractice for which physicians, too, could be responsible—and held the power to leverage these when discipline was nigh. They closed ranks when accusations were made, precluding the possibility of recourse let alone justice when women were harmed or died. When case details were egregious enough to warrant action and disciplining, LHVs' supervising physicians would need to first concretely establish culpability. Even when they were convinced of another provider's malfeasance, though, many described themselves as largely powerless to act. Not only were physicians largely estranged from the Labour Room and the darker aspects of its operations but the evidence needed to substantiate claims was misreported, disputed, or altogether denied. (The hospital's reporting and surveillance instruments required frontline medical personnel self-assess and report on the results of the treatments they themselves had provided.) The reporting obfuscations and denials needed for vulnerable personnel to sidestep allegations of wrongdoing, and the sanctioning that could follow, all but guaranteed the production of partial hospital accounts (see De Brouwere et al. 2013; Gouda et al. 2017; Kingori and Gerrets 2016; Melberg et al. 2018). Nightside practices were thereby cast into the domain of public secrets—namely, that which is "open to experience but absent from public speech and scientific texts" (Taussig 1999 in Geissler 2013, 13). There were also the pressures placed on physicians and patients by the hospital's administration to withdraw complaints; not only were collegiality, trust, and reputations at stake, but LHVs were protected by their union and exceedingly hard to reprimand, suspend and fire, let alone replace.

CONCLUSION

My work relies on a still small but richly elaborative precedent of hospital ethnographies that pull into view medicine's precarities and trace their after-effects (Berry 2008; Chadwick 2017; Livingston 2012; Pinto 2004; Sadler et al. 2016). It is an even smaller number, though, that prioritize inquiry and theorization not only of medical misdeeds, mismanagement, and malpractice but also the iatrogenesis that results (Chabrol 2018; Greenhalgh 2001; Kehr 2018; Metzl 2010; C. Smith 2013; Smith-Oka 2013; Strong 2016; Stevenson 2014). Embedded in our critical relay are questions engaged even less-often—namely, of intentionality, accountability, culpability, and complicity. As qualifiers, these emerge in the ways our interlocutors speak back to the conditions of care, its failures, its imperilments, and purposeful lapses. They serve to indict health systems and authorities. By contrast, hospital ethnographies can be more cautious, leaning into analysis that assumes providers' competency and altruism, rather than more vigorously evaluate wrongdoing or even illegality, insofar as illegality accords with clinical, juridical-criminal, and indigenous registers all. When gaps and harms arise, these can be attributed to "blind spots" (see Keshavjee 2014) rather than a biopolitics that thrives on misconduct. By contrast, nightside ethnography deliberately seeks out these sharper edges, and nightside medicine refers to diverse, often overlapping, and sometimes undeniably intentional practices and processes, ranging from patient under-management and neglect to providers' "off-label" reworking of protocols (Towghi 2013) to medical mismanagement and malpractice. My chapter challenges hospital ethnographers to better account for wrongdoing and injustice, whether they represent a steady norm or are infrequent and unusual acts. Whether exploring nightside medicine's more mundane or most spectacular forms, we should never fail to interrogate the circumstances that serve as its foundations, and create the opportunities by which wrongdoing can flourish.

The risks and damages bound up with medicine at the DHQ should serve as a necessary cautionary tale, giving us pause as we consider the wealth of program, policy, and interventions that unequivocally predicate improvements in women's maternal health on their use of biomedical providers and facilities, especially in settings defined by precarity. Indeed, medicine's dangers require a fundamental repositioning of maternal health debates away from a disproportionately heavy emphasis on patient- and community-side factors, to critical re-appraisal of institutional settings, and the social texture and clinical efficacy of the obstetric services provided therein (see Clark 2016). However, closely focused, system-challenging hospital ethnography—especially that which zeroes in on iatrogenesis—can come to be seen by our health care interlocutors and health system stakeholders as a hostile act. The evidences we gather on iatrogenesis and its multiplex sources hold the power to not only affirm and corroborate patients' claims but they also establish culpability.

Hospital ethnographers are uniquely positioned to generate the bottom-up evidence needed for upstream accountability and compel health systems to more deeply consider the darker *and* brighter innovations that see patients through to harm or save their lives. Because ethnography differs from clinical audits by nature of its sustained attention to medicine's sociological features, our findings hold the power to challenge and thereby also enrich the evaluative criteria typically used by health systems and interventions, and assessments of the same. Verbal autopsies and obstetric and facility audits would benefit from additional etiological factors and measures, such as they are used to gauge policy or programming success, and expanded evaluation of the medical and nonmedical forces at work in medical practices and outcomes.

However, our witnessing and ethnographies of nightside practices will never be easy or even safe so long as we work alone. Until anthropology surpasses its undeserved reputation as an "anecdotal" and "storytelling" social science, ethnographers should continue to strategically capitalize on the legitimacy afforded by teamwork with epidemiologists, clinicians, and statisticians. When achieving a burden of proof is an urgent or fraught process, interdisciplinary collaboration allows us the vital opportunity to enmesh our ethnography with positivist methodologies and triangulate, test, and confirm our findings in both social and clinical terms. By working across disciplines to disentangle the tightly coiled correlations that comprise iatrogenesis, our goals are dual: to identify its sources and the seriousness of its scope.

The benefits of collaborative approaches, so long as anthropology's methodological and analytic boundaries are neither breached nor degraded, are several. Not only will our evidence be less vulnerable to interdisciplinary challenge or dismissal, but we will also be better positioned to mobilize our findings to reach diverse audiences, benefit varied stakeholders, and impel action. Nightside ethnography holds the power to counterbalance under-calculations and obfuscations, and help re-align health recording and evaluation systems to better capture and reduce the widest range of risks present in hospital settings. But for necessary change to come, and our potential as ethnographer-witnesses and advocates both to be ethically fulfilled, our ethnographies need to more fully reflect medicine's manifold social and clinical hazards, and the circumstances giving them rise.

Afterword

Claire Wendland

INSTITUTIONS THINK, Mary Douglas argued many years ago. Institutions decide, adjudicate, triage. Douglas claimed that individuals "have no other way to make the big decisions except within the scope of institutions they build"—institutions that make consequential judgments with efficiency and grant them legitimacy (Douglas 1986, 128). We delegate to institutions the unbearable decisions about who will be encouraged to flourish and who will be left to die.

Outside observers have had great difficulty gaining access to hospitals, medicine's most sacred and secret institutions. Lofty commitments to patient privacy are often used to protect hospitals and their workers. Insider accounts of hospitals are typically incomplete, strongly biased toward particular interests. Outsider accounts are both rare and valuable. Those assembled in this edifying and often devastating collection reveal aspects of biomedicine's global circulations and local manifestations, as the volume's editors note. These accounts also reveal hospitals to be not just thinking institutions but testing, triaging, and changing ones.

TESTING

Hospitals can become spaces in which religious, social, and political ideals are tested. Testing often—but not always—leads to reinforcement of dominant ideologies. Davis-Floyd (1992) described childbirth in hospitals as a rite of passage that affirmed American ideas about science, technology, and patriarchy. In a study of soldiers recuperating at Walter Reed, the flagship United States Veterans Administration hospital, Wool (2015) showed that intimate care from a wife or girlfriend was elevated to a stamp of heteronormative masculinity rather than a marker of dependency; ideas about masculinity that might have been threatened by soldiers' debilities were shored up against those threats. In this volume, Hannig describes how religious authority and medical authority prop one another up in an Ethiopian fistula hospital, as a doctor's knowledge is both divinely sanctioned and proof of the goodness of God. Hoke's chapter on maternity care in Peru shows the mutual constitution of social stratification and medical authority: healthcare providers, mostly nonindigenous, hold power over rural indigenous women and their families because they function as agents of the state, controlling access to social insurance programs.

Testing does not always lead to a reinforcement of the status quo. Hospitals are also places where narratives about the causes of illness can be challenged, and sometimes changed (Hamdy 2012; Langwick 2008; Mulemi 2014; Street 2014). New narratives of causation can open up possibilities that were foreclosed by older ones. Both Olsen's chapter on epilepsy in Ghana and that by Amoussouhoui and colleagues on Buruli-ulcer care in Benin show that hospital practices can reduce the stigma of some afflictions. Notably, in each case the success of new destigmatizing narratives depends on health workers who find patients where they are—whether through drop-in, open-ended consultations or outreach to prayer camps—rather than fitting patients into the everyday machinery of the hospital and its spaces and policies.

Hospitals also test the degree to which states are responsible for their citizens' medical care. Smith-Oka and Hurd describe a Mexican system in which national policies reflect collective ideals, but their actual enactment in frayed and ill-supplied hospitals by burned-out staff can work counter to those ideals. Strong describes the damage to hospitals and communities that accrues as Tanzanian medical leaders abandon the language of nation-building in favor of a watered-down development discourse. In each case, the whittling away of a commitment to quality care for all citizens engenders protest.

Triaging

Hospitals turn life-and-death triage decisions into matters of ordinary bureaucracy and mundane practice, as this volume's chapters about cancer care in France and in Guatemala reveal clearly. In theory, health care in both countries is a human right. In practice, as Sargent explains, bureaucracy and logistics make it a right hard to access for West African immigrants in Paris, as it is for the rural Mayans that Chary and Rohloff describe in Guatemala. When staff, money, and supplies are inadequate to provide treatment for everyone, institutional procedures ensure that not everyone can get it. For a time during my own work in a large referral center in Malawi, the institution's policy was never to initiate antiretroviral therapy in hospitalized patients, who were judged "too sick" to start treatment. Overtly, this policy was justified by the dangers of immune reconstitution syndrome, which strikes about one in six seriously ill patients who begin antiretroviral therapy, and among those kills about one in twenty (Müller et al. 2010). Tacitly, it was also a way to handle the mismatch between overwhelming numbers of immune-compromised people who could benefit from antiretroviral drugs and minimal stocks of those medications.

Triage can be less deadly. Instead of leaving some people to die, institutions can leave some to suffer. In a rural hospital in which I worked in the United States, after-hours anesthesia was restricted to emergencies. But laboring women who knew an anesthesiologist well could privately arrange for one to be on call to provide a labor epidural. In effect, the combination of official policy and unofficial practice meant that hospital workers (nurses and doctors) could get labor anesthesia for their own childbirths while the great majority of patients, who lacked such social ties, could not. This informal triage system allowed thin on-call staffing to continue. Had every laboring woman been able to ask for an epidural, the hospital would have needed to employ more anesthesiologists. Several of the chapters in this volume demonstrate similar institutional mechanisms, processes that metabolize social inequalities into biological ones.

Because more care does not necessarily mean better care, triage mechanisms that restrict access to medical treatment do not always worsen health outcomes. Georges explains that immigrant women in Greece, left to the care of midwifery students while nonimmigrant Greek women seek out doctors, have much lower rates of cesarean delivery, and presumably also much lower rates of the complications that attend it. Varley's work in Pakistan makes clear that over-intervention and over-attention can be as harmful as neglect. In obstetrics, this point is well documented and widely accepted—at least outside hospitals. Over-intervention, and its consequences for social and health inequities, begs for analysis in other arenas of medical care.

Yet social triage is also quite evidently harmful to people already rendered vulnerable in other ways. Chary and Rohloff show that lab slips, referrals across town, and prescriptions to be filled are an obstacle-lined maze through which patients must run to have a chance at cancer treatment in Guatemala. If they fail at the complex, expensive, and time-consuming project, they have demonstrated insufficient commitment to the cause of their own cure and can be shunted to the back of the line. Those who fail are disproportionately poor, rural, and indigenous. Hospital triage works more invisibly if those who do not get necessary care can be blamed for it. Blaming is easier when those blamed are already on the social margins.

Victim-blaming has another function: when biomedical action fails, as it often does, criticism of patients can shift focus away from the limits of medical institutions and workers. Several chapters in this volume show how hospitals shield their practitioners by finding fault with patients. Patients who seek out non-sanctioned "alternative" healers for fistula treatment are likely to be blamed for their own failure to improve, Hannig describes. Patients can be cast as impediments to their own healing, shows Mattingly, if they are depressed, unmotivated, or lack the stable family situations that allow steady provision of invisible but vital care. Clinicians are not the only ones who attribute medical failure to nonmedical actors. Sobo's research on families with sick children reveals that parents have many ways of shoring up the authority of medicine, even holding children's unpredictable bodies responsible for unexpected treatment results.

Mary Douglas's work on the decision-making functions of institutions appeared in print at a time when neoliberal political-economic policies were newly ascendant: shrinking states, maximizing profit-making opportunities, shredding social safety nets. More than three decades on, anthropologists are well aware that neoliberal policies require the construction of undeserving citizens, understood as liabilities to social prosperity and threats to their own physical well-being. Hospitals are among the institutions that make such judgments easy, as many of the chapters in this volume show.

But blame does not always, or necessarily, work to absolve the already powerful by holding the less powerful accountable for their own injuries. Criticism can circulate within medical hierarchies. Senior nurses in Tanzania, as Strong notes, lament the younger generation's lack of work ethic and the seductions of "globalization" in the form of cell phones; supervisors and low-level health workers who spoke to Varley blame one another for lethal practices in Pakistan. Blame can go upwards in the power structure too. It can be leveled at institutions—including hospitals—that function to enrich the few while providing a charade of care and concern. It can be laid at the feet of inequitable political and economic systems.

CHANGING

Janzen reminds us that hospitals are "corporate" structures, existing independent of the individuals who hold office within them, attempting to ensure their own permanence. Permanence is, however, an elusive goal. Hospitals change as the world in which they are embedded changes. When change happens fast, exigency can allow a sudden shift in perception that can lead to new institutional practices and new explanations for suffering and death.

For many years I have been writing about people learning and working, living and dying within Malawian hospitals (and clinics and health centers). I have contrasted those institutions, whether implicitly or explicitly, with the various rural and urban hospitals in which I worked as a doctor in the United States. Especially in terms of improvisation and political orientation, I wrote, Malawian hospitals were *different*. I wrote of those observable differences as if they were stable. They were not.

One difference was the role of improvisation (Livingston 2012; Wendland 2010). Supplies in Malawi were erratic. Staffing was uneven and rarely adequate. Standard protocols, while they existed, had to be modified on the fly to match available people and things, including diagnostic tools and therapeutic options. Where a good clinician in an American hospital had to know and adhere to best-practice guidelines, a good clinician in a Malawian hospital had to be able to improvise and experiment. One might only be able to access certain kinds of treatment by enrolling in a research project or seeking out care at a nongovernmental site, whether private or nonprofit. Even within hospitals, people made do with homemade remedies and consulted nonmedical healers.

The other key difference between the Malawian hospitals and American hospitals I knew best was their orientation to politics. American medical professionals rarely spoke publicly about health or medical care as political issues. Many construed medicine as apolitical, a technical rather than social good. Hospitals were not often in the news. In Malawi, hospital care—or the lack of it—was a hot-button political issue, as was public health. Journalists wrote regular exposés about the inadequacies of national referral hospitals, exposés in which they routinely quoted outraged medical staff. Much as Smith-Oka and Hurd described for Mexican clinicians, Malawian doctors and nurses went on strike not just for better wages but for working conditions that would allow them to do their jobs. Political diagnoses were not uncommon: some doctors explained that the country's shocking toll of road traffic accidents had to do with corrupt vehicle licensing and certification, and some nurse-midwives attributed a dreadful rate of maternal deaths to national policies that prioritized fines for out-of-hospital birth over training adequate numbers of skilled staff.

In 2020, as the coronavirus pandemic swept the globe, the striking contrasts I once saw between Malawian and American hospitals suddenly seemed much diminished. Both improvisation and political diagnosis quickly became hallmarks of hospital work in the United States too—and, by many accounts, of hospitals in other wealthy nations.

Improvisation made COVID care possible. Hallways were rapidly made into wards, clinics divided into "clean" and "dirty" spaces, lobbies converted overnight into triage zones. Health officials in Ireland, Spain, New York, and elsewhere organized heterogeneous arrays of public and private hospitals that had been competitors into coordinated networks that shared staff, supply chains, and other key infrastructures. Telemedicine projects decades in the making were implemented within weeks. Clinical trials began on short notice while sick people sought access to investigational therapies. An obstetrics resident in Wisconsin circulated advice on social media about how to make personal protective equipment with old transparency films, autoclave wrap, and cord. A hospitalist physician in Kentucky won plaudits from her colleagues by making face shields from two-liter soft-drink bottles. Hospitals mobilized eager volunteers to sew cloth masks for patients, visitors, and health personnel: they were far from perfect but much better than nothing. "Standard protocols" changed nearly every day, as respirators, masks, gowns and medications ran short. Clinicians exchanged provisional treatment guidelines for COVID-19 pneumonia across state and national borders, between private and public hospitals—then modified and recirculated them. Anticoagulants? Antimalarials? Prone posture? CPAP masks instead of ventilators? Two or more patients to a single ventilator? It was time to experiment, to improvise, as "ironclad emergency medical practices . . . dissolved almost overnight" (Dwyer 2020). Some of these improvised approaches probably killed people. Others became new standards.

Political diagnoses too were suddenly common in places where they had once been rare. In the United States, doctors and nurses and other staff, working hard to meet a disastrous challenge, found time to level fierce public critiques at federal leadership: why did we still have so few coronavirus tests? Where were the nation's stockpiles of critical equipment? How many people would die because the tests, the ventilators, the anesthesiologists, the protective gear ran short? Claims that "we are all in this together" rang hollow. The triage that had stretched across years and decades, comfortably invisible to those not injured by it, became much more difficult to overlook when compressed into the space of a few months. Why were Black and Brown communities suffering so many more deaths? How many people died because nursing-home workers and airplane cleaners were paid so poorly that they could not afford to leave work when they were sick? How many people died because health care is constructed around profit? Or because health insurance is connected, in the United States, with full-time employment, so that when a pandemic is complicated by massive unemployment the effects are synergistic?

Medical anthropologists, historians, and other keen observers of our biosocial worlds have long suspected that metastatic stage-IV capitalism is lethal (Beckfield and Krieger 2009; Hart 2010; Wallace et al. 2020). It has nonetheless seemed unstoppable, its infiltration into all social connective tissues and every part of the global circulatory system too advanced to treat. The relentlessness of its spread is powered by a model of *homo economicus* in which public good—if it exists at all—must not infringe upon private rapacity, a model in which heroism, altruism, and even community-mindedness are no more than foolish aberrations. Mary Douglas marveled at the power of institutions to reinforce this model. "Only by deliberate bias and by an extraordinarily disciplined effort," she wrote, "has it been possible to erect a theory of human behavior whose formal account of reasoning only considers the self-regarding motives" (Douglas 1986, 128). We could collectively chart other courses, she argued. But only if we understood institutions as communal sites in which we humans think together, instituting ideas—about who we are, how things work, what is of value, what is just—that we then imagine to be "natural."

At the moment I write, many of our key institutions are changing rapidly, and the prognosis for our collective biopolitical life is uncertain. Almost certainly, every hospital and health system described in this volume continues to grapple right now with the terrible effects of a pandemic, just as every country in which these ethnographers worked is facing economic injury and its downstream political and social effects. Some governments and hospitals that had seemed well prepared are in lethal disarray. Some hospitals and governments are facing grave challenges with unexpected resilience (Dalglish 2020). By the time the book is in print, perhaps ethnographers and historians and others will be assessing the pandemic's aftermath. The world will be forever changed. Hospitals will still think, and they will still triage. But they will be changed, too: they have been already. We just do not know, now, whether those changes will entail a brutal reinforcement of the status quo or its upheaval.

References

Aberese-Ako, Matilda. 2016. "'I Won't Take Part!': Exploring the Multiple Identities of the Ethnographer in Two Ghanaian Hospitals." *Ethnography* 18, no. 3: 300–321.

Abu-Lughod, Lila. 1991. "Writing Against Culture." In *Recapturing Anthropology*, edited by Richard G. Fox, 137–162. Santa Fe, NM: School of American Research Press.

Achilles, Kiwanuka. 2010. "Image of Nursing Profession as Viewed by Secondary School Students in Ilala District, Dar es Salaam." *Dar es Salaam Medical Students' Journal* 12–18.

Adams, Richard. 1994. "Guatemalan Ladinization and History." *The Americas* 50, no. 4: 527–43.

Adams, Vincanne. 2001. "The Sacred in the Scientific: Ambiguous Practices of Science in Tibetan Medicine." *Cultural Anthropology* 16, no. 4: 542–575.

Adjei, Patrick, et al. 2013. "Beliefs on Epilepsy in Northern Ghana." *Epilepsy and Behavior* 29:316–321.

Adoukonou, T. 2015. "Aspects Socioculturels de l'Epilepsi dans une Communaute Rurale au Nord Benin en 2011." *Bulletin de la Societe de Pathologie Exotique* 108, no. 2015: 133–138.

Agbo, Ines Elvire, Roch Christian Johnson, Ghislain Emmanuel Sopoh, and Mark Nichter. 2019. "The Gendered Impact of Buruli Ulcer on the Household Production of Health and Social Support Networks: Why Decentralization Favors Women." *PLoS Neglected Tropical Diseases* 13, no. 4.

Allotey, P., and D. Reidpath. 2007. "Epilepsy, Culture, Identity and Well-Being: A Study of the Social, Cultural, and Environmental Context of Epilepsy in Cameroon." *Journal of Health Psychology* 12, no. 3: 431–443.

American Academy of Pediatrics Committee on Drugs. 2014. "Off-Label Use of Drugs in Children." *Pediatrics* 133:563–567.

Amoussouhoui, Arnaud Setondji, Roch Christian Johnson, Ghislain Emmanuel Sopoh, Ines Elvire Agbo, Paulin Aoulou, Jean-Gabin Houezo, Albert Tingbe-Azalou, Micah Boyer, and Mark Nichter. 2016. "Steps Toward Creating a Therapeutic Community for Inpatients Suffering from Chronic Ulcers: Lessons from Allada Buruli Ulcer Treatment Hospital in Benin." *PLoS Neglected Tropical Diseases* 10, no. 7.

Andaya, Elise. 2009. "The Gift of Health: Socialist Medical Practice and Shifting Material and Moral Economies." *Medical Anthropology Quarterly* 23, no. 4: 357–374.

Andersen, Helle Max. 2004. "'Villagers': Differential Treat in a Ghanaian Hospital." *Social Science and Medicine* 59:2003–2012.

Anderson, Warwick. 2009. "Modern Sentinel and Colonial Microcosm: Science, Discipline, and Distress at the Philippine General Hospital." *Philippine Studies* 57, no. 2: 153–177.

Appadurai, Arjun. 1991. "Global Ethnoscapes: Notes and Queries for a Transnational Anthropology." In *Interventions*, edited by Richard G. Fox, 191–210. Santa Fe, NM: School of American Research.

Appadurai, Arjun. 1996. *Modernity at Large*. Minneapolis: University of Minnesota Press.

Appiah, Kwame. 2006. *Cosmopolitanism*. New York: Norton.

Archundia-García, Abel. 2011. "El Movimiento Médico en 1964–1965." *Revista de Especialidades Médico-Quirúrgicas* 16, no. 1: S28–S31.

Aujoulat, Isabelle, Christian Johnson, Claude Zinsou, Augustin Guédénon, and Françoise Portaels. 2003. "Psychosocial Aspects of Health Seeking Behaviours of Patients with Buruli Ulcer in Southern Benin." *Tropical Medicine & International Health* 8, no. 8: 750–759.

Austad, Kirsten, Anita Chary, Sandy Mux Xocop, Sarah Messmer, Nora King, Lauren Carlson, and Peter Rohloff. 2018. "Barriers to Cervical Cancer Screening and the Cervical Cancer Care Continuum in Rural Guatemala: A Mixed-Method Analysis." *Journal of Global Oncology* July (4): 1–10.

Auyero, Javier. 2012. *Patients of the State: The Politics of Waiting in Argentina*. Durham, NC: Duke University Press Books.

Bajpai, Vikas. 2014. "The Challenges Confronting Public Hospitals in India, Their Origins, and Possible Solutions." *Advances in Public Health* 2014:21–27.

Balibar, Etienne. 2012. "Civic Universalism and Its Internal Exclusions: The Issue of Anthropological Difference." *Boundary* 39, no. 1: 207–229.

Bardes, Charles L. 2009. "Defining "Patient-Centered Medicine." *Health Aff (Millwood)* 28, no. 4: w555–w565.

Barogui, Yves Thierry, Ghislain Emmanuel Sopoh, Roch Christian Johnson, Janine de Zeeuw, Ange Dodji Dossou, Jean Gabin Houezo, Annick Chauty et al. 2014. "Contribution of the Community Health Volunteers in the Control of Buruli Ulcer in Benin." *PLoS Neglected Tropical Diseases* 8, no. 10.

Barry, Andrew, Thomas Osborne, and Nikolas Rose, eds. 1996. *Foucault and Political Reason*. London: Taylor & Francis Group.

Beck, Ulrich. 1992. *Risk Society: Towards a New Modernity*. London: Sage.

Beckfield, Jason, and Nancy Krieger. 2009. "Epi + demos + cracy: Linking Political Systems and Priorities to the Magnitude of Health Inequities—Evidence, Gaps, and a Research Agenda." *Epidemiologic Reviews* 31, no. 1: 152–177.

Benagiano, G., and B. Thomas. 2003. "Safe Motherhood: The FIGO Initiative." *International Journal of Gynecology and Obstetrics* 82:263–274.

Benedict, Peter. 1976. "Aspects of the Domestic Cycle in a Turkish Provincial Town." In *Mediterranean Family Structures*, edited by J. G. Peristiany, 219–242. Cambridge: Cambridge University Press.

Berglund, S. 2012. "'Every Case of Asphyxia Can Be Used as a Learning Example': Conclusions from an Analysis of Substandard Obstetrical Care." *Journal of Perinatal Medicine* 40, no. 1: 9–18.

Bernard, H., Russell, Amber Wutich, and Gery Ryan. 2017. *Analyzing Qualitative Data: Systematic Approaches*. Newberry Park, CA: Sage.

Berry, Nicole S. 2008. "Who's Judging the Quality of Care? Indigenous Maya and the Problem of 'Not Being Attended.'" *Medical Anthropology* 27, no. 2: 164–189.

Berry, Nicole. 2010. *Unsafe Motherhood*. New York: Berghahn Books.

Bhabha, Homi K. 1994. *The Location of Culture*. New York: Routledge.

Bhabha, Homi K. 2017. "Spectral Sovereignty, Vernacular Cosmopolitans, and Cosmopolitan Memories." In *Cosmopolitanisms*, edited by Bruce Robbins and Paulo Horta, 141–152. New York: New York University Press.

Biehl, Joao. 2005. *Vita*. Berkeley: University of California Press.

Biehl, Joao. 2016. "Theorizing Global Health." *Medicine, Anthropology, Theory* 3, no. 2: 127–142.

Biershenk, Thomas, and Jean-Pierre Olivier de Sardan, eds. 2014. *States at Work: Dynamics of African Bureaucracies.* Leiden: E. J. Brill.

Boddy, Janice. 1998. "Remembering Amal." In *Pragmatic Women and Body Politics,* edited by Margaret Lock and Patricia Kaufert. Cambridge: Cambridge University Press.

Bottles, Kent. 2012. "Physician Leaders Should Embrace Patient Engagement/Activation." *Physician Executive* 38, no. 6: 68–70.

Bourdieu, Pierre. 1977. *Outline of a Theory of Practice.* Translated by Richard Nice. Cambridge, United Kingdom: Cambridge University Press.

Bourdieu, Pierre. 1986. *Distinction: A Social Critique of the Judgement of Taste.* Cambridge, MA: Harvard University Press.

Bourgois, P. 2010. "Recognizing Invisible Violence: A Thirty-year Ethnographic Retrospective." In *Global Health in Times of Violence,* edited by B. Rylko-Bauer, L. Whiteford, and P. Farmer, 17–40. Santa Fe, NM: School for Advanced Research Press.

Boylston, Tom. 2012. "The Shade of the Divine: Approaching the Sacred in an Ethiopian Orthodox Christian Community." PhD diss., London School of Economics.

Brhlikova, Petra, et al. 2009. "Intrapartum Oxytocin (Mis)use in South Asia." *Journal of Health Studies* 2:33–50.

Briggs, Charles, and Clara Mantini-Briggs. 2016. *Tell Me Why My Children Died.* Durham, NC: Duke University Press.

Bringa, Tone. 1995. *Being Muslim the Bosnian Way.* Princeton, NJ: Princeton University Press.

Brown, Hannah. 2012. "Hospital Domestics: Care Work in a Kenyan Hospital." *Space and Culture* 15, no. 1: 18–30.

Brunson, Emily K. 2013. "How Parents Make Decisions about Their Children's Vaccinations." *Vaccine* 31, no. 46: 5466–5470.

Calderón Sanchez, G. Amilcar. 2012. *Historia General de Nuñoa: Ensayos.* Lima, Peru: Editorial San Marcos.

Camacho, A. V., M. D. Castro, and R. Kaufman. 2006. "Cultural Aspects Related to the Health of Andean Women in Latin America: A Key Issue for Progress toward the Attainment of Millennium Development Goals." *International Journal of Obstetrics and Gynecology and Obstetrics* 94 no. 3: 357–363.

Campbell, J. K. 1964. *Honour, Family and Patronage.* Oxford: Oxford University Press.

Caraveli, Anna. 1986. "The Bitter Wounding." In *Gender and Power in Rural Greece,* edited by Jill Dubisch, 169–194. Princeton, NJ: Princeton University Press.

Carey, Matthew, and Morten Axel Pedersen. 2017. "Introduction: Infrastructures of Certainty and Doubt." *Cambridge Journal of Anthropology* 35, no. 2:18–29.

Carpenter, Mick. 2003. "On the Edge: The Fate of Progressive Modernization in Greek Health Policy." *International Political Science Review* 24, no. 2: 257–272.

Carpio, Carmen, and Natalia Santiago Bench. 2015. *The Health Workforce in Latin America and the Caribbean.* Washington, DC: The World Bank.

Case, Spencer. 2014. "Cultural Perspectives on Traditional and Medical Treatments for Mental Health Problems in Ghana." M.S. Thesis. Georgetown University.

Castaneda, Claudia. 2002. *Figurations: Child, Bodies, Worlds.* Durham, NC: Duke University Press.

Castro, A., and V. Savage. 2019. "Obstetric Violence as Reproductive Governance in the Dominican Republic." *Medical Anthropology* 38, no. 2: 123–136.

CEDAW (Committee on the Elimination of Discrimination against Women). 2013. Concluding Observations on the Seventh Periodic Report of Greece Adopted by the Committee at Its 54th Session (11 February–March 2013).

Central Intelligence Agency. 2020. "The World Factbook." Last updated March 15, 2020.

Chabal, Patrick, and Jean-Pascal Daloz. 1999. *Africa Works: Disorder as Political Instrument*. London: International Africa Institute; Oxford: James Currey; Bloomington: Indiana University Press.

Chabrol, Fanny. 2018. "Viral Hepatitis and a Hospital Infrastructure in Ruins in Cameroon." *Medical Anthropology* 37, no. 8: 645–658.

Chadwick, Rachelle. 2017. "Ambiguous Subjects: Obstetric Violence, Assemblage and South African Birth Narratives." *Feminism & Psychology* 27, no. 4: 489–509.

Chang, Bernard S., and Daniel Lowenstein. 2003. "Epilepsy." *New England Journal of Medicine* 349:1257–1266.

Chapkis, Wendy, and Richard J. Webb. 2008. *Dying to Get High: Marijuana as Medicine*. New York: New York University Press.

Chary, Anita. 2015. "Hysterectomies and Healer Shopping: Cervical Cancer and Therapeutic Anarchy in Guatemala." In *Privatization and the New Medical Pluralism: Shifting Healthcare Landscapes in Maya Guatemala*, edited by A. Chary & P. Rohloff, 107–124. Lanham, MD: Lexington Press.

Chary, Anita. 2017. *"A Poor Woman's Disease": An Ethnography of Cervical Cancer and Global Health in Guatemala*. Doctoral diss., Anthropology: Washington University in St. Louis, Missouri.

Chary, Anita, David Flood, Kirsten Austad, Jessica Hawkins, Katia Cnop, Boris Martínez, Waleska López, and Peter Rohloff. 2018. "Accompanying Indigenous Maya Patients with Complex Medical Needs: A Patient Navigation System in Rural Guatemala." *Healthcare: The Journal of Delivery Science and Innovation* 6, no. 2: 144–149.

Chary, Anita, David Flood, Kirsten Austad, Jillian Moore, Nora King, Boris Martínez, Pablo Garcia, Waleska Lopez, Shom Dasgupta-Tsikinas, and Peter Rohloff. 2016. "Navigating Bureaucracy: Accompanying Indigenous Maya Patients with Complex Healthcare Needs in Guatemala." *Human Organization* 75 (4, Winter): 305–14.

Chary, Anita, and Peter Rohloff, eds. 2015. *Privatization and the New Medical Pluralism: Shifting Healthcare Landscapes in Maya Guatemala*. Lanham, MD: Lexington Books.

Chatjouli, Aiglaia. 2015. "(In)fertility and ART Drugs. Making Sense of ART Drug Consumption and the Art of Achieving Motherhood." In *(In)Fertile Citizens: Anthropological and Legal Challenges of Assisted Reproductive Technologies*, edited by Venetia Kantsa, Giulia Zanini, and Lina Papadoupoulou. University of the Aegean.

Cheliotis, Leonidas. 2016. "Punitive Inclusion: The Political Economy of Irregular Migration on the Margins of Europe." *European Journal of Criminology* 1–22.

Chuwa, Leonard Tumaini. 2014. *African Indigenous Ethics in Global Bioethics: Interpreting Ubuntu*. Vol. 1. Springer.

Clark, Jocalyn. 2016. "The Global Push for Institutional Childbirths—in Unhygienic Facilities." *BMJ* 352: 3 pages.

Clarke, Adele, et al. 2010. *Biomedicalization. Technoscience, Health and Illness in the U.S.* Durham, NC: Duke University Press.

Clifford, James. 1992. "Traveling Cultures." In *Cultural Studies*, edited by Larry Grossberg, 96–116. London: Routledge.

Clifford, James. 1997. *Routes*. Cambridge, MA: Harvard University Press.

Cohen, Nissim. 2012. "Informal Payments for Health Care—the Phenomenon and Its Context." *Health Economics, Policy and Law* 7:285–308.

Coleman, Rosalind, et al. 2002. "The Treatment Gap and Primary Health Care for People with Epilepsy in Rural Gambia." *Bulletin of the World Health Organization* 80:378–383.

Colen, Shelee. 1986. "With Respect and Feelings." Voices of West Indian Childcare and Domestic Workers in New York City. In *All American Women: Lines that Divide, Ties that Bind*, edited by Johnnetta B. Cole. New York: Free Press.

Collier, Jane. 1997. *From Duty to Desire*. Princeton, NJ: Princeton University Press.

Colombotos, John, and Nikos Fakiolas. 1993. "The Power of Organized Medicine in Greece." In *The Changing Medical Profession: An International Perspective*, edited by F. Hafferty and J. McKinlay, 138–149. New York: Oxford University Press.

Comaroff, Jean, and John Comaroff. 1997. *Of Revelation and Revolution: The Dialectics of Modernity on a South African Frontier*. Vol. II. Chicago: University of Chicago Press.

Cooper, Barbara M. 2006. *Evangelical Christians in the Muslim Sahel*. Bloomington: Indiana University Press.

Corbin J., and A. Strauss. 1985. "Managing Chronic Illness at Home: Three Lines of Work." *Qualitative Sociology* 8, no. 3: 224–247.

Cutileiro, Jose. 1971. *A Portuguese Rural Society*. Oxford: Oxford University Press.

Dalglish, Sarah L. 2020. "COVID-19 Gives the Lie to Global Health Expertise." *The Lancet* 395, no. 10231:1189.

Dastur, F. D. 2016. "Public Health—The 'Black Hole' in Indian Medical Services." *Journal of the Association of Physicians of India* 64:70–72.

Davis, Dána-Ain. 2019. "Obstetric Racism: The Racial Politics of Pregnancy, Labor, and Birthing." *Medical Anthropology* 38, no. 7: 560–573.

Davis, John. 1973. *Land and Family in Pisticci*. London: Athlone.

Davis, Sara L. 2017. "The Uncounted: Politics of Data and Visibility in Global Health." *The International Journal of Human Rights* 21, no. 8: 1144–1163.

Davis-Floyd, Robbie. 1992. *Birth as an American Rite of Passage*. Berkeley: University of California Press.

Davis-Floyd, Robbie. 2018. "The Technocratic, Humanistic, and Holistic Paradigms of Birth and Health Care." In *Ways of Knowing about Birth: Mothers, Midwives, Medicine, and Birth Activism*, edited by Robbie Davis-Floyd et al., 3–40. Long Grove, IL: Waveland Press.

Davis-Floyd, Robbie, and Melissa Cheyney, eds. 2019. *Birth in Eight Cultures*. Long Grove, IL: Waveland Press.

Dawson, Angela J., et al. 2014. "Task Shifting and Sharing in Maternal and Reproductive Health in Low-Income Countries: A Narrative Synthesis of Current Evidence." *Health Policy and Planning* 29, no. 3: 396–408.

De Brouwere, Vincent at al. 2013. "Maternal Death Reviews." *Lancet* 381:1718–1719.

de-Graft Aikins, Ama. 2015. "Mental Illness and Destitution in Africa." In *The Culture of Mental Illness and Psychiatric Practice in Africa*, edited by A. Akyeampong, Allan Hill, and Arthur Kleinman, 112–143. Bloomington: Indiana University Press.

del Valle Escalante, Emilio. 2009. *Maya Nationalisms and Postcolonial Challenges in Guatemala: Colonality, Modernity, and Identity Politics*. Santa Fe, NM: School for Advanced Research Press.

DeMello e Souza, Cecilia. 1994. "C-Sections as Ideal Births: The Cultural Constructions of Beneficence and Patients' Rights in Brazil." *Cambridge Quarterly of Healthcare Ethics* 3:358–366.

Development Goals. 2006. *International Journal of Obstetrics and Gynecology and Obstetrics*, 94(3), 357–363.

Devinsky, O., J.H.P. Cross, L. Laux, E. Marsh, I. Miller, R. Nabbout, I. E. Scheffer, E. A. Thiele, and S. Wright, for the Cannabidiol in Dravet Syndrome Study Group. 2017. "Trial of Cannabidiol for Drug-Resistant Seizures in the Dravet Syndrome." *New England Journal of Medicine* 376, no. 21: 2011–2020.

Devries, Raymond, et al., eds. 2001. *Birth by Design: Pregnancy, Maternity Care and Midwifery in North America and Europe*. New York: Routledge.

Diaz-Tello, Farah. 2016. "Invisible Wounds: Obstetric Violence in the United States." *Reproductive Health Matters* 24, no. 47: 56–64.

Diniz, Simone, and A. S. Chacham. 2004. "'The Cut Above' and 'the Cut Below': The Abuse of Cesareans and Episiotomy in Sao Paulo, Brazil." *Reproductive Health Matters* 12, no. 23: 100–110.

Dixon, Lydia Zacher. 2015. "Obstetrics in a Time of Violence: Mexican Midwives Critique Routine Hospital Practices." *Medical Anthropology Quarterly* 29, no. 4: 437–454.

D'Oliveira, Ana F., Simone G. Diniz, and Lilia B. Schraiber. 2002. "Violence against Women in Health-Care Institutions: An Emerging Problem." *Lancet* 359, no. 9318: 1681–1685.

Donham, Donald L. 1999. *Marxist Modern*. Berkeley: University of California Press.

Douglas, Mary. 1986. *How Institutions Think*. Syracuse, NY: Syracuse University Press.

du Bouley, Juliette. 1974. *Portrait of a Greek Mountain Village*. Oxford: Oxford University Press.

Dubisch, Jill. 1991. "Gender, Kinship and Religion: 'Reconstructing' the Anthropology of Greece." In *Contested Identities: Gender and Kinship in Modern Greece*, edited by P. Loizos and E. Papataxiarchis, 29–46. Princeton, NJ: Princeton University Press.

Dubisch, Jill. 1995. *In a Different Place*. Princeton, NJ: Princeton University Press.

Duncan, Whitney. 2018. *Transforming Therapy: Mental Health Practice and Cultural Change in Mexico*. Nashville, TN: Vanderbilt University Press.

Dwyer, Jim. 2020. "What Doctors on the Front Lines Wish They'd Known a Month Ago." *The New York Times*, April 14, 2020.

Ecks, Stefan, and Ian Harper. 2013. "Public-Private Mixes: The Market for Antituberculosis Drugs in India." In *When People Come First: Critical Studies in Global Health*, edited by João Biehl and Adriana Petryna, 252–275. Princeton, NJ: Princeton University Press.

Economou, Charalampos, et al. 2017. "Greece: Health System Review." *Health Systems in Transition* 19, no. 5: 1–166.

Emanuel, Ezekiel J., and Linda L. Emanuel. 1992 "Four Models of the Physician-Patient Relationship." *Jama* 267, no. 16: 2221–2226.

Ence, Nic. 2006. "Tuberculosis: Perceptions in Mampong, Ghana." B.A. Thesis. Brigham Young University.

Enciso, Angélica L. 2014. "Miles de Médicos Demandan no Criminalizar su Actividad." *La Jornada,* June 23, 2014.

England, Roger. 2007. "The Dangers of Disease Specific Programs for Developing Countries." *BMI* 335, no. 7619: 565–565.

Epstein, Ronald M., and Richard L. Street. 2011. "The Values and Value of Patient-centered Care." *Annals of Family Medicine* 9:100–103.

Erickson, Susan. 2008. "Getting Political." *Lancet* 371, no. 9620: 1229–1230.

Ewig, Christina. 2010. *Second-Wave Neoliberalism*. College Station, PA: Pennsylvania State University Press.

Excelsior. 2014. "#YoSoy17: La Muerte del Joven que Desató un Movimiento Nacional." *Excelsior,* June 23, 2014.

Farmer, Paul. 2005. *Pathologies of Power*. Berkeley: University of California Press.

Fassin, Didier. 2011. *Humanitarian Reason*. Berkeley: University of California Press.

Faubion, James. 1993. *Modern Greek Lessons: A Primer in Historical Constructivism*. Princeton, NJ: Princeton University Press.

Fealy, Gerard M. 2004. "'The Good Nurse': Visions and Values in Images of the Nurse." *Journal of Advanced Nursing* 46, no. 6: 649–656.

Ferguson, James. 2006. *Global Shadows*. Durham, NC: Duke University Press.

Ferlay, J., H. R. Shin, F. Bray, et al. 2012. "GLOBOCAN 2012, Cancer Incidence and Mortality Worldwide: IARC Cancer Base No. 10." Lyon, France: International Agency for Research on Cancer.

Fikree, Fariyal F., Ali M. Mir, and Inaam-ul Haq. 2006. "She May Reach a Facility but Will Still Die! An Analysis of Quality of Public Sector Maternal Health Services, District Multan, Pakistan." *Journal of the Pakistan Medical Association* 56:156–163.

Finkler, Kaja. 2001. *Physicians at Work, Patients in Pain*. Durham, NC: Carolina Academic Press.

Finkler, Kaja. 2004. "Biomedicine Globalized and Localized: Western Medical Practices in an Outpatient Clinic of a Mexican Hospital." *Social Science & Medicine* 59:2037–2051.

Finkler, Kaja. 2008. "Can Bioethics Be Global and Local, or Must It Be Both?" *Journal of Contemporary Ethnography* 37, no. 2: 155–179.

Finkler, Kaja, Cynthia Hunter, and Rick Iedema. 2008. "What Is Going On? Ethnography in Hospital Spaces." *Journal of Contemporary Ethnography* 37, no. 2: 246–250.

Finkler, Kaja, and Sjaak van der Geest. 2004. "Hospital Ethnography." *Social Science & Medicine* 59, no. 10:1995–2001.

Fletcher, Anita. 2015. "Stigma and Quality of Life at Long-Term Follow-Up after Surgery for Epilepsy in Uganda." *Epilepsy and Behavior* 52:128–138.

Foley, Ellen. 2008. "Neoliberal Reform and Health Dilemmas." *Medical Anthropology Quarterly* 22, no. 3:257–273.

Foucault, Michel. 1994. *The Birth of the Clinic: An Archaeology of Medical Perception*. Translated by A. M. Sheridan Smith. New York: Vintage Books.

Francke, Pedro. 2013. *Peru's Comprehensive Health Insurance and New Challenges for Universal Coverage*. UNICO Study Series No. 11. Washington, DC: World Bank.

Frankenberg, Ronald, Ian Robinson, and Amber Delahooke. 2000. "Countering Essentialism in Behavioural Social Science: The Example of 'the Vulnerable Child' Ethnographically Examined." *Sociological Review* 48, no. 4:586–611.

Frenk, Julio, Jaime Sepúlveda, Octavio Gómez-Dantés, and Felicia Knaul. 2003. "Evidence-Based Health Policy: Three Generations of Reform in Mexico." *Lancet* 362:1667–1671.

Friedman, Daniel, and Joseph I. Sirven. 2017. "Historical Perspective on the Medical Use of Cannabis for Epilepsy: Ancient Times to the 1980s." *Epilepsy & Behavior* 70 (Part B):298–301.

Fujita, Noriko, Xavier R. Perrin, Joséf A. Vodounon, Michel K. Gozo, Yasuyo Matsumoto, Sanae Uchida, and Yasuo Sugiura. 2012. "Humanised Care and a Change in Practice in a Hospital in Benin." *Midwifery* 28, no. 4: 481–488.

Fund for Peace. 2020. *Fragile States Index*. Washington, DC: The Fund for Peace.

Gadamer, Hans Georg. 1975. *Truth and Method*. London: Continuum International Publishing Group.

Geissler, P. W. 2013. "Public Secrets in Public Health: Knowing Not to Know While Making Scientific Knowledge." *American Ethnologist* 40, no. 1: 13–34.

Geissler, Paul W., Richard Rottenburg, and Julia Zenker, eds. 2012. *Rethinking Biomedicine and Governance in Africa: Contributions from Anthropology*. Bielefeld, Germany: Transcript Verlag.

George, Asha. 2007. "Persistence of High Maternal Mortality in Koppal District, Karnataka, India: Observed Service Delivery Constraints." *Reproductive Health Matters* 15, no. 30: 91–102.

Georges, Eugenia. 1996. "Fetal Ultrasound Imaging and the Production of Authoritative Knowledge in Greece." *Medical Anthropology Quarterly* (ns), 10, no. 2: 1–19.

Georges, Eugenia. 2008. *Bodies of Knowledge*. Nashville, TN: Vanderbilt University Press.

Georges, Eugenia, and Rae Dallenbach. 2019. "Divergent Meanings and Practices of Childbirth in Greece and New Zealand." In *Birth in Eight Cultures*, edited by Robbie Davis-Floyd and Melissa Cheyney, 129–164. Long Grove, IL: Waveland Press.

Geschiere, Peter. 2013. *Witchcraft, Intimacy and Trust*. Chicago: University of Chicago Press.

Geschiere, Peter, and Roitman, J. 1997. *The Modernity of Witchcraft: Politics and the Occult in Postcolonial Africa*. Charlottesville, VA: University of Virginia Press.

Ghana Ministry of Health. 2015. *Ghana's Fight Against Epilepsy*. Accra: Ministry of Health.

Gibson, Diana. 2004. "The Gaps in the Gaze in South African Hospitals." *Social Science and Medicine* 59:2013–2024.

Giddens, Anthony. 1991. *The Consequences of Modernity*. Cambridge: Polity Press.

Gilmour, Jean A. 2006. "Hybrid Space: Constituting the Hospital as a Home Space for Patients." *Nursing Inquiry* 13, no. 1:16–22.

Gimlin, Debra. 2007. "What Is 'Body work'? A review of the literature." *Sociology Compass*, 353–370.

Ginsburg, Faye, and Rapp, Rayna. 1995. "Introduction: Conceiving the New World Order." In *Conceiving the New World Order: The Global Politics of Reproduction*, edited by Faye Ginsburg and Rayna Rapp, 1–17. Berkeley: University of California Press.

Glaser, Barney G., and Anselm Strauss. 1967. *The Discovery of Grounded Theory*. New York: Aldine de Gruyter.

Good, Byron. 1994. *Medicine, Rationality, and Experience*. Cambridge: Cambridge University Press.

Good, Mary-Jo Delvecchio, Cara James, Byron Good, and Anne Becker. 2002. "The Culture of Medicine and Racial, Ethnic, and Class Disparities in Healthcare." In *Unequal Treatment*, edited by Brian Smedley, Adrienne Stith, and Alan Nelson, 594–625. Washington, DC: National Academy Press.

Gottschalk, Louis A., and Goldine C. Gleser. 1969. *The Measurement of Psychological States Through Analysis of Verbal Behavior*. Berkeley: University of California Press.

Gouda, Hebe E., et al. 2017. "New Challenges for Verbal Autopsy: Considering the Ethical and Social Implications of Verbal Autopsy Methods in Routine Health Information Systems." *Social Science & Medicine* 184:65–74.

Government of Gilgit-Baltistan and UNICEF. 2017. *Gilgit-Baltistan Final Report: Monitoring the Situation of Children and Women, Multiple Indicator Cluster Survey 2016–2017*. Gilgit: Planning and Development Department.

Greene, Jessica, and Judith H. Hibbard. 2012. "Why Does Patient Activation Matter? An Examination of the Relationships between Patient Activation and Health-Related Outcomes." *Journal of General Internal Medicine* 27, no. 5: 520–526.

Greenhalgh, Susan. 2001. *Under the Medical Gaze*. Berkeley: University of California Press.

Groupement Hospitalier de Territoire Plaine de France Centres Hospitaliers de Saint-Denis et de Gonesse. Rapport d'activite 2018. Accessed October 1, 2018. http://www.ch.stdenis.fr.

Grünebaum, Amos, et al. 2015. "Home Birth Is Unsafe. For: The Safety of Planned Homebirths: A Clinical Fiction. Against: Safe for Whom?" *BJOG Debate* 122, no. 9: 1235.

Guerra-Reyes, Lucia. 2016. "Implementing a Culturally Appropriate Birthing Policy: Ethnographic Analysis of the Experiences of Skilled Birth Attendants." *Journal of Public Health Policy*, 37, no. 3, 353–68.

Gupta, Akhil. 1997. *Anthropological Locations*. Berkeley: University of California Press.

Gupta, Akhil. 2012. *Red Tape*. Durham, NC: Duke University Press Books.

Gupta, Akhil, and James Ferguson. 1997. *Culture, Power, Place: Explorations in Critical Anthropology.* Durham, NC: Duke University Press

Gutschow, Kim. 2016. "Going 'Beyond the Numbers': Maternal Death Reviews in India." *Medical Anthropology* 35, no. 4: 322–337.

Hamdy, Sherine F. 2008. "When the State and Your Kidneys Fail: Political Etiologies in an Egyptian Dialysis Ward." *American Ethnologist* 35, no. 4: 553–569.

Hamdy, Sherine. 2012. *Our Bodies Belong to God.* Berkeley: University of California Press.

Hamlin, Catherine, with John Little. 2001. *The Hospital by the River.* Oxford: Monarch Books.

Hanna, Bridget, and Arthur Kleinman. 2013. "Unpacking Global Health." In *Reimagining Global Health*, edited by Paul Farmer et al., 15–32. Berkeley: University of California Press.

Hannig, Anita. 2013. "The Pure and the Pious: Corporeality, Flow, and Transgression in Ethiopian Orthodox Christianity." *Journal of Religion in Africa* 43, no. 3: 297–328.

Hannig, Anita. 2014. "Spiritual Border Crossings: Childbirth, Postpartum Seclusion, and Religious Alterity in Amhara, Ethiopia." *Africa* 84 (2): 294–313.

Hannig, Anita. 2017. *Beyond Surgery.* Chicago: University of Chicago Press.

Hanson, C., J. Cox, G. Mbaruku, et al. 2015. "Maternal mortality and distance to facility-based obstetric care in rural southern Tanzania: a secondary analysis of cross-sectional census data in 226 000 households." *Lancet Global Health* 3, no. 7: e387–e395.

Hart, Gillian. 2010. "D/developments after the Meltdown." *Antipode* 41(S1): 117–141.

Hautefeuille, Michel. 2011. "Les communautés thérapeutiques." *Psychotropes* 17, no. 3: 5–8.

Henderson, Sara, and Alan Petersen, eds. 2001. *Consuming Health: The Commodification of Health Care.* New York: Routledge.

Herzfeld, Michael. 1997. *Cultural Intimacy: Social Poetics in the Nation-State.* New York, London: Routledge.

Hetherington, Kregg. 2011. *Guerrilla Auditors.* Durham, NC: Duke University Press.

Hionidou, Violetta. 2020. Abortion and Contraception in Modern Greece, 1830-1967: Medicine, Sexuality and Popular Culture. Cham, Switzerland: Palgrave.

Hoben, Allan. 1970. "Social Stratification in Traditional Amhara Society." In *Social Stratification in Africa*, edited by Arthur Tuden and Leonard Plotnicov, 187–224. New York: Free Press.

Horne, J., 2014. "The Salary You Need to Buy a Home Here in San Diego." *Union Tribune.* San Diego, CA. May 22.

Horsley, Philomena A. 2008. "Death Dwells in Spaces: Bodies in the Hospital Mortuary." *Anthropology & Medicine* 15, no. 2: 133–146.

Howes-Mischel, Rebecca. 2016. "'With This You Can Meet Your Baby': Fetal Personhood and Audible Heartbeats in Oaxacan Public Health." *Medical Anthropology Quarterly* 30, no. 2: 186–202.

Huicho, Luis, E. R. Segura, C. A. Huayanay-Espinoza, J. Niño de Guzman, M. C. Restrepo-Mendez, Y. Tam, A. J. D. Barros, and C. G. Victora. 2016. "Child Health and Nutrition in Peru with an Anti-poverty Political Agenda: A Countdown to 2015 Country Case Study." *Lancet Global Health* 4:414–426.

Hull, Elizabeth. 2017. *Contingent Citizens.* London: Bloomsbury.

Illich, Ivan. 1976. *Limits to Medicine—Medical Nemesis.* New York: Pantheon Books.

INEGI. 2017. "México en Cifras." *Instituto Nacional de Estadística y Geografía,* Accessed March 20, 2017. http://www.beta.inegi.org.mx/app/areasgeograficas/?ag=21.

Inhorn, Marcia. 1996. *Infertility and Patriarchy.* Philadelphia: University of Pennsylvania Press.

Inhorn, Marcia C. 2004. "Privacy, Privatization, and the Politics of Patronage: Ethnographic Challenges to Penetrating the Secret World of Middle Eastern, Hospital-Based in Vitro Fertilization." *Social Science & Medicine* 59:2095–2108.

Inhorn, Marcia. 2006. "Making Muslim Babies: IVF and Gamete Donation in Sunni versus Shi'a Islam." *Culture, Medicine, and Psychiatry* 30, no. 4: 427–450.

Institute of Medicine Committee on Quality of Health Care in America. 2001. *Crossing the Quality Chasm: A New Health System for the 21st Century.* Washington DC: National Academy Press.

Jacay, Sheilah. 2012. "The Operation of Biopower and Biopolitics in the Implementation Process of Reproductive Health Policies in Peru." Master's thesis, University of Waikato, Hamilton, NZ.

Jackson, Michael. 1998. *Minima Ethnographica.* Chicago: University of Chicago Press.

Jafarey, S., I. Kamal, A. F. Qureshi, and F. Fikree. 2008. "Safe Motherhood in Pakistan." *International Journal of Gynecology & Obstetrics* 102, no. 2: 179–185.

Jafarey, Sadiqua N. and Arjumand Rabbani. 2014. "Maternal Mortality in Pakistan." *JSOGP* 4, no. 3: 133–136.

Jaffré, Yannick. 2012. "Towards an Anthropology of Public Health Priorities: Maternal Mortality in Four Obstetric Emergency Services in West Africa." *Social Anthropology/Anthropologie Sociale* 20, no. 1: 3–18.

Jaffré, Yannick, and Siri Suh. 2016. "Where the Lay and the Technical Meet: Using an Anthropology of Interfaces to Explain Persistent Reproductive Health Disparities in West Africa." *Social Science & Medicine* 156:175–183.

Jaffré, Yannick, and Alain Prual. 1994. "Midwives in Niger: An Uncomfortable Position Between Social Behaviours and Health Care Constraints." *Social Science & Medicine* 38, no. 8: 1069–1073.

Janzen, John M. 1978. *Quest for Therapy.* Berkeley: University of California Press.

Janzen, John M. 2015. "Divergent Legitimations of Post-State Health Institutions in Western Equatorial Africa." *Working Paper Series 14, SPP 1448, Adaptation & Creativity in Africa.* University of Halle-Wittenberg. Halle/Saale, Germany.

Janzen, John. 2017. "Science in the Moral Space of Health and Healing Paradigms in Western Equatorial Africa." In *African Medical Pluralism,* edited by W. C. Olsen and C. Sargent, 90–109. Bloomington: Indiana University Press.

Janzen, John M. 2019. *Health in a Fragile State.* Madison: University of Wisconsin Press.

Jeffery, Patricia, and Roger Jeffery. 2010. "Only When the Boat Has Started Sinking: A Maternal Death in Rural North India." *Social Science & Medicine* 71:1711–1718.

Jeffrey, Patricia, and Petra Brhlikova. 2009. "Tracing Pharmaceuticals in South Asia: Use and Abuse of Oxytocin: Millennium Development Goals 4 and 5 in South Asia: Draft Working Paper." School of Social & Political Science and Centre for South Asian Studies, University of Edinburgh.

Jewkes, Rachel, Naeemah Abrahams, and Zudumo Mvo. 1998. "Why Do Nurses Abuse Patients? Reflections from South African Obstetric Services." *Social Science & Medicine* 47, no. 11: 1781–1795.

Jilek-Aall, Louise. 1997. "Psychosocial Study of Epilepsy in Africa." *Social Science and Medicine* 45:783–790.

Jordan, Brigitte. 1993. *Birth in Four Cultures.* New York: Waveland.

Juan López, Mercedes, Adolfo Martínez Valle, and Nelly Aguilera. 2015. "Reforming the Mexican Health System to Achieve Effective Health Care Coverage." *Health Systems & Reform* 1, no. 3: 181–188.

Jusadanis, Gregory. 1992. *Belated Modernity and Aesthetic Culture.* Minneapolis: University of Minnesota Press.

Kahn, Susan Martha. 2000. *Reproducing Jews.* Durham, NC: Duke University Press.

Kaitelidou, Daphne, et al. 2012. "Understanding the Oversupply of Physicians in Greece: The Role of Human Resources Planning, Financing Policy, and Physician Power." *International Journal of Health Services* 42, no. 4: 719–738.

Kaitelidou, Daphne, et al. 2013. "Informal Payments for Maternity Health Services in Public Hospitals in Greece." *Health Policy* 109:23–30.

Kalyvas, Stathis N. 2015. *Modern Greece: What Everyone Needs to Know.* New York: Oxford University Press.

Kamwangamalu, Nkonko M. 1999. "Ubuntu in South Africa: A sociolinguistic perspective to a Pan-African concept." *Critical Arts* 13, no. 2: 24–41.

Kariuki, Symon, et al. 2014. "Clinical Features, Proximate Causes, and Consequences of Active Convulsive Epilepsy in Africa." *Epilepsia* 55:76–85.

Kaufman, Sharon. 2005. *And a Time to Die: How American Hospitals Shape the End of Life.* New York: Scribner.

Kehr, Janina. 2018. "Colonial Hauntings: Migrant Care in a French Hospital." *Medical Anthropology* 37, no. 8: 659–673.

Keshavjee, Salman. 2014. *Blind Spot.* Berkeley: University of California Press.

Khuri, Fuad. 1975. *From Village to Suburb.* Chicago: University of Chicago Press.

Kilroy-Marac, Katie. 2019. *An Impossible Inheritance.* Berkeley: University of California Press.

Kingori, P., and R. Gerrets. 2016. "Morals, Morale and Motivations in Data Fabrication: Medical Research Field Workers Views and Practices in Two Sub-Saharan African Contexts." *Social Science & Medicine* 166:150–159.

Klassen, Pamela E. 2011. *Spirits of Protestantism.* Berkeley: University of California Press.

Kleinman Arthur. 1998. *The Illness Narratives.* New York: Basic Books.

Kleinman, Arthur. 2009. "Caregiving: The Odyssey of Becoming More Human." *The Lancet* 373:292–293.

Kleinman, Arthur. 2012. "Caregiving as Moral Experience." *The Lancet* 380:3550–3551.

Kleinman, Arthur, and Peter Benson. 2006. "Anthropology in the Clinic: The Problem of Cultural Competency and How to Fix It." *PLoS Medicine* 3, no. 10.

Knight, H. E., A. Self, and S. H. Kennedy. 2013. "Why Are Women Dying When They Reach Hospital on Time? A Systematic Review of the 'Third Delay.'" *PloS One* 8, no. 5: e63846.

Kofi, Antwi. 1996. "Role of Ashanti Mampong District Hospital in the Primary Health Care Delivery System in the Sekyere West District, Ashanti Region." B.A. thesis, University of Ghana, Legon.

Kofu, Jesse. 4 March 2016. "6 Suspended as Twins Die at a Hospital." *The Citizen.* https://www.thecitizen.co.tz/news/6-suspended-as-twins-die-at-a-hospital /1840340-3103254-format-xhtml-v2211uz/index.html.

Kohn, Linda T., Janet M. Corrigan, and Molla S. Donaldson, eds. 2000. *To Err is Human: Building a Safer Health System.* For the Committee on Quality of Health Care in America, Institute of Medicine ed. Washington, DC: National Academy Press.

Kotobi, Laurence, Stephanie Larchanche, and Zahia Kessar. 2013. "Enjeux et Logiques du Recours à l'Interprétariat en Milieu Hospitalier: Une Recherche-action Autour de l'Annonce d'une Maladie Grave.' *Migrations Santé* 146–147:53–80.

Kristoffersen, Margareth, and Febe Friberg. 2017. "Relationship-based Nursing Care and Destructive Demands." *Nursing Ethics* 24, no. 6, 663–674.

Laine, Christine, and Frank Davidoff. 1996. "Patient-Centered Medicine: A Professional Evolution." *Jama* 275, no. 2: 152–156.

Langwick, Stacey. 2008. "Articulate(d) Bodies: Traditional Medicine in a Tanzanian Hospital." *American Ethnologist* 35, no. 3: 428–39.

Larchanche, Stephanie. 2012. "Intangible Obstacles: Health Implications of Stigmatiza-
    tion, Structural Violence, and Fear among Undocumented Immigrants in France."
    Social Science and Medicine 74, no. 6: 858–863.

Larme, Ann. 1998. "Environment, Vulnerability and Gender in Andean Medicine."
    Social Science and Medicine 47, no. 8, 1005–1015.

Larme, Ann, and Leatherman, Thomas. 2003. "Why Sobreparto? Women's Work,
    Health, and Reproduction in Two Districts in Southern Peru." In *Medical Pluralism in
    the Andes*, edited by J. Koss- Chioino, T. L. Leatherman, and C. Greenway, 191–208
    New York: Routledge.

Last, Murray. 1986. "Introduction." In *The Professionalization of African Medicine*, edited by
    Murray Last and G. L. Chavunduka, 1–29. Manchester: University of Manchester Press.

Lawrence, Christopher M. 2007. *Blood and Oranges*. New York: Berghahn Books.

Lee, Martin A. 2012. *Smoke Signals*. New York: Scribner.

Lee, Ellie, Jan Macvarish, and Jennie Bristow. 2010. "Risk, Health and Parenting Cul-
    ture." *Health, Risk & Society* 12, no. 4: 293–300.

Levine, Donald. 1965. *Wax and Gold*. Chicago: University of Chicago Press.

Liaschenko, Joan, and Elizabeth Peter. 2004. "Nursing Ethics and Conceptualizations
    of Nursing: Profession, Practice, and Work." *Journal of Advanced Nursing* 46, no. 5:
    488–495.

Lison-Tolosano, Carmelo. 1966. *Belmonte de los Caballeros*. Oxford: Oxford University
    Press.

Little, John. 2010. *Catherine's Gift*. Oxford: Monarch Books.

Livingston, Julie. 2012. *Improvising Medicine*. Durham, NC: Duke University Press.

Lock, Margaret. 2002. *Twice Dead*. Berkeley: University of California Press.

Lock, Margaret, and Vinh-Kim Nguyen. 2010. *An Anthropology of Biomedicine*. New
    York: Wiley.

Lock, Margaret, and Kaufert, Patricia, eds. 1998. *Pragmatic Women and Body Politics*.
    Cambridge: Cambridge University Press.

Long, Debbi, Cynthia Hunter, and Sjaak van der Geest. 2008. "When the Field Is a
    Ward or a Clinic: Hospital Ethnography." *Anthropology & Medicine* 15, no. 2: 71–78.

Lorgeoux, Jeanny, and Jean-Marie Bockel. 2013. "Afrique est Notre Avenir. Commis-
    sion des Affaires Etrangeres, de la Defense et des Forces Armees."

Lupton, Deborah. 1997. "Consumerism, Reflexivity and the Medical Encounter." *Social
    Science and Medicine* 45:373–381.

Maa, Edward, and Paige Figi. 2014. "The Case for Medical Marijuana in Epilepsy."
    Epilepsia 55 no. 6: 783–786.

Mahon, Maureen. 2000. "Visible Evidence of Cultural Producers." *Annual Review of
    Anthropology* 29:467–492.

Malara, Diego Maria. 2011. "Le tradizioni terapeutiche della Chiesa Ortodossa Etiope."
    In *Il Corno d'Africa: Tra medicina politica e storia*, edited by Beatrice Nicolini and Irma
    Taddia, 55–81. Aprilia, Italy: Novalogos.

Malara, Diego Maria, and Tom Boylston. 2016. "Vertical Love: Forms of Submission
    and Top-Down Power in Orthodox Ethiopia." *Social Analysis* 60, no. 4: 40–57.

Makoye, Kizito. 3 August 2017. "Trust the Nurse? Not Everyone Does in Tanzania."
    https://www.reuters.com/article/us-tanzania-health-nursing/trust-the-nurse-not
    -everyone-does-in-tanzania-idUSKBN1AJ1IG

Malchau, Susanne. 2007. "'Angels in Nursing': Images of Nursing Sisters in a Lutheran
    Context in the Nineteenth and Twentieth Centuries." *Nursing Inquiry* 14, no. 4,
    289–298.

Mander, Rosemary. 2004. *Cesarean*. New York: Routledge.

Manderson, Lenore, and Pascale Allotey. 2003. "Cultural Politics and Clinical Competence in Australian Health Services." *Anthropology & Medicine* 10, no. 1: 71–85.

Manzi, Fatuma, Joanna Armstrong Schellenberg, Guy Hutton, Kaspar Wyss, Conrad Mbuya, Kizito Shirima, Hassan Mshinda, Marcel Tanner, and David Schellenberg. 2012. "Human Resources for Health Care Delivery in Tanzania: A Multifaceted Problem." *Human Resources for Health* 10, no. 3: 1–10.

Marcus, George. 1999. *Critical Anthropology Now.* Santa Fe, NM: School of American Research Press.

Martin, Helle Max. 2009. *Nursing Contradictions.* Diemen, The Netherlands: AMB Publishers.

Mathews, Holly F., Nancy J. Burke, and Eirini Kampriani, eds. 2015. *Anthropologies of Cancer in Transnational Worlds.* New York: Routledge.

Mattingly, Cheryl. 2008. "Reading Minds in a Cultural Borderland." *Ethos* 36, no. 1: 136–54.

Mattingly, Cheryl. 2010. *The Paradox of Hope.* Berkeley: University of California Press.

Mattingly, Cheryl. 2014. *Moral Laboratories.* Berkeley: University of California Press.

McCaskie, T. C. 1995. *State and Society in Pre-Colonial Asante.* Cambridge: Cambridge University Press.

McKay, Ramah. 2018. *Medicine in the Meantime.* Durham, NC: Duke University Press.

McMullin, Juliet. 2016. "Cancer." *Annual Review of Anthropology* 45:251–266.

McMullin, Juliet, and Diane Weiner, eds. 2008. *Confronting Cancer.* Santa Fe. NM: School for Advanced Research.

Mechanic, David. 2008. *The Truth about Health Care.* New Brunswick, NJ: Rutgers.

Meiring, A., and N. C. van Wyk. 2013. "The Image of Nurses and Nursing as Perceived by the South African Public." *African Journal of Nursing and Midwifery* 15, no. 2, 3–15.

Melberg, Andrea, et al. 2018. "Policy, Paperwork and 'Postographs': Global Indicators and Maternity Care Documentation in Rural Burkina Faso." *Social Science & Medicine* 215: 28–35.

Men, C., B. Meessen, M. Van Pelt, W. Van Damme, and H. Lucas. 2012. "I Wish I Had AIDS": A Qualitative Study on Access to Health Care Services for HIV/AIDS and Diabetic Patients in Cambodia." *Health, Culture and Society* 2, no. 1: 23–39.

Messay Kebede. 1999. *Survival and Modernization.* Lawrenceville, NJ: Red Sea Press.

Metcalf, Peter. 2001. "Global 'Disjuncture' and the 'Sites' of Anthropology." *Cultural Anthropology* 16:165–182.

Metz, Brent. 2006. *Ch'orti'-Maya Survival in Eastern Guatemala.* Albuquerque: University of New Mexico Press.

Metzl, Jonathan. 2010. *The Protest Psychosis.* Boston, MA: Beacon Press.

Ministerio de Salud. 2005. *Norma tecnica para la atencion del partovertical con adecuacion intercultural.* Lima: Ministerio de Salud.

Ministerio de Salud. 2009. *Plan Estrategico Nacional Para la Reduccion de al Mortalidad Materna y Perinatal 2009–2015.* Lima: Ministerio de Salud.

Ministerio de Salud Pública y Asistencia Social (MSPAS). 2015. *VI Encuesta Nacional de Salud Materno Infantil.* Guatemala City, Guatemala: Ministerio de Salud Pública y Asistencia Social.

Miranda, Jaime J., Yamin, Alicia E. 2004. "Reproductive Health without Rights in Peru." *Reproductive Health and Rights* 363, no. 9402: 68–69.

Mishtal, Joanna. 2010. "Neoliberal Reforms and Privatisation of Reproductive Health Services in Post-Socialist Poland." *Reproductive Health Matters* 18, no. 36: 56–66.

Mishtal, Joanna. 2019. "Reproductive Governance and the (Re)definition of Human Rights in Poland." *Medical Anthropology* 38:182–194.

Mol, Annemarie, Ingunn Moser, and Jeannette Pols, eds. 2010. *Care in Practice. On Tinkering in Clinics, Homes and Farms.* Transcript-Verlag.

Montagu, Dominic, et al. 2017. "Where Women Go to Deliver: Understanding the Changing Landscape of Childbirth in Africa and Asia." *Health Policy and Planning* 32, no. 8: 1146–1152.

Morse, L. L., and B. P. Stoner. 1986. *Utilization and Effectiveness of Health Services in an Andean Community.* Unpublished manuscript, University of Indiana, Bloomington, IN.

Mossialos, E., S. Allin, K. Karras, and K. Davaki. 2005. "An Investigation of Ceasarean Sections in Three Greek Hospitals." *The European Journal of Public Health* 15, no. 3: 288–295.

Mselle, Lillian, Karen Marie Moland, Abu Mvungi, Bjorg Evjen-Olsen, and Thecla W. Kohi. 2013. "Why Give Birth in Health Facility? Users' and Providers' Accounts of Poor Quality of Birth Care in Tanzania." *BMC Health Services Research* 13:174, 1–12.

Mulemi, Benson. 2008. "Patients' Perspectives on Hospitalization: Experiences from a Cancer Ward in Kenya." *Anthropology and Medicine* 15, no. 2: 177–191.

Mulemi, Benson. 2010. *Coping with Cancer and Adversity.* Leiden: African Studies Centre.

Mulemi, Benson. 2014. "Technologies of Hope: Managing Cancer in a Kenyan Hospital." *In Making and Unmaking Public Health in Africa,* edited by R. J. Prince and R. Marsland, 162–183. Athens, OH: Ohio University Press.

Müller, Monika, Simon Wandel, Robert Colebunders, Suzanna Attia, Hansjakob Furrer, and Matthias Egger for IeDEA Southern and Central Africa. 2010. "Immune Reconstitution Inflammatory Syndrome in Patients Starting Antiretroviral Therapy for HIV Infection." *Lancet Infectious Diseases* 10, no. 4: 251–261.

Mumtaz, Zubia, et al. 2014. "Improving Maternal Health in Pakistan: Toward a Deeper Understanding of the Social Determinants of Poor Women's Access to Maternal Health Services." *American Journal of Public Health* 104 (S1): S17–S24.

Musa, Jonathan. 7 November 2018. "Doctor, Four Nurses Suspended in Mwanza Over Infant's Death." In *The Citizen.* https://www.thecitizen.co.tz/news/Doctor—four -nurses-suspended-in-Mwanza-over-infant-s-death-/1840340-4841504-format -xhtml-90mxi5z/index.html.

Mwangoka, Mussa. 24 April 2016. "Council Fires 7 Healthworkers, Suspends 3 Others." *The Citizen.* https://www.thecitizen.co.tz/news/1840340-3173912-oydsouz/index.html.

National Bureau of Statistics (NBS) and ICF Macro. 2011. *Tanzania Demographic and Health Survey 2010.* Dar es Salaam, Tanzania: NBS and ICF Macro.

Ngugi, Anthony, et al. 2013. "Prevalence of Active Convulsive Epilepsy in Sub-Saharan Africa and Associated Risk Factors." *Lancet Neurology* 12: 253–263.

Nguyen, Vinh-Kim. 2010. *The Republic of Therapy.* Durham, NC: Duke University Press Books.

Nichter, M. 2005. *Understanding the Patient's Experience of Illness.* Oakstone Medical Publishing.

Nichter, Mark. 2008. *Global Health.* Tucson: University of Arizona Press.

Nichter M., A. Amoussouhoui, F. Mou, E. Koka, P. K. Awah, E. Mbah, J. T. Koin, and M. Boyer. 2015. "Buruli Ulcer Outreach Education: An Exemplar for Community-Based Tropical Disease Interventions." Presentation at The 9th European Congress on Tropical Medicine and International Health. Basel, Switzerland.

Nichter, Mark, Gordon Trockman, and Jean Grippen. 1985. "Clinical Anthropologist as Therapy Facilitator: Role Development and Clinician Evaluation in a Psychiatric Training Program." *Human Organization* 44, no. 1: 72–80.

Nijamnshi, Alfred. 2009. "General Public Knowledge, Attitudes, and Practice with Respect to Epilepsy in the Batibo Health District, Cameroon." *Epilepsy and Behavior* 14:83–88.

Nikolentzos, A., and N. Mays. 2008. "Can Existing Theories of Health Care Reform Explain the Greek Case?" *Journal of European Social Policy* 18, no. 2:163–176.

Nisar, N., et al. 2017. "Maternal Mortality in Pakistan: Is There Any Metamorphosis towards Betterment?" *Journal of the Ayub Medical College Abbottabad* 29, no. 1: 118–122.

Nwani, P. O., et al. 2013. "Illness Concept among People with Epilepsy and Their Caregivers and Preferred Treatment Methods in a Suburban Community in Southwest Nigeria." *West African Journal of Medicine* 32:26–30.

Obeng, Cecilia. 2007. "Perceptions of Epilepsy in a Traditional Society." In *HIV/AIDS, Illness, and African Well-Being*, edited by Toyin Falola and Matthew Heaton, 95–115. Rochester: University of Rochester Press, 2007.

Observatoire Régional de Santé (ORS). 2013. La santé des femmes en Ile-de-France. www.ors-idf.org.

O'Connor, Anne-Marie, and William Booth. 2010. "Mexico's Medical Workers on the Front Lines of the Drug War." *Washington Post*, November 19, 2010.

OECD. (2017). *OECD Review of Health Systems: Peru*. Paris: OECD Publishing.

Olsen, William C. 2017. "Body and *Sunsum*: Stroke in Asante." In *African Medical Pluralism*, edited by William C. Olsen and Carolyn Sargent, 50–68. Bloomington: Indiana University Press.

Olsen, William C. 2019. "The Intention of Evil." In *Engaging Evil*, edited by William C. Olsen and Thomas Csordas, 254–274. Oxford: Berghahn Books.

Olsen, William C., and Carolyn Sargent. 2017. "Introduction." In *African Medical Pluralism*, edited by William Olsen and Carolyn Sargent, 1–30. Bloomington: Indiana University Press.

Olwig, Karen, and Kirsten Hastrup. 1997. *Siting Culture*. London: Routledge.

O'Neill, Brian Juan. 1987. *Social Inequality in a Portuguese Hamlet*. Cambridge: Cambridge University Press.

Padilla, Lizbeth. 2018. "La Inseguridad Pega a la Salud: Médicos Abandonan Centros de Salud de la Sierra De Chihuahua." *Animal Político*, August 18, 2018.

Palacios, Eduardo. 2013. "Comemoración para el Día Mundial de Cáncer." Presentation at the Congreso del Programa Nacional para la Prevención de las Enfermedades Crónicas No Transmisibles y Cáncer. Guatemala City, Guatemala: February 5.

Papagaroufali, Eleni. 1990. "Greek Women in Politics: Gender Ideology and Practice in Neighborhood Groups and the Family." PhD diss., Columbia University.

Papagaroufali, Eleni, and Eugenia Georges. 1993. "Greek Women in the Europe of 1992: Brokers of European Cargos and the Logic of the West." In *Perilous States: Conversations on Culture, Race and Nation*, edited by G. Marcus, 235–54. Chicago: University of Chicago Press.

Parsons, Talcott. 1951. *The Social System*. London: Collier-MacMillan Limited, Free Press of Glencoe.

Paxson, Heather. 2004. *Making Modern Mothers*. Berkeley: University of California Press.

Peters, Emyrs. 1990. *The Bedouin of Cyrenaica*. Cambridge: Cambridge University Press.

Petryna, Adriana. 2002. *Life Exposed*. Princeton, NJ: Princeton University Press.

Pezzia, Carla. 2015. "Engaging Mental Health Care in a Disengaged System." In *Privatization and the New Medical Pluralism*, edited by A. Chary and P. Rohloff, 91–106. Lanham, MD: Lexington Press.

Pfeiffer, James. 2003. "International NGOs and Primary Health Care in Mozambique: The Need for a New Model of Collaboration." *Social Science and Medicine* 56, no. 4:725–38.

Pfeiffer, James, and Rachel Chapman. 2010. "Anthropological Perspectives on Structural Adjustment and Public Health." *Annual Review of Anthropology* 39:149–65.

Physicians for Human Rights (PHR). 2007. *Deadly Delays*. Cambridge, MA: Physicians for Human Rights.

Pinto, Sarah. 2004. "Development without Institutions: Ersatz Medicine and the Politics of Everyday Life in Rural North India." *Cultural Anthropology* 19, no. 3: 337–364.

Pigg, Stacy Leigh. 1996. "The Credible and the Credulous: The Question of 'Villagers' Beliefs' in Nepal." *Cultural Anthropology* 11, no. 2: 160–201.

Pluschke, Gerd, and Katharina Röltgen. 2019. *Buruli Ulcer*. New York: Springer.

Pope, Catherine, Sue Ziebland, and Nicholas Mays. 2000. "Qualitative Research in Health Care: Analysing Qualitative Data." *BMJ: British Medical Journal* 320, no. 7227: 114.

Praspaliauskiene, Rima. 2016. "Enveloped Lives: Practicing Health and Care in Lithuania." *Medical Anthropology Quarterly* 30, no. 4: 582–598.

Prata, Ndola, et al. 2009. "Saving Maternal Lives in Resource-Poor Settings: Facing Reality." *Health Policy* 89:131–148.

Pratilas, Georgios, Alexandros Sotiridis and Konstantinos Dinas. 2019. "Is High Use of Cesarean Section Sometimes Justified?" *Lancet* 10192:25–26.

Prentice, Rachel. 2013. *Bodies in Formation*. Durham, NC: Duke University Press.

Preux, Pierre-Marie. 2005. "Epidemiology and Aetiology of Epilepsy in Sub-Saharan Africa." *Lancet Neurology* 4:21–31.

Price, L. 1987. "Ecuadorian Illness Stories." In *Cultural Models in Language and Thought*, edited by D. Holland and N. Quinn, 313–342. Cambridge, UK: Cambridge University Press.

Prince, Ruth. 2018. "Death, Detachment, and Moral Dilemmas of Care in a Kenyan Hospital." In *A Companion to the Anthropology of Death*, edited by Antonius C.G.M. Robbin, 445–460. Hoboken, NJ: Wiley Blackwell.

Prince, Ruth, and Rebecca Marsland, Eds. 2014. *Making and Unmaking Public Health in Africa*. Athens: Ohio University Press.

Psimmenos, Iordanis, and Koula Kasimati. 2003. "Immigration Control Pathways: Organizational Culture and Work Values of Greek Welfare Officers." *Journal of Ethnic and Migration Studies* 29, no. 2: 337–373.

Pupillo, Elisabetta. 2014. "Knowledge and Attitudes towards Epilepsy in Zambia." *Epilepsy and Behavior* 34:42–46.

Quansah, Emmanuel, and T. K. Karikari. 2016. "Neuroscience-related Research in Ghana: A Systematic Evaluation of Direction and Capacity." *Metabolic Brain Disease* 31:11–24.

Quinn, Naomi, ed. 2005. *Finding Culture in Talk: A Collection of Methods*. New York: Palgrave Macmillan.

Rabinowitz, Dan. 1997. *Overlooking Nazareth*. Cambridge: Cambridge University Press.

Rafael, F., et al. 2010. "Sociocultural and Psychological Features of Perceived Stigma Reported by People with Epilepsy in Benin." *Epilepsia* 51:1061–1088.

Reich, Jennifer A. 2014. "Neoliberal Mothering and Vaccine Refusal: Imagined Gated Communities and the Privilege of Choice." *Gender and Society* 28, no. 5: 679–704.

Reyes-Foster, Beatriz. 2018. *Psychiatric Encounters*. New Brunswick, NJ: Rutgers University Press.

Rice, Tom. 2010. "Learning to Listen: Auscultation and the Transmission of Auditory Knowledge." *Journal of the Royal Anthropological Institute* 16 (S1): S41–S61.

Rivkin-Fish, Michele. 2005. *Women's Health in Post-Soviet Russia*. Bloomington: Indiana University Press.

Rivkin-Fish, M. 2005. "Bribes, Gifts and Unofficial Payments: Rethinking Corruption in Post-Soviet Russian Health Care." In *Corruption*, edited by C. Shore and D. Haller, 47–64. London: Pluto Press.

Robbins, Bruce. 2017. "Comparative Cosmopolitanisms." In *Cosmopolitanisms*, edited by Bruce Robbins and Paulo Horta, 246–264. New York: New York University Press.

Robbins, Bruce, and Paulo Horta. 2017. "Introduction." In *Cosmopolitanisms*, edited by Bruce Robbins and Paulo Horta, 1–20. New York: New York University Press.

Roberts, Elizabeth F. S. 2012. *God's Laboratory*. Berkeley: University of California Press.

Rohatynskyj, Marta. 2001. "My Friend Amsatou Barry." *Anthropology and Humanism* 26, no. 1: 59–70.

Rondet, Claire, Annabelle Lapostolle, Marion Soler, Francesca Grillo, Isabelle Parizot, and Pierre Chauvin. 2014. "Are Immigrants and Nationals Born to Immigrants at Higher Risk for Delayed or No Lifetime Breast and Cervical Cancer Screening? The Results from a Population-Based Survey in Paris Metropolitan Area in 2010." *PLoS ONE* 9, no. 1: e7048. https://doi.org/10.1371/journal.pone.0087046.

Rondet, Claire, Marion Soler, Virginie Ringa, Isabelle Parizot, and Pierre Chauvin. 2013. "The Role of a Lack of Social Integration in Never Having Undergone Breast Cancer Screening: Results from a Population-based, Representative Survey in the Paris Metropolitan Area in 2010." *Preventive Medicine* 57:251–406.

Ronsmans, C., and W. J. Graham. 2016. "Maternal Mortality: Who, When, Where, and Why." *Lancet* 368, no. 9542: 1189–1200.

Rose, Nikolas. 2007. *The Politics of Life Itself*. Princeton, NJ: Princeton University Press.

Rosen, Lawrence. 1984. *Bargaining for Reality*. Chicago: University of Chicago Press.

Rosenberg, Charles. 1987. *The Care of Strangers*. New York: Basic Books.

Russo, Ethan B. 2017. "Cannabis and Epilepsy: An Ancient Treatment Returns to the Fore." *Epilepsy and Behavior* 70 (Part B): 292–297.

Sadler, Michelle, Mario J.D.S. Santos, Dolores Ruiz-Berdun, Gonzalo Leiva Rojas, Elena Skoko, Patricia Gillen, and Jette A. Clausen. 2016. "Moving beyond Disrespect and Abuse: Addressing the Structural Dimensions of Obstetric Violence." *Reproductive Health Matters* 24, no. 47: 45–55.

Saint-Martin, D. 2004. *Building the New Managerialist State*. Oxford: Oxford University Press.

Salmi, Anna-Maria. 2003. "Health in Exchange: Teachers, Doctors, and the Strength of Informal Practices in Russia." *Culture, Psychiatry and Medicine* 27:109–130.

Sambala, Evanson Z., Sara Cooper, and Lenore Manderson. 2020. "Ubuntu as a Framework for Ethical Decision Making in Africa: Responding to Epidemics." *Ethics & Behavior* 30, no. 1: 1–13.

Samuel Jeannie. 2015. "Struggling with the State: Rights-based Governance of Reproductive Health Service Delivery in Puno, Peru." Doctoral diss., University of Toronto, Toronto, ON.

Samuel, Jeannie. 2016. "The Role of Civil Society in Strengthening Intercultural Maternal Health Care in Local Health Facilities: Puno, Peru." *Global Health Action* 9, no. 1: 33355.

Sandelowski, Margarete. 2000. *Devices & Desires*. Chapel Hill, NC: University of North Carolina Press.

Sandelowski, Margaret. 2002. "Visible Humans, Vanishing Bodies, and Virtual Nursing: Complications of Life, Presence, Place, and Identity." *Advanced Nursing Science* 24, no. 3: 58–70.

Sargent, Carolyn, and Laurence Kotobi. 2017. "Austerity and Its Implications for Immigrant Health in France." *Social Science and Medicine* 187:259–267.

Sargent, Carolyn, and Peter Benson. 2019. "Cancer and Precarity: Rights and Vulnerabilities of West African Immigrants in France." In *Structural Vulnerability and Cancer Treatment, Prevention, and Research in Global Health*, edited by Julie Armin, Nancy Burke, and Laura Eichenberger, 21–47. Santa Fe, NM: School for Advanced Research.

Scheper-Hughes, Nancy. 2002. *Death Without Weeping.* Berkeley: University of California Press.

Scheper-Hughes, Nancy, and Mariana Leal Ferreira. 2007. "Dombá's Spirit Kidney: Transplant Medicine and Suyá Indian Cosmology." In *Disability in Local and Global Worlds*, edited by Benedicte Ingstad and Susan Reynolds Whyte, 149–185. Berkeley: University of California Press.

Shah, Safia, et al. 2016. "Unregulated Usage of Labor-Inducing Medication in a Region of Pakistan with Poor Drug Regulatory Control: Characteristics and Risk Patterns." *International Health* 8:89–95.

Shapiro, Johanna. 2018. "'Violence' in Medicine: Necessary and Unnecessary, Intentional and Unintentional." *Philosophy, Ethics, and Humanities in Medicine* 13, no. 7: 8 pages.

Sheikh, Kabir, Michael Kent Ranson, and Lucy Gilson. 2014. "Explorations on People Centredness in Health Systems." *Health Policy and Planning* 29, no. Suppl 2: ii1.

Sheikh, Kabir, Asha George, and Lucy Gilson. 2014. "People-Centred Science: Strengthening the Practice of Health Policy and Systems Research." *Health Research Policy and Systems* 12, no. 1: 19.

Skalkidis, Y., E. Petridou, E. Papathoma, K. Revinthi, D. Tong, and D. Trichopoulos. 1996. "Are Operative Deliveries in Greece Socially Conditioned?" *International Journal of Qualitative Health Care* 8, no. 2: 159–165.

Smedley, Brian, Adrienne Stith, and Alan Nelson. 2002. *Unequal Treatment.* Washington, DC: National Academy Press.

Smith, Catherine. 2013. "Doctors That Harm, Doctors That Heal: Reimagining Medicine in Post-Conflict Aceh, Indonesia." *Ethnos: Journal of Anthropology* 80, no. 2: 272–291.

Smith, Michael G. 1974. *Corporations and Society.* London: Duckworth.

Smith-Oka, Vania. 2009. Unintended Consequences: Exploring the Tensions between Development Programs and Indigenous Women in Mexico in the Context of Reproductive Health. *Social Science and Medicine* 68:2069–77.

Smith-Oka, Vania. 2013. "Managing Labor and Delivery among Impoverished Populations in Mexico: Cervical Examinations as Bureaucratic Practice." *American Anthropologist* 115, no. 4: 595–607.

Sobo, E. J. 2004. "Pediatric Nurses May Misjudge Parent Communication Preferences." *Journal of Nursing Care Quality* 19, no. 3: 253–262.

Sobo, E. J. 2005. "Parents' Perceptions of Pediatric Day Surgery Risks: Unforeseeable Complications, or Avoidable Mistakes?" *Social Science & Medicine* 60, no. 10: 2341–2350.

Sobo, E. J. 2009. *Culture and Meaning in Health Services Research.* Walnut Creek, CA: Left Coast Press.

Sobo, Elisa J. 2011. "Medical Anthropology in Disciplinary Context: Definitional Struggles and Key Debates (or Answering the Cri Du Coeur)." In *A Companion to Medical Anthropology*, edited by Merrill Singer and Pamela I. Erickson, 9–20. West Sussex, UK: Wiley Blackwell.

Sobo, E. J. 2016. "What Is Herd Immunity, and How Does It Relate to Pediatric Vaccination Uptake? US Parent Perspectives." *Social Science and Medicine* 165:187–195.

Sobo, E. J. 2017. "Parent Use of Cannabis for Intractable Pediatric Epilepsy: Everyday Empiricism and the Boundaries of Scientific Medicine." *Social Science and Medicine* 190:190–198.

Sobo, E. J. 2021. "Cultural Conformity and Cannabis Care for the Iatrogenic and Idiosyncratic Complications of Intractable Pediatric Epilepsy." *Anthropology & Medicine* 28, no. 2:205–222. https://doi.org/10.1080/13648470.2021.1893583.

Sobo, Elisa J., Glenn Billman, Lilian Lim, J. Wilken Murdock, Elvia Romero, Donna Donoghue, William Roberts, and Paul S. Kurtin. 2002. "A Rapid Interview Protocol Supporting Patient-Centered Quality Improvement." *Joint Commission Journal on Quality Improvement* 28, no. 9: 498–509.

Sorensen, Roslyn, and Rick Iedema. 2009. "Emotional Labour: Clinicians' Attitudes to Death and Dying." *Journal of Health Organization and Management* 23, no. 1: 5–22.

Soto Laveaga, Gabriela. 2013. "Shadowing the Professional Class: Reporting Fictions in Doctors' Strikes." *Journal of Iberian and Latin American Research* 19, no. 1: 30–40.

Soto Laveaga, Gabriela. 2015. "Building the Nation of the Future, One Waiting Room at a Time: Hospital Murals in the Making of Modern Mexico." *History and Technology* 31, no. 3: 275–294.

Souliotis, Kyriakos, et al. 2016. "Informal Payments in the Greek Health Sector amid the Financial Crisis: Old Habits Die Hard." *European Journal of Health Economics* 17, no. 2: 159–170.

Stephenson, P. A., et al. 1993. "Patterns of Use of Obstetrical Interventions in 12 Countries." *Paediatric and Perinatal Epidemiology* 7:45–54.

Stevenson, Lisa. 2014. *Life Beside Itself.* Berkeley: University of California Press.

Strauss A., and J. Corbin. 1994. "Grounded Theory Methodology: An Overview." In *Handbook of Qualitative Research*, edited by N. K. Denzin and Y. S. Lincoln, 273–285. Thousand Oaks, CA: Sage.

Strauss, Anselm, and Juliet Corbin. 1998. *Basics of Qualitative Research*, 2nd ed. Thousand Oaks, CA: Sage.

Street, Alice. 2009. "Failed Recipients: Extracting Blood in a Papua New Guinean Hospital." *Body & Society* 15, no. 2: 193–215.

Street, Alice. 2014. *Biomedicine in an Unstable Place.* Durham, NC: Duke University Press.

Street, Alice, and Simon Coleman. 2012. "Introduction: Real and Imagined Spaces." *Space and Culture* 15, no. 1: 4–17.

Strong, Adrienne A. 2016. "Working in Scarcity: Effects on Social Interactions and Biomedical Care in Rukwa, Tanzania." *Social Science & Medicine* 172:217–224.

Strong, Adrienne. 2018. "Causes and Effects of Occupational Risk Exposure for Healthcare Workers on the Maternity Ward of a Tanzanian Hospital." *Human Organization* 77, no. 3, 273–286.

Strong, Adrienne. 2020. *Documenting Death: Maternal Mortality and the Ethics of Care in Tanzania.* Berkeley: University of California Press.

Stumo, Samya. 2015. *"For Their Own Good": An Ethnography of Health Experience in the Southern Peruvian Andes.* Undergraduate honors thesis, University of Massachusetts. Amherst, MA.

Sullivan, Noelle. 2012. "Enacting Spaces of Inequality: Placing Global/State Governance within a Tanzanian Hospital." *Space and Culture* 15, no. 1: 57–67.

Tambiah, Stanley J. 1990. *Magic, Science, and Religion and the Scope of Rationality.* Cambridge: Cambridge University Press.

Tanzania National Archives (TNA). 1990. Medical Department Files, Accession No. HE 1172/67 *Medical Development Plan.*

Tarimo, Edith, Gustav Moyo, Happy Masenga, Paul Magesa, and Dafroza Mzava. 2018. "Performance and Self-Perceived Competencies of Enrolled Nurse/Midwives: A Mixed Methods Study from Rural Tanzania." *BMC Health Services Research* 18, no. 277: 1–14. https://doi.org/10.1186/s12913-018-3096-8.

Thornber, Karen. 2018. "World Literature and Health Humanities: Translingual Encounters Brain Disorders." In *Territories and Trajectories: Cultures in Circulation*, edited by Diana Sorensen, 163–185. Raleigh-Durham, NC: Duke University Press.

Ticktin, Miriam. 2011. *Casualties of Care: Immigration and the Politics of Humanitarianism in France*. Berkeley: University of California Press.

Towghi, Fouzieyha. 2013. "Normalizing Off-Label Experiments and the Pharmaceutical-ization of Homebirths in Pakistan." *Ethnos, Journal of Anthropology* 79, no. 1: 108–137.

Towghi, Fouzieyha. 2018. "Haunting Expectations of Hospital Births Challenged by Traditional Midwives." *Medical Anthropology* 37, no. 8: 674–687.

Trostle, James. 2005. *Epidemiology and Culture*. Cambridge: Cambridge University Press.

Tsing, Anna. 2005. *Friction: An Ethnography of Global Connections*. Princeton, NJ: Princeton University Press.

Tsoukalas, Constantinos. 1991. "Enlightened" Concepts in the "Dark": Power and Freedom, Politics, and Society. *Journal of Modern Greek Studies* 9:1:22.

Twigg, Julia. 2000. Carework as a Form of Bodywork. *Ageing and Society* 20:38.

Ureste, Manu. 2016. "YoSoyMédico17 Convoca Otra Marcha Nacional el 23 de Octubre, Tras Recorte a Salud." *Animal Político*, September 15, 2016.

USAID. 2015. "Guatemala Health System Assessment 2015." https://www.usaid.gov/sites/default/files/documents/1862/Guatemala-HSA%20_ENG-FULL-REPORT-FINAL-APRIL-2016.pdf.

Van der Geest, Sjaak, and Kaja Finkler. 2004. "Hospital Ethnography: An Introduction." *Social Science and Medicine* 59:1995–2001.

Van Dyke, Miriam E., et al. 2020. "Trends in County-Level COVID-19 Incidence in Counties with and without a Mask Mandate—Kansas." *CDC Morbidity and Mortality Weekly Report* 69, no. 47: 1777–1781.

Van Hollen, Cecilia. 1998. "Moving Targets: Routine IUD Insertion in Maternity Wards in Tamil Nadu, India." *Reproductive Health Matters* 6, no. 11: 98–105.

Varley, Emma. 2016. "Abandonments, Solidarities and Logics of Care: Hospitals as Sites of Sectarian Conflict in Gilgit-Baltistan." Special Issue "The Clinic in Crisis": *Culture, Medicine, and Psychiatry* 40, no. 2: 159–180.

Varley, Emma. 2019. "Against Protocol: The Politics and Perils of Oxytocin (Mis)Use in a Pakistani Labor Room." Special Issue: "The Hospital in South Asia." *Puruṣārtha* 36:105–130.

Varley, Emma, and Saiba Varma. 2019. "Attending to the Dark Side of Medicine." *Anthropology News* 60, no. 2: e197–e202.

Velogiannis-Moutsopoulos, L., and Bartsocas, C. S. 1989. Medical Genetics in Greece. In *Human Genetics: A Cross-Cultural Perspective*, edited by D. Wertz and J. Fletcher, 209–234. Heidelberg: Springer.

Vogelstein, Fred. 2015. "Boy, Interrupted." *Wired* (July).

Waldheim, Carlos, and Mynor Villeda. 2014. "Registro Hospitalario del Instituto y Hospital de Cancerología de Guatemala, año 2011." *Revista Médica Colegio de Médicos y Cirujanos de Guatemala* 151:8–14.

Wallace, Rob, Alex Liebman, Luis Fernando Chaves, and Rodrick Wallace. 2020. "COVID-19 and Circuits of Capital." *Monthly Review* 72, no. 1.

Walter, Brenda. 2014. "Listening to Ghosts: Haunted Hospitals, Spectral Patients, and the Monstrous in Modern Medicine." *Trespassing Journal* 4:51–62.

Warner, Joel. 2014. "Charlotte's Web: Untangling One of Colorado's Biggest Cannabis Success Stories." *Westword.com*, December 3.

Watts, A. E. 1989. "A Model for Managing Epilepsy in a Rural Community in Africa." *BMJ* 29, no. 8: 805–807.

Weber, Max, 1980. *The Theory of Social and Economic Organization.* London: Collier MacMillan.

Wendland, Claire. 2010. *A Heart for the Work.* Chicago: University of Chicago Press.

Wendland, Claire. 2014. "The Anthropology of African Biomedicine." In *Medical Anthropology in Global Africa*, edited by Kathryn Rhine, John M. Janzen, Glenn Adams, and Heather Aldersey, 45–53. Lawrence: University of Kansas, Publications in Anthropology.

Wendland, Claire L. 2016. "Estimating Death: A Close Reading of Maternal Mortality Metrics in Malawi." In *Metrics*, edited by Vincanne Adams, 57–81. Durham, NC: Duke University Press.

Werbner, Pnina. 2008. "Introduction: Toward a New Cosmopolitan Anthropology." In *Anthropology and the New Cosmopolitanism*, edited by Pnina Werbner, 1–32. Oxford: Berg.

Whittaker, Andrea, and Heng Leng Chee. 2015. "Perceptions of an 'International Hospital' in Thailand by Medical Travel Patients: Cross-Cultural Tensions in a Transnational Space." *Social Science & Medicine* 124:290–297.

Whyte, Susan Reynolds. 1995. "Constructing Epilepsy." In *Disability and Culture*, edited by Benedicte Ingstad and Susan Reynolds Whyte, 226–245. Berkeley: University of California Press.

Wind, Gitte. 2008. "Negotiated Interactive Observation: Doing Fieldwork in Hospital Settings." *Anthropology & Medicine* 15, no. 2: 79–89.

Winkler, Andrea. 2010. "Belief Systems of Epilepsy and Attitudes Toward People Living with Epilepsy in a Rural Community in Northern Tanzania." *Epilepsy and Behavior* 19:596–601.

Wirrell, Elaine C. 2013. "Predicting Pharmacoresistance in Pediatric Epilepsy." *Epilepsia* 54 (Suppl. S2): 19–22.

Wool, Zoë. 2015. *After War.* Durham, NC: Duke University Press.

World Health Organization (WHO). 2012. "Traitement de l'infection à mycobacterium ulcerans (ulcère de Buruli): recommandations à l'intention des agents de santé."

World Health Organization (WHO). 2015. *Information Kit on Epilepsy.* New York: WHO.

World Health Organization (WHO). 2015.*WHO Statement on Cesarean Section Rates.* WHO/RHR/15.02.

World Health Organization (WHO). 2016. *Time to Respond: A Report on the Global Implementation of Maternal Death Surveillance and Response.* Geneva: World Health Organization.

World Health Organization (WHO). 2020. *COVID-19 Dashboard.*

Wynne, Brian. 1996. "May the Sheep Safely Graze? A Reflexive View of the Expert-Lay Knowledge Divide." In *Risk, Environment and Modernity: Towards a New Ecology*, edited by Scott Lash, Bronislaw Szerszynski, and Brian Wynne, 44–83. London: Sage.

Zacher Dixon, Lydia. 2015. "Obstetrics in a Time of Violence: Mexican Midwives Critique Routine Hospital Practices." *Medical Anthropology Quarterly* 29, no. 4: 437–454.

Zaman, Shahaduz. 2008. "Native among the Natives: Physician Anthropologist Doing Hospital Ethnography at Home." *Journal of Contemporary Ethnography* 37, no. 2: 135–154.

Zamorano, Abigail S., Joaquín Barnoya, Eduardo Gharzouzi, Camaryn Chrisman Robbins, and David Mutch. 2017. "Compliance after Treatment Is a Major Barrier to the Optimal Treatment of Cervical Cancer in Guatemala." Presented at the Western Association of Gynecologic Oncologists Annual Meeting.

Notes on Contributors

WILLIAM C. OLSEN is a medical anthropologist whose research is based in the Asante zone of western, central Ghana for more than thirty years. His publications include *Evil in Africa*, *African Medical Pluralism*, and *Engaging Evil*.

CAROLYN SARGENT is a medical anthropologist who has conducted research in West Africa (Benin, Mali), Jamaica, and France. Her publications include *African Medical Pluralism, Reproduction, Globalization and the State, Medical Anthropology: Handbook of Theory and Method*, and *Maternity, Medicine and Power*. She is professor of anthropology at Washington University in St. Louis.

ANITA CHARY is chief resident physician of emergency medicine at the Massachusetts General Hospital, Brigham and Women's Hospital. She is also a clinical fellow at Harvard Medical School and a researcher at Wuqu' Kawoq, Maya Health Alliance, Guatemala.

EUGENIA GEORGES is professor of anthropology at Rice University in Houston, Texas.

ANITA HANNIG is associate professor of anthropology at Brandeis University in Waltham, Massachusetts.

MORGAN K. HOKE is assistant professor of anthropology at the University of Pennsylvania.

KAYLA J. HURD is a PhD candidate in anthropology at the University of Notre Dame in Indiana.

JOHN M. JANZEN is emeritus professor of anthropology at the University of Kansas.

ROCH CHRISTIAN JOHNSON is professor of public health at the Centre Interfacultaire de Formation et de Recherche en Environnement et Développement, Université d'Abomey Calavi, Benin.

THOMAS L. LEATHERMAN is professor of anthropology at the University of Massachusetts.

CHERYL MATTINGLY is professor of anthropology at the University of Southern California.

MARK NICHTER is regents professor emeritus of anthropology in the Mel and Enid Zuckerman College of Public Health and the Department of Family Medicine at the University of Arizona. He is also adviser to the Stop Buruli International Consortium.

PETER ROHLOFF is assistant professor of medicine and global health Equity, Brigham and Women's Hospital, Harvard Medical School.

VANIA SMITH-OKA is associate professor of anthropology, University of Notre Dame in Indiana.

ELISA J. SOBO is professor of anthropology at San Diego State University in California.

GHISLAIN EMMANUEL SOPOH is professor of public health, Institut Régional de Santé Publique, Université d'Abomey Calavi, Benin.

ADRIENNE E. STRONG is assistant professor of anthropology at the University of Florida.

SAMYA R. STUMO was a data analyst at the ThinkWell Organization.

EMMA VARLEY is associate professor of anthropology at Brandon University in Manitoba, Canada.

CLAIRE WENDLAND is professor of anthropology and of obstetrics & gynecology at the University of Wisconsin.

Index